ANATOMY, PHYSIOLOGY, AND PATHOLOGY

A Practical, Illustrated Guide to the Human Body for Students and Practitioners

Third Edition

Ruth Hull

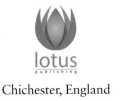

lotus
publishing

Chichester, England

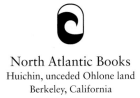

North Atlantic Books
Huichin, unceded Ohlone land
Berkeley, California

This third edition published in 2024 by
Lotus Publishing
Apple Tree Cottage, Inlands Road, Nutbourne, Chichester, PO18 8RJ, and
North Atlantic Books
Huichin, unceded Ohlone land
Berkeley, California

Illustrations Amanda Williams, Vicky Slegg
Pathology Photographs Wellcome Trust Photo Library, Shutterstock.com
Text Design Medlar Publishing Solutions Pvt Ltd., India
Cover Design Chris Fulcher
Printed and Bound Replika Press Pvt Ltd., India

Anatomy, Physiology, and Pathology: A Practical, Illustrated Guide to the Human Body for Students and Practitioners, Third Edition is sponsored and published by North Atlantic Books, an educational nonprofit based on the unceded Ohlone land Huichin (Berkeley, CA), that collaborates with partners to develop cross-cultural perspectives, nurture holistic views of art, science, the humanities, and healing, and seed personal and global transformation by publishing work on the relationship of body, spirit, and nature.

North Atlantic Books' publications are distributed to the US trade and internationally by Penguin Random House Publishers Services. For further information, visit our website at www.northatlanticbooks.com.

MEDICAL DISCLAIMER: The following information is intended for general information purposes only. Individuals should always see their healthcare provider before administering any suggestions made in this book. Any application of the material set forth in the following pages is at the reader's discretion and is their sole responsibility.

British Library Cataloging-in-Publication Data
A CIP record for this book is available from the British Library
ISBN 978 1 913088 39 2 (Lotus Publishing)
ISBN 978 1 62317 970 0 (North Atlantic Books)

Library of Congress Cataloging-in-Publication Data
Names: Hull, Ruth, author.
Title: Anatomy, physiology and pathology, third edition: a practical, illustrated
    guide to the human body for students and practitioners / Ruth Hull.
Description: Third edition. | Chichester, England : Lotus Publishing ;
    Berkeley, California : North Atlantic Books, 2023. | "This second
    edition published in 2021 and reprinted in 2023"--Title page verso. |
    Includes bibliographical references and index.
Identifiers: LCCN 2023005927 (print) | LCCN 2023005928 (ebook) |
    ISBN 9781623179700 (trade paperback) | ISBN 9781623179717 (ebook)
Subjects: MESH: Anatomy | Physiological Phenomena | Pathologic Processes |
    Signs and Symptoms | Outline
Classification: LCC QP34.5 (print) | LCC QP34.5 (ebook) | NLM QS 18.2 |
    DDC 612--dc23/eng/20230620
LC record available at https://lccn.loc.gov/2023005927
LC ebook record available at https://lccn.loc.gov/2023005928

Contents

Bring a new dimension to learning with Augmented Reality (AR)

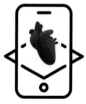

Deepen your understanding with AR, including 3D models, videos, audio, and links to further reading materials. Figures featuring AR will be indicated with the icon to the right.

1. Download the app "**Ludenso Explore**" to your phone or tablet.
2. Select the book from the reading list and launch the title.
3. Point the camera to the book page indicated on the top of your screen.
4. Explore 3D models by clicking on the labels, rotating and zooming.
5. Bring the 3D models out into your surroundings, by clicking on the "content" button and selecting the 3D model.

Introduction

This book is for anyone studying to be a healthcare professional. It presents all the information necessary to gain a thorough understanding of the subject in a clear, accurate, and easily absorbed format. We have tried to strike a balance between a friendly, informal tone, and serious academic content.

We hope you will enjoy using this book and would welcome any feedback, good or bad, which will help us to improve it in subsequent editions.

Picture Credits

We would like to thank the following for granting permission to reproduce copyright material in this book:

Pages 24, 27, Shutterstock.com

Page 38, CarlsonStockArt.com

Pages 74–84, Wellcome Trust Photo Library, Shutterstock.com

Page 117, Sobotta: Atlas der Anatomie des Menschen, 22nd edition © Elsevier GmbH, Urban & Fischer Verlag Munchen

Pages 118, 120, Wellcome Trust Photo Library

Pages 121, 122, Shutterstock.com

Page 144, Sobotta: Atlas der Anatomie des Menschen, 22nd edition © Elsevier GmbH, Urban & Fischer Verlag Munchen

Pages 186–188, Wellcome Trust Photo Library

Pages 194–196, Sobotta: Atlas der Anatomie des Menschen, 22nd edition © Elsevier GmbH, Urban & Fischer Verlag Munchen

Pages 224, 225, 233, 234, Sobotta: Atlas der Anatomie des Menschen, 22nd edition © Elsevier GmbH, Urban & Fischer Verlag Munchen

Pages 238–240, Wellcome Trust Photo Library

Pages 259–261, Wellcome Trust Photo Library

Page 280, Sobotta: Atlas der Anatomie des Menschen, 22nd edition © Elsevier GmbH, Urban & Fischer Verlag Munchen

Page 287, Wellcome Trust Photo Library

Pages 291, 294, 295, Sobotta: Atlas der Anatomie des Menschen, 22nd edition © Elsevier GmbH, Urban & Fischer Verlag Munchen

Page 300, Wellcome Trust Photo Library

Pages 308, 309, 313, Sobotta: Atlas der Anatomie des Menschen, 22nd edition © Elsevier GmbH, Urban & Fischer Verlag Munchen

Pages 320 and 322, Wellcome Trust Photo Library

Page 340, Shutterstock.com

Page 341, Wellcome Trust Photo Library

Pages 377, 388, 358, 361, 362, Sobotta: Atlas der Anatomie des Menschen, 22nd edition © Elsevier GmbH, Urban & Fischer Verlag Munchen

Pages 364–368, Wellcome Trust Photo Library

Page 368, Shutterstock.com

Page 384, Wellcome Trust Photo Library

Page 442, Sobotta: Atlas der Anatomie des Menschen, 22nd edition © Elsevier GmbH, Urban & Fischer Verlag Munchen

Page 446, Wellcome Trust Photo Library

Additional Material

The publisher would like to thank Dr. Daniel Quemby, MBBS (Hons), BSc (Hons), BSc Med Sci, MRCS, FRCA, medical doctor, anesthetist, and expedition doctor for his kind permission to use some additional material that has been included in Chapters 4 and 5. This material first appeared in *The Concise Book of Muscles, 4th ed.*, also published by Lotus Publishing.

A Note on American and British Spellings

This book uses US spelling conventions, and some of the technical ones may be unfamiliar to students from the UK or elsewhere. A list of these is provided below. Students should be aware of these different spellings as they may encounter them in their future studies or work.

The list doesn't include examples of the simple s/z difference, such as in "mineralised" and "catalysed" (UK) versus "mineralized" and "catalyzed" (US). And some of the more common words—e.g., the American "millimeter, " "gray," and "odor" versus the British "millimetre," "grey," and "odour"—are likewise not included here.

For the most part, the differences in spelling are minor; for example, "ae" in the British "anaemia" and "haemoglobin" versus just "e" in the US "anemia" and "hemoglobin." Or "oe" in the British "oestrogen" and "oesophagus" versus just "e" in the American "estrogen" and "esophagus."

There is an exception, however, where the most common term in the US is an entirely different word from the one most commonly used in the UK: "epinephrine" is the preferred American form for what the British mostly call "adrenaline." The same difference is seen with "norepinephrine" and "noradrenaline." This book uses "epinephrine" and "norepinephrine," but in places readers will see "adrenaline" and "noradrenaline" also, as a reminder.

BRITISH/AMERICAN SPELLING DIFFERENCES OF TECHNICAL TERMS

British term	US term
adrenaline	epinephrine
aetiology	etiology
aluminium	aluminum
amenorrhoea	amenorrhea
anaemia	anemia
anaesthetise	anesthetize
bacteraemia	bacteremia
caecum	cecum
coeliac	celiac
diarrhoea	diarrhea
dyslipidaemia	dyslipidemia
dysmenorrhoea	dysmenorrhea
dyspnoea	dyspnea

BRITISH/AMERICAN SPELLING DIFFERENCES OF TECHNICAL TERMS

British term	US term
faeces	feces
foetus, foetal	fetus, fetal
galactorrhoea	galactorrhea
goitre	goiter
gonorrhoea	gonorrhea
gynaecologist	gynecologist
gynaecomastia	gynecomastia
haematoma	hematoma
haematuria	hematuria
haemoglobin	hemoglobin
haemophilia	hemophilia
haemopoiesis	hemopoiesis
haemoptysis	hemoptysis
haemorrhage, haemorrhagic	hemorrhage, hemorrhagic
haemorrhoids	hemorrhoids
haemostasis	hemostasis
humour	humor
hypercholesterolaemia	hypercholesterolemia
hyperglycaemia	hyperglycemia
hypertriglyceridaemia	hypertriglyceridemia
hypocalcaemia	hypocalcemia
hypoglycaemia	hypoglycemia
ileocaecal	ileocecal
ischaemia, ischaemic	ischemia, ischemic
leukaemia	leukemia
lymphoedema	lymphedema
mould	mold
myxoedema	myxedema
noradrenaline	norepinephrine
oedema	edema
oesophageal	esophageal
oesophagitis	esophagitis
oesophagus	esophagus
oestradiol	estradiol
oestriol	estriol
oestrogen, oestrogenic	estrogen, estrogenic
oestrone	estrone
onychogryphosis	onychogryposis
oxyhaemoglobin	oxyhemoglobin
seborrhoea	seborrhea
septicaemia	septicemia
sulphur	sulfur
thalassaemia	thalassemia
tumour	tumor

1

Before You Begin

Introduction

If someone asked you to name an organ superior to the bladder, would you understand exactly what they meant? Before you even begin to look at the structure and function of the body, let's learn a few of the basic anatomical terms and their meanings.

What is **anatomy**? Anatomy is the study of the *structure* of the body. It looks at what the body is made of—for example, bones and organs.

What is **physiology**? Physiology is the study of the *functions* of the body. It looks at how the body works—for example, how the blood is pumped around the body.

What is **pathology**? Pathology is the study of the *diseases* of the body. It looks at what can go wrong in the body.

Anatomical position

The anatomical position is a basic position that can always be used as a reference point. It allows you to describe or name areas of the body in terms of a specific reference that all anatomists will know. This avoids any confusion.

The person in figure 1.1 is standing in the **anatomical position**:

- Head facing forward
- Feet parallel
- Arms hanging by the side
- Most importantly, palms facing forward.

The front of the body (where the face is) is called the **anterior** or **ventral**, and the back of the body is the **posterior** or **dorsal**. These terms can also be used to indicate when something is in front of or behind something else. For example, the heart is anterior to the spine and the spine is posterior to the heart.

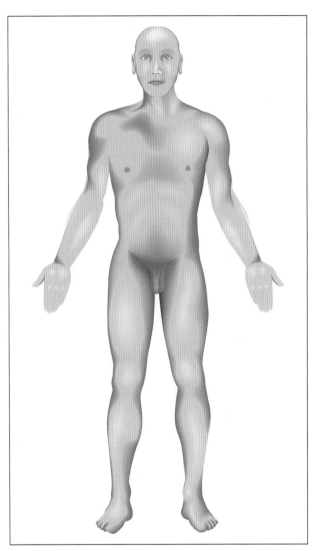

Figure 1.1 *Anatomical position*

Directional terms

Imagine a line running right through the center of the body: between your eyes, through the middle of your nose and mouth, down through the center of your neck, chest, stomach, and pelvis, and ending between your feet. This is the **midline** or **median line**. It is an imaginary line that acts as a reference for many anatomical terms, including those describing certain movements, such as adduction (which you will learn about later).

In relation to the midline are the following directional terms:

DIRECTIONAL TERMS	
Term	**Direction**
Superior	toward the head, above
Inferior	away from the head, below
Medial	toward the midline, on the inner side
Lateral	away from the midline, on the outer side
Proximal	closer to its origin or point of attachment of a limb
Distal	farther from its origin or point of attachment of a limb
Superficial	toward the surface of the body
Deep	away from the surface of the body
Peripheral	at the surface or outer part of the body
Anterior	at the front of the body, in front of
Posterior	at the back of the body, behind
Cephalad	toward the head, above
Cranial	of or relating to the skull (can also mean toward the head or cranium)
Caudal	away from the head, below
Ventral	at the front of the body, in front of
Dorsal	at the back of the body, behind

Here are a few examples to help you get used to the anatomical terms:

The nose is **superior** to the mouth.
The mouth is **inferior** to the nose.
The nose is **medial** to the ears.
The ears are **lateral** to the nose.
The elbow is **proximal** to the wrist (the arm's point of attachment is the shoulder).

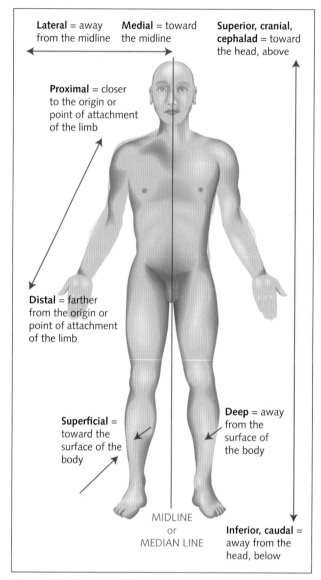

Figure 1.2 *Directional terms*

The wrist is **distal** to the elbow (the arm's point of attachment is the shoulder).
The skin is **superficial** to the muscles.
The muscles are **deep** to the skin.
The hands and feet are at the **periphery** of the body.

Terms relating to movement are covered in chapter 4.

Anatomical Regions and Body Cavities

When studying the body it makes sense to divide it into smaller areas or regions. This enables us to discuss parts of the body without having to continually describe where they are. The body can be divided into:

- **Anatomical regions:** These relate to specific areas of the body. For example, the neck is the cervical region. When we discuss cervical nerves or cervical vertebrae we are talking about the nerves and vertebrae of the neck.
- **Body cavities:** These are spaces in the body that contain and protect the organs of the body. For example, the cranial cavity contains the brain.

Anatomical regions

Study tips

Certain facts in anatomy simply have to be memorized and this is especially true for the anatomical regions of the body. The following charts will help you learn the correct terminology for each region.

Learn one chart at a time and touch the areas on your body as you memorize the words.

Make flash cards. On the front of the card will be the anatomical term. On the back of the card will be the area described. Use these cards in a study group.

GENERAL	
Term	**Region described**
Cutaneous	Skin

REGIONS OF THE HEAD AND NECK	
Term	**Region described**
Cephalic	Head
Cranial	Skull
Facial	Face
Frontal	Forehead
Ophthalmic/orbital	Eye
Otic	Ear
Buccal	Cheek
Nasal	Nose
Occipital	Back of head
Cervical	Neck

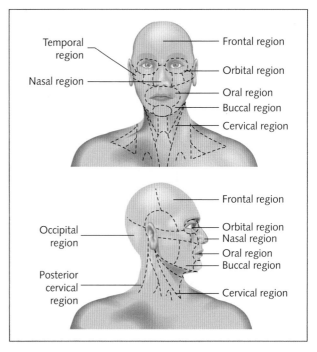

Figure 1.3 *Anatomical regions of the head and neck*

REGIONS OF THE TRUNK	
Term	**Region described**
Thoracic	Chest
Costal	Ribs
Pericardial	Heart
Mammary	Breast
Abdominal	Abdomen
Umbilical	Navel
Dorsal	Back
Lumbar	Lower back
Coxal	Hip
Pelvic	Pelvis
Inguinal	Groin
Pubic	Pubis
Perineal	Area between anus and urethral opening

REGIONS OF THE ARM	
Term	**Region described**
Acromial	Shoulder
Scapular	Shoulder blade
Axillary	Armpit
Brachial	Arm, upper limb
Cubital	Elbow or forearm
Antecubital	Front of the elbow
Olecranal	Back of the elbow
Antebrachial	Forearm
Carpal	Wrist
Manus	Hand
Palmar/metacarpal	Palm, inner surface of the hand
Digital/phalangeal	Fingers (also refers to toes)

REGIONS OF THE LEG	
Term	**Region described**
Gluteal	Buttock
Crural	Leg, lower limb
Femoral	Thigh
Patellar	Front of the knee
Popliteal	Hollow behind the knee
Sural	Calf
Tarsal	Ankle
Pedal	Foot
Calcaneal	Heel
Plantar	Sole of the foot
Digital/ phalangeal	Toes (also refers to fingers)

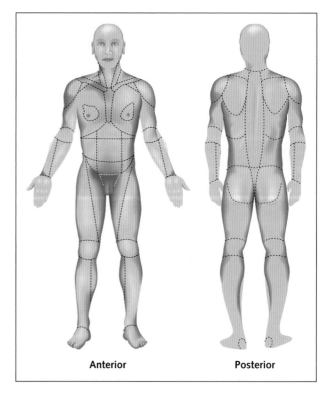

Anterior   **Posterior**

Figure 1.4 *Anatomical regions*

Body cavities

Body cavities are spaces within the body that contain and protect the internal organs. There are two main cavities:

1. The **dorsal** cavity (at the back of the body)
2. The **ventral** cavity (at the front of the body).

These are subdivided as follows:

DORSAL CAVITY	
Cranial cavity	Contains the brain and is protected by the bony skull (cranium)
Spinal cavity/ canal	Contains the spinal cord and is protected by the vertebrae

VENTRAL CAVITY	
Thoracic cavity	Contains the trachea, two bronchi, two lungs, the heart, and the esophagus, and is protected by the ribcage; it is separated from the abdominal cavity by the diaphragm
Abdominopelvic cavity, consisting of the:	
Abdominal cavity	Contains the stomach, spleen, liver, gall bladder, pancreas, small intestine, and most of the large intestine, covered by a serous membrane called the peritoneum; the abdominal cavity is mainly protected by the muscles of the abdominal wall and partially by the ribcage and diaphragm
Pelvic cavity	Contains a portion of the large intestine, the urinary bladder, and the reproductive organs; it is protected by the pelvic bones

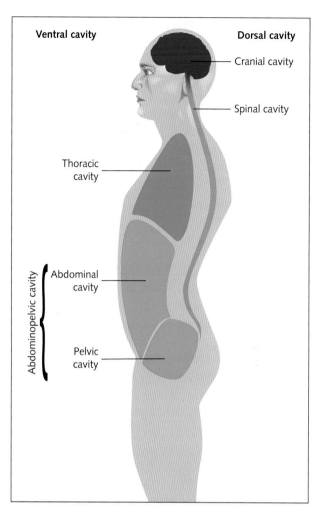

Figure 1.5 *Body cavities*

Note: For ease of learning, blood vessels, lymphatic vessels, lymph nodes, and nerves have not been included in these charts. When learning about the body cavities it is important to know the following terms:

- **Parietal:** Relating to the inner walls of a body cavity
- **Visceral:** Relating to the internal organs of the body.

Dividing the Body

The body is often divided by:

- **Planes:** These are imaginary lines used to cut the body or organs into sections. They can be used anywhere on the body or on any organ.
- **Quadrants:** These are imaginary lines that specifically divide the abdominopelvic cavity into four parts so that it is easier to locate the organs found in this large cavity.

Planes

Anatomists often divide the body or an organ into sections so that they can study its internal structures. These sections are made along imaginary flat surfaces called **planes**, which are as follows:

- **Sagittal plane:** Divides the body vertically into right and left portions

- **Frontal/coronal plane:** Divides the body vertically (longitudinally) into posterior and anterior portions
- **Transverse plane (cross-section):** Divides the body horizontally into inferior and superior portions
- **Oblique plane:** Divides the body at an angle between the transverse plane and the frontal/sagittal plane.

Quadrants

The abdominopelvic cavity is large and contains many organs. It is, therefore, helpful to divide it into smaller regions that can be named according to their relative positions. These regions are **quadrants** and include the right upper quadrant (RUQ), the left upper quadrant (LUQ), the right lower quadrant (RLQ), and the left lower quadrant (LLQ).

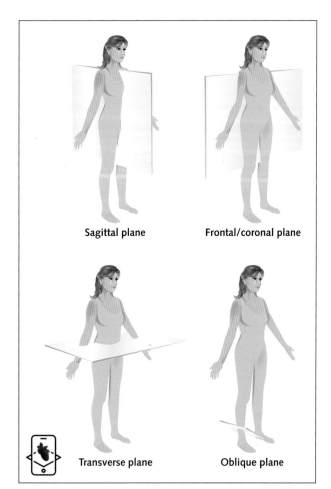

Sagittal plane   Frontal/coronal plane

Transverse plane   Oblique plane

Figure 1.6 *Planes*

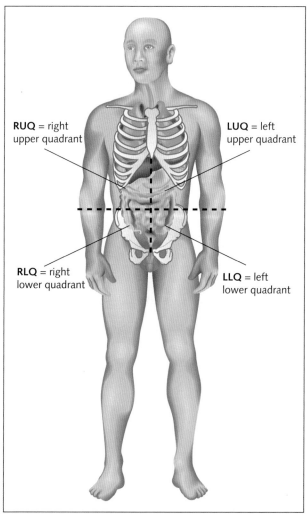

RUQ = right upper quadrant   **LUQ** = left upper quadrant

RLQ = right lower quadrant   **LLQ** = left lower quadrant

Figure 1.7 *Quadrants*

NEW WORDS	
Anatomical position	Position in which the body is standing erect with the feet parallel, the arms hanging down by the side, and the face and palms facing forward
Anatomy	The study of the structure of the body
Anterior	At the front of the body, in front of
Caudal	Away from the head, below
Cephalad	Toward the head, above
Coronal plane	Divides vertically (longitudinally) into anterior and posterior portions
Cranial	Toward the head, above
Cross-section	Divides horizontally into inferior and superior portions
Deep	Away from the surface of the body
Distal	Farther from its origin or point of attachment of a limb
Dorsal	At the back of the body, behind
Frontal plane	Divides vertically (longitudinally) into anterior and posterior portions
Inferior	Away from the head, below
Lateral	Away from the midline, on the outer side
Medial	Toward the midline, on the inner side
Median line	Line through the middle of the body

NEW WORDS	
Midline	Line through the middle of the body
Oblique plane	Divides at an angle between a transverse plane and a frontal or sagittal plane
Parietal	Relating to the inner walls of a body cavity
Pathology	The study of the diseases of the body
Peripheral	At the surface or outer part of the body
Physiology	The study of the functions of the body
Plane	Imaginary flat surface that divides the body or organs into parts
Posterior	At the back of the body, behind
Proximal	Closer to its origin or point of attachment of a limb
Quadrant	A region of the abdominopelvic cavity
Sagittal plane	Divides vertically into right and left portions
Superficial	Toward the surface of the body
Superior	Toward the head, above
Transverse plane	Divides horizontally into inferior and superior portions
Ventral	At the front of the body, in front of
Visceral	Relating to the internal organs of the body

Multiple-Choice Questions

1. Superficial means:
   a. Toward the center of the body
   b. Toward the surface of the body
   c. Toward the head
   d. Toward the feet

2. The front of the body is referred to as:
   a. Dorsal
   b. Proximal
   c. Superficial
   d. Ventral

3. In the anatomical position the palms are:
   a. Facing backward
   b. Facing forward
   c. In front of the body
   d. Behind the body

4. The shoulders are _____ to the neck.
   a. Medial
   b. Superior
   c. Lateral
   d. Superficial

5. The skeleton is _____ to the skin.
   a. Proximal
   b. Distal
   c. Superficial
   d. Deep

6. The knee is _____ to the thigh.
   a. Proximal
   b. Distal
   c. Superficial
   d. Deep

7. The imaginary line that divides the body horizontally into superior and inferior portions is called the:
   a. Sagittal plane
   b. Frontal plane
   c. Transverse plane
   d. Oblique plane

8. The feet are _____ to the knees.
   a. Caudal
   b. Cephalad
   c. Medial
   d. Lateral

9. Anatomy is the study of the:
   a. Diseases of the body
   b. Structure of the body
   c. Function of the body
   d. None of the above

10. The study of how the heart works forms part of:
    a. Anatomy
    b. Pathology
    c. Physiology
    d. Herbology

11. Imaginary straight lines used to divide the body into sections are called:
    a. Planes
    b. Cavities
    c. Quadrants
    d. Regions

12. The left upper quadrant is commonly referred to as the:
    a. RUQ
    b. LUQ
    c. RLQ
    d. LLQ

13. Oblique planes cut the body:
    a. At angles to the other planes
    b. Perpendicular to the other planes
    c. Parallel to the other planes
    d. None of the above

14. The right lower quadrant is found in the:
    a. Thoracic cavity
    b. Spinal cavity
    c. Cranial cavity
    d. Abdominopelvic cavity

15. Sagittal planes divide the body into:
    a. Superior and inferior portions
    b. Right and left portions
    c. Anterior and posterior portions
    d. Angles

Note to Students

Now that you have a basic idea of anatomical language, it is time to start looking at the body in more depth. The following chapter describes the organization of the body and introduces you to the different systems that you will need to learn. Each of these systems is then covered in depth in its own chapter.

As you work through this book you will find the following:

- **Infoboxes:** These boxes will help you put your learning into perspective and bring it to life for you.
- **New words:** You may want to memorize these new words to help you improve your vocabulary.
- **In the classroom:** These are simple ideas and exercises that can be used in a classroom environment or with a group of friends in a study group.
- **Study tips:** These will help you revise previous sections that are important to what you are currently learning and will also give you simple techniques to help you grasp a topic.
- **Red flags:** Red flag signs or symptoms alert you to possible health conditions that need to be investigated by a medical doctor.
- **Review and multiple-choice questions:** By covering these at the end of every chapter you will be able to see how well you have understood the topic. Answers are on p. 410.

Anatomy and physiology is a fascinating subject and easy to learn because *you* are everything you need to know—simply look at yourself when learning the subject. Think about what is going on inside your body and learn about yourself!

Learning Pathology

Defining pathology as the study of diseases is a very simplistic view of what pathology really is. Pathology is not only studying diseases, but also their causes, signs, and symptoms—it is putting together all the pieces of a puzzle so that a complete picture can be revealed and understood. Unfortunately, learning pathology cannot be rushed. It can't be done "parrot-fashion" or straight from a book. So take some time to learn it slowly and you will enjoy it. Take time to:

- **Learn what is "normal":** If you learn your anatomy and physiology well and know what is considered healthy, then you will be able to recognize when something is wrong.
- **Look for the difference:** Each time you learn about a new disease, try to find what makes that disease different from another one that is similar. What one thing do you find odd, different, or distinctive (and therefore memorable)?
- **Analyze the causes:** Spend time analyzing the underlying causes of the disease. In doing this you will not only come to understand the disease process better, you will also be revising your basic anatomy and physiology.
- **Think about the effects:** Again, spend time actually thinking about what it must be like to have the disease you are studying. How would having that disease affect your day-to-day life and your mental health? Get to know what it must be like to live with the disease and you will get to know the disease.
- **Talk to people:** Most people have an ailment or condition of some kind and, as William Osler (1849–1919) said, "To study the phenomena of diseases without books is to sail an uncharted sea, while to study books without patients is not to go to sea at all."

Important vocabulary

Rippey (1994, p. 1) wrote, "To understand pathology it is necessary to learn a new language," and this section covers a few of the more common terms you will need to know.

To begin with, every disease comes with a list of signs and symptoms. It is important that you know the difference:

- **Sign:** Signs can be detected by someone next to the patient. For example, skin rashes, lumps, and high blood pressure.
- **Symptom:** Symptoms are felt by the patient. Examples include pain, fatigue, anxiety, and thirst.

It is also necessary to know how much of the body is affected by the condition:

- **Localized:** If only a specific organ or area is affected then it is said to be localized. For example, rosacea on the cheeks.

- **Systemic:** If the whole body is involved the condition is said to be systemic. For example, influenza.

Here are some examples to help you understand the difference:

- A sprained ankle is localized inflammation because only the ankle is affected, while rheumatoid arthritis is systemic inflammation because many joints are affected.
- A urinary tract infection is a localized infection, while septicemia is systemic.

Diseases are viewed and treated differently depending on whether they are acute or chronic:

- **Acute:** Acute diseases generally begin suddenly and are short-lived. They are resolvable. For example, chickenpox or a broken bone.
- **Chronic:** Chronic diseases, on the other hand, are persistent and not always resolvable. For example, diabetes mellitus or rheumatoid arthritis.

The following signs accompany a range of diseases and are indicative of underlying disorders that require further investigation:

- **Cachexia:** This term refers to muscle wasting. Cachexic people lose not only fat but also muscle, and they look as if they are "wasting away." Their weight loss is usually accompanied by fatigue and a loss of appetite. Cachexia is common in chronic diseases, especially cancer, tuberculosis, and AIDS.
- **Cyanosis:** Cyanosis is a bluish discoloration of the skin or mucous membranes. It usually represents low oxygen levels in the blood and should be investigated. Someone having an acute asthma attack may become cyanotic, or an individual with a chronic respiratory disease such as emphysema may be cyanotic.
- **Fever:** A fever is an elevated body temperature (>100°F, or 37.8°C). If a person presents with a fever it is important to find its cause. Acute fevers often indicate an infection, while chronic fevers can be indicative of chronic disease such as cancer.
- **Inflammation:** Inflammation is a common immune response to injury or invasion and is characterized by localized swelling, warmth, redness, pain, and sometimes loss of movement.
- **Jaundice:** Jaundice is not a disease, but it is a sign that there is an underlying disorder that needs to be investigated. Jaundice is the yellowing of the skin or whites of the eyes and is caused by high levels of bilirubin in the bloodstream. It can result from liver disease, blockage of bile ducts, or excessive breakdown of red blood cells.
- **Edema:** This is the excessive accumulation of interstitial fluid in body tissues. It results in swelling and puffiness. Edema may be localized—for example, swelling at a site of injury—or it may be more generalized. Causes of edema can range from local injuries to heart or kidney disorders.
- **Pallor:** Pallor is a lack of color, or paleness. It can be difficult to distinguish unless you know the person's "healthy" skin color and so is best assessed by looking at a person's conjunctiva and skin creases. Pallor is common in conditions such as anemia and shock.

Finally, when discussing diseases doctors often talk about the etiology, diagnosis, prognosis, and pathogenesis of the disease:

- **Etiology**—the cause or origin of the disease
- **Diagnosis**—the identification or process of naming the disease
- **Prognosis**—the doctor's opinion of how the disease will progress and what its most likely outcome will be for the patient
- **Pathogenesis**—how a disease process is set up in the body, including the cause and mechanisms of the disease.

The following paragraph will hopefully help you put these new words into context:

Mark went to his doctor because he had a small but angry rash (**sign**) on the palms of his hands (**localized**). The doctor asked him if the rash was a new, sudden rash (**acute**) or if he had had it for a couple of months (**chronic**). Then the doctor tried to find out what caused the rash (the **etiology**): perhaps contact with a chemical, or stress? He also asked Mark if he had any accompanying itching or pain (**symptoms**). Eventually the doctor told Mark he had contact dermatitis (**diagnosis**) caused by the new hand soap he was using. He explained how the chemicals caused an inflammatory response in his skin (**pathogenesis**) and then told Mark that if he stopped using the soap his rash should clear up quickly (**prognosis**).

Stress and Mental Health

Mental, emotional, and physical health are deeply intertwined and cannot be separated. When homeostasis is threatened, or perceived to be threatened, our body reacts to that stressor in a number of different ways:

- **The fight-flight-freeze response—epinephrine and norepinephrine:** When put under short-term stress, such as being physically threatened, our autonomic nervous system responds with a "fight-flight-freeze response." Part of this response is the stimulation of the adrenal medulla, which secretes epinephrine and norepinephrine into the blood system. These two hormones prepare the body to either fight or flee a situation by causing changes in the body that result in more oxygen and glucose in the blood and a faster circulation of blood to the brain, muscles, and heart. Occasionally, a person may freeze in response to a situation.

- **Long-term stress—cortisol:** To help you deal with long-term stress, such as the death of a loved one, glucocorticoids like cortisol are secreted by the adrenal cortex. Glucocorticoids help protect the body from the long-term effects of stress, but they also depress the immune system.

- **Stress mediators:** In addition to the hormones mentioned above, the body also releases neurotransmitters, cytokines, and growth factors to help the body mediate stress. Importantly, the immune system is stimulated and this often results in an inflammatory response (hence allergies and autoimmune diseases can be aggravated by stress).

In the classroom

As you work your way through this book, take time to discuss the impact stress has on each system of the body.

As a therapist, it is important to be aware of the impact that a newly diagnosed illness, an unpleasantly disabling condition, or a terminal disease can have on an individual's mental and emotional state. Similarly, physical signs and symptoms can be suggestive of underlying emotional conditions that need to be addressed. The table below highlights a few common conditions.

DISORDER	PSYCHOLOGICAL SIGNS AND SYMPTOMS	SOMATIC SIGNS AND SYMPTOMS
Alcohol abuse	Depression Anxiety Behavior changes Restlessness Alcoholic dementia	Physical injuries due to falls, accidents, or fighting Liver disease Thiamin (vitamin B_1) deficiency Peripheral neuropathy Gastrointestinal problems
Anxiety	Worry Irritability Apprehension Poor concentration	Fatigue Insomnia Headaches Palpitations Tremors Dizziness Sweating Breathlessness Chest pain Urinary frequency Diarrhea

DISORDER	PSYCHOLOGICAL SIGNS AND SYMPTOMS	SOMATIC SIGNS AND SYMPTOMS
Depression	Low mood Loss of interest Loss of enjoyment Low self-esteem Pessimism/negativity Guilt Suicidal thoughts	Fatigue Insomnia Appetite and weight changes Loss of libido
Post-traumatic stress disorder (PTSD)	Recurrent memories (flashbacks) Nightmares Emotional blunting Anxiety Depression	Insomnia Avoidance of situations similar to how/where trauma occurred Alcohol or drug misuse
Substance (drug) abuse	Addiction Depression Anxiety Personality changes Psychiatric disturbances	Overdosage Behavior changes Problems linked to route of administration, e.g., infections such as hepatitis or HIV in intravenous users, local abscesses or thrombi developing at site of use in intravenous users, erosion of nasal septum in chronic cocaine use) Cardiac disorders Toxic psychosis

2

Organization of the Body

Introduction

The body is a complex and intricate machine. When you break it down into its smallest parts and put it together again you will be fascinated at how clever it really is. You may also feel a little overwhelmed. For example, it's mind-boggling to think that you started your life as an egg, an egg formed inside your mother, an egg formed when your mother was an embryo inside her mother—in other words, you started your life inside your grandmother!

Your body is also composed of trillions of cells, yet you lose billions of those cells every day, and your body keeps replacing them. In addition, did you know that every human cell, except for mature red blood cells, is potentially capable of forming a complete human being? In this chapter you'll get a look into this incredible world. We look firstly at the organization of the body and how it all fits together, and then we look at exactly what makes up the body: cells. We will then discover how cells function, divide, and unite to form tissues such as skin, muscles, and nerves.

Student objectives

By the end of this chapter you will be able to:

- Identify the different levels of organization of the body
- Describe the basic chemical make-up of the body
- Describe the structure and function of cells and discuss how they reproduce
- Identify the major tissues that make up the body and be able to describe their structure, function, and location
- Identify the major systems of the body.

Infobox

Anatomy and physiology in perspective

You may be asking yourself why you should study the chemistry of the body. There is one simple answer. You are made up of thousands of tiny chemicals continuously reacting with one another. What you put into your body (everything you eat or drink) and what you put on top of it (such as creams or lotions) are also made up of chemicals. These chemicals react with those in your body and change it. Now, isn't it worth knowing a little about chemistry?

Levels of Structural Organization of the Body

Look at yourself: you are an organism, a living individual who breathes, moves, eats, and functions. But do you know what you are really made of?

Figure 2.1 below summarizes the different levels of structural organization of the body.

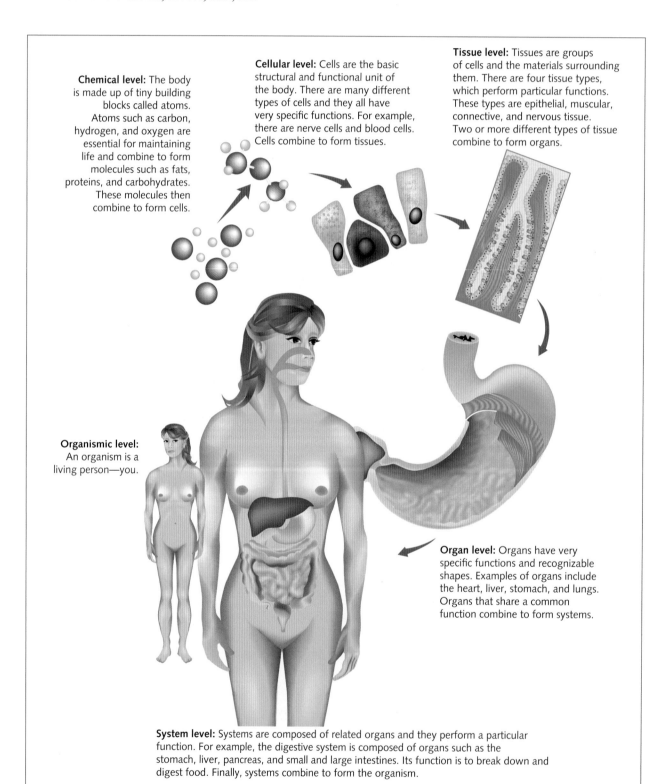

Chemical level: The body is made up of tiny building blocks called atoms. Atoms such as carbon, hydrogen, and oxygen are essential for maintaining life and combine to form molecules such as fats, proteins, and carbohydrates. These molecules then combine to form cells.

Cellular level: Cells are the basic structural and functional unit of the body. There are many different types of cells and they all have very specific functions. For example, there are nerve cells and blood cells. Cells combine to form tissues.

Tissue level: Tissues are groups of cells and the materials surrounding them. There are four tissue types, which perform particular functions. These types are epithelial, muscular, connective, and nervous tissue. Two or more different types of tissue combine to form organs.

Organismic level: An organism is a living person—you.

Organ level: Organs have very specific functions and recognizable shapes. Examples of organs include the heart, liver, stomach, and lungs. Organs that share a common function combine to form systems.

System level: Systems are composed of related organs and they perform a particular function. For example, the digestive system is composed of organs such as the stomach, liver, pancreas, and small and large intestines. Its function is to break down and digest food. Finally, systems combine to form the organism.

Figure 2.1 *Levels of structural organization of the body*

Chemical Organization of the Body

In order to understand what our bodies are made of and how they work, it helps to have a basic knowledge of chemistry. Chemistry is the study of matter, of its structures and interactions. Matter is anything that occupies space (has volume) and has mass (weight), and all living and non-living things consist of matter. Everything around you is made of matter!

So take a look at what is around you. The chair you are sitting on is made of matter. Perhaps it is a wooden chair? If it is made from wood, then what is that wood made from? What can it be broken down into? Wood can be broken down into a number of different components, one of which is cellulose. Cellulose can be broken down into smaller "building blocks," or molecules, of glucose. Glucose can be broken down into even smaller building blocks of carbon, hydrogen, and oxygen. These are elements. Sitting there, thinking what your chair is made of and what smaller and smaller building blocks you can break it down into is basically thinking "like a chemist."

Atoms and elements

The chart below shows the common elements found in the body.

ELEMENTS OF THE BODY	
Element	**Role in the body**
There are four major elements in the body, which make up 96% of the body's mass. They are:	
Oxygen	A component of water and organic molecules and essential to cellular respiration, a process in which cellular energy, adenosine triphosphate (ATP), is produced
Carbon	The main component of all organic molecules (e.g., carbohydrates, lipids, proteins, and nucleic acids)
Hydrogen	A component of water, all foods, and organic molecules; also influences the pH of body fluids
Nitrogen	A component of all proteins and nucleic acids
There are nine lesser elements in the body, which make up 3.9% of the body's mass. They are:	
Calcium	Found in bones and teeth; also necessary for muscle contraction, nerve transmission, release of hormones, and blood clotting
Phosphorus	Found in bones and teeth as well as in nucleic acids and many proteins; also forms part of ATP
Potassium	Necessary for many chemical reactions within the cell; also important for nerve impulses and muscle contraction
Sulfur	A component of some vitamins and many proteins
Sodium	Necessary for many chemical reactions in the extracellular fluid (fluid outside of the cell); also plays a role in water balance, nerve impulses, and muscle contraction
Chlorine	Necessary for many chemical reactions in the extracellular fluid
Magnesium	Found mainly in bone and necessary for the activity of more than 300 enzymes in the body
Iodine	Necessary for the synthesis of thyroid hormones
Iron	A component of the hemoglobin molecule, which transports oxygen within red blood cells
There are thirteen other elements in the body that are present in such small quantities that they are known as trace elements. They make up 0.1% of the body's mass and are:	
Aluminum, boron, chromium, cobalt, copper, fluorine, manganese, molybdenum, selenium, silicon, tin, vanadium, and **zinc**	

Let's get back to the elements carbon, hydrogen, and oxygen. Can they be broken down further? Yes—into atoms. The atoms themselves can be broken down into subatomic particles called **protons, neutrons**, and **electrons**, which are also made of smaller particles. However, we are going to stop our deconstruction of wood at atoms because **atoms are the smallest units of matter that retain the properties of that matter.**

Think about a gold wedding ring for a moment. Break that ring into the smallest pieces you possibly can and it will still be gold. If you keep breaking down that shiny, malleable, bright gold into even smaller pieces you will eventually get atoms. All the atoms will be the same, they will all have the same number of protons and hence the same chemical properties—this means that gold is an element. **Elements are substances made up of only one type of atom.** An atom of gold will always have 79 protons in it. If you take away one proton it will no longer be gold—it will in fact be platinum. If you add one proton to the atom of gold it will become mercury. Strange, isn't it?

Hopefully you can now see that it is the atom that has the properties of a particular element. It is the atom that is the most basic unit of the element. If you break an atom of gold into protons, neutrons, and electrons and mix these with the protons, neutrons, and electrons from silver, you will simply have piles of protons, neutrons, and electrons—no gold or silver.

The number of protons in the nucleus of the atom defines the element, and never changes. The electrons, however, can be attracted to other atoms and interact (bond) with them. To be able to predict how elements will interact with one another it is necessary to know how many protons and electrons each element has. Luckily for us, this is depicted in the periodic table (below). The periodic table displays chemical elements arranged from left to right and top to bottom in order of increasing atomic number (number of protons). It helps chemists quickly predict the properties and behavior of an element.

Structure of atoms

Take a look at the atom of carbon in the diagrams opposite. At the center of the atom is a **nucleus** of protons and neutrons. Moving around the nucleus in circles, known as **electron shells**, are electrons. The protons have a positive charge and the electrons have a negative charge and so the two are attracted to each other, and it is through this attraction that

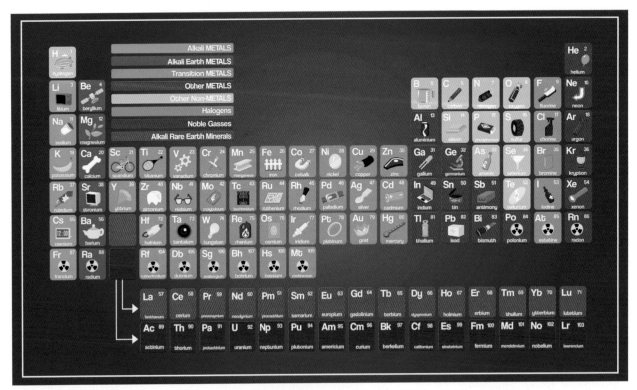

Figure 2.2 *The periodic table*

the electrons are bound to the nucleus. The neutrons don't have a charge—they are neutral.

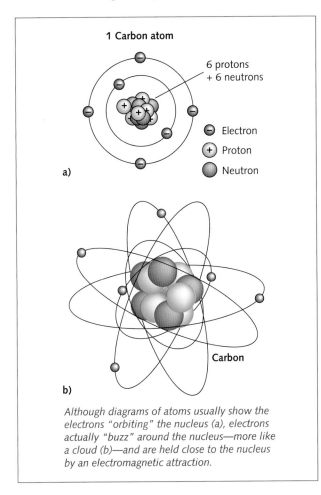

1 Carbon atom

6 protons
+ 6 neutrons

- Electron
+ Proton
Neutron

a)

Carbon

b)

Although diagrams of atoms usually show the electrons "orbiting" the nucleus (a), electrons actually "buzz" around the nucleus—more like a cloud (b)—and are held close to the nucleus by an electromagnetic attraction.

The number of shells an atom has depends on how many electrons it has. The first shell, closest to the nucleus, can hold only 2 electrons. The second shell can hold a maximum of 8 electrons, and the third can hold up to 18. Electron shells are always filled from the one nearest the nucleus outward, and the outermost shell of an atom is called the **valence shell**.

To know whether or not an element is going to bond with another element, you need to know how many electrons are in its valence shell. If an atom has eight electrons in its valence shell it will be chemically stable. If it doesn't have eight electrons, then it will easily bond with other atoms. Try to think of valence electrons as being social creatures who always want to be part of a group of eight friends! This rule applies to most atoms, except for hydrogen and helium because they only have one shell—remember, the first shell can hold only two electrons. Helium has two electrons in this shell and so is stable and does

not bond easily with other atoms. Hydrogen, on the other hand, has only one electron in this shell and so readily bonds with other atoms—hydrogen is always looking for a friend!

When atoms bind with one another, it is the distribution of their valence electrons that determines the chemical bonds that are formed. There are three types of chemical bonds: **ionic bonds, covalent bonds,** and **hydrogen bonds**. Before looking at these chemical bonds, it is important to take note of how the atoms have achieved their stable valence shells—have they given up or gained electrons, or have they shared electrons? Atoms that give up or gain electrons become **ions**, while atoms that share electrons combine with one another to form **molecules**.

Ions

Although the number of protons (**atomic number**) of an atom can never change, the number of electrons can change. An atom can lose or gain another electron and this will change the charge of the atom. **A "charged" atom is called an ion.**

Let us look at carbon again. When neutral, carbon has six protons and six electrons. Each electron in this atom is attracted to a proton and so the atom is nicely "balanced." However, carbon can lose an electron to another atom and so have six protons but only five electrons. Because protons hold a positive charge and there is one more proton than the number of electrons, the carbon will now have a net positive charge. **A positive ion is called a cation.** If the atom has more electrons than protons in the atom, it will have a net negative charge, and **a negative ion is called an anion.**

> ## Atoms and elements in a nutshell
>
> - Atoms are the smallest unit of matter.
> - Elements consist of uniquely structured atoms.
> - The four major elements in the body are carbon, hydrogen, oxygen, and nitrogen.

Molecules and compounds

When atoms share electrons they combine to form molecules. A molecule can be composed of two atoms of the same element, for example an oxygen molecule, or it can be composed of atoms of different elements, for example water (containing hydrogen and oxygen). **Molecules containing atoms of two or more different elements are called compounds.**

Most of the chemicals in the body exist in the form of compounds (see the chart on p. 28, "Major Compounds of the Body").

Molecules and compounds in a nutshell

- Water is the solvent in body fluids.
- Carbohydrates are the fuel of the body.
- Fats have many roles, such as insulation, protection, and energy storage.
- Proteins are the building blocks of the body.
- Nucleic acids build our genes.
- ATP gives our cells energy.
- Nutrients are needed for growth, maintenance, and repair.

Infobox

Anatomy and physiology in perspective

Free radicals are atoms or groups of atoms with an unpaired electron in their valence shell. This means they are "electrically charged" and therefore highly reactive. In the body, free radicals are unstable, highly reactive atoms that can destroy nearby molecules. Consuming antioxidants such as vitamins C and E can help inactivate some oxygen-derived free radicals.

Chemical bonds

As mentioned above, atoms are always seeking to have a full valence shell and so often combine with one another. In doing so, they form chemical bonds. There are three types of bonds:

1. **Ionic bonds:** In ionic bonds the electrons from one atom are fully transferred to the outer shell of another atom. This leaves the atoms with an "imbalanced" number of electrons and protons and so the atoms are now charged—they are now **ions** and are held together through an electrostatic attraction.

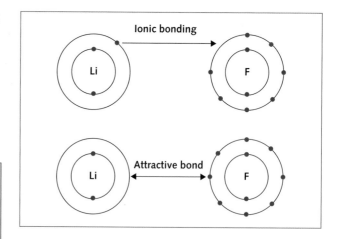

2. **Covalent bonds:** In covalent bonds two atoms share pairs of electrons and form molecules.

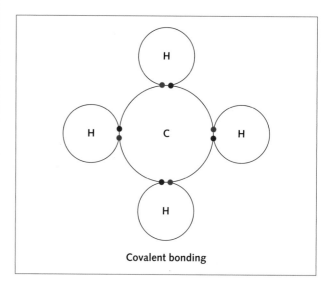

Covalent bonding

3. **Hydrogen bonds:** Hydrogen bonds form between hydrogen atoms and other atoms because of the attraction of oppositely charged molecules, rather than the actual sharing or transfer of electrons. Hence they are weak bonds that do not bind atoms into molecules. Hydrogen bonds link water molecules together.

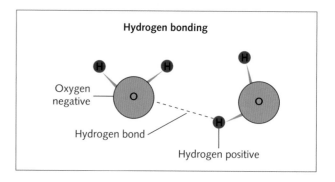

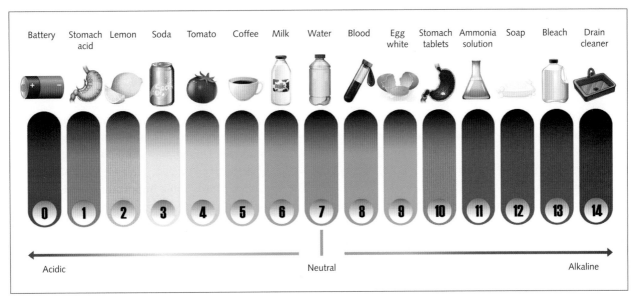

Figure 2.3 *The pH scale*

The pH scale: Acids, bases, and salts

Most chemical reactions in the body can occur only when the fluid in which these reactions take place is at a specific pH.

pH is a measure of the concentration of hydrogen ions (H^+) in a solution: the higher the concentration of hydrogen ions, the lower the pH and the more acidic it is. Alkalis contain hydroxide ions (OH^-), which in solution will react with free hydrogen ions to form water, thereby lowering the concentration of hydrogen ions, raising the pH and making the solution alkaline.

Let us look at some examples. Lemon juice is acidic. When it dissolves in water it separates, or dissociates, into hydrogen ions and anions. It also has specific acid properties, such as a sour, sharp, "acidic" taste. Bleach, on the other hand, is alkaline. When dissolved in water it dissociates into hydroxide ions and cations, and has specific alkaline properties such as a soapy, slimy texture.

Salts, on the other hand, are substances that when dissolved in water dissociate into cations and anions, none of which are hydrogen ions or hydroxide ions. Salts play a vital role in the body. Potassium chloride, for example, dissociates into positive and negative ions able to carry electrical currents in nerve and muscle tissues. This is why it is called an electrolyte. Salts also form essential elements in blood, lymph, and interstitial fluid. Acids and bases can react with one another to form salts.

The pH of a fluid greatly influences the biological reactions that can take place within it and it is therefore vital that the body maintains its fluids at the correct pH. Most enzymes in our bodies work only at a specific pH. Pepsin, for example, can digest proteins only in an environment with a very low pH—that's why we have stomach acid. Blood is slightly alkaline and if it becomes too acidic a dangerous condition called acidosis will occur. In order to maintain the pH of our bodies, we have many homeostatic mechanisms in place, e.g., buffer systems. Buffer systems involve weak acids and bases that are able to convert strong acids and bases into weaker ones by adding or removing hydrogen ions. Our lungs and kidneys also help maintain pH.

pH is measured on a scale from 0 to 14, with zero being very acidic (contains more H^+), 14 being alkaline (contains more OH^-), and 7 being neutral.

Nutrients

Nutrients are found in the food we eat and are essential for the growth, maintenance, and repair of the body. Essential nutrients include macronutrients (carbohydrates, proteins, fats, essential minerals, and water) and micronutrients (vitamins and trace minerals). Some macronutrients are discussed in the chart below, "Major Compounds of the Body." Other nutrients include:

- **Vitamins:** Organic compounds required in minute amounts. They are essential for the normal functioning of the body and they help convert food into energy; help form tissues such as bones, muscles, nerves, blood, and skin; and help the body resist infection. There are two groups of vitamins:

- Fat-soluble vitamins: A, D, E, and K are stored by the body in the liver and fatty tissues
- Water-soluble vitamins: B and C are not stored by the body and are easily lost through excretion. They are also more sensitive to the effects of storing and cooking

- **Minerals:** Play a role in body growth and maintenance and form bones, teeth, hair, nails, red blood cells, body fluids, hormones, and enzymes. They are categorized as follows:
  - Macro minerals: Calcium, phosphorus, sodium, potassium, chloride, magnesium—essential minerals needed daily
  - Trace minerals: Iron, zinc, copper, fluoride, iodine, selenium, cobalt, molybdenum, manganese
- **Essential fatty acids (EFAs):** Fats that cannot be synthesized by the body and are vital for the proper functioning of the body. They are necessary for brain and nerve function, the cardiovascular and immune systems, the hormones, and the joints of the body.
- **Free radicals:** Highly unstable, reactive molecules that damage cells and are implicated in many diseases and aging.
- **Antioxidants:** Substances that combat or neutralize free radicals. They include vitamins E and C and beta-carotene, and the minerals selenium, zinc, manganese, and copper.

The appendix details some important sources and functions of nutrients.

Infobox

....

Anatomy and physiology in perspective

One molecule you will learn about in the following chart is DNA. DNA fingerprinting can be used to identify a child's parents or to convict criminals. Only a minute quantity of DNA is needed—for example, from a single drop of blood or a strand of hair.

MAJOR COMPOUNDS OF THE BODY

Inorganic compounds: *These compounds generally do not contain the element carbon and are usually simpler and smaller than organic compounds:*

Compound	Elements present	Role in the body
Water	Hydrogen, oxygen	This is the most abundant substance in the body because it is the *solvent* in body fluids, meaning that different materials and substances can dissolve in it
Water has many important functions in the body, including:		
Maintaining body temperature	Water can absorb and give off large amounts of heat without its temperature changing too much; it is therefore able to maintain a normal internal temperature despite hot sun, cold winds, and other external changes	
Acting as a lubricant	Water acts as a lubricant where internal organs touch and slide over one another or where bones, ligaments, and tendons meet and rub together; it also lubricates the gastrointestinal tract so that food can easily move through it and feces out of it	
Providing cushioning	Water creates a protective cushion around certain organs; e.g., it forms cerebrospinal fluid, which cushions the brain and protects it from external trauma	
Being a "universal solvent"	Water can dissolve or suspend many different substances and is therefore an ideal medium in which chemical reactions can take place; it can also transport substances such as nutrients, respiratory gases, and waste around the body	

MAJOR COMPOUNDS OF THE BODY

Organic compounds: *These are compounds that **contain the element carbon**. Carbon is a very useful element because it reacts easily to form large molecules that do not dissolve easily in water. These molecules build body structures and also break down to give off energy when the body needs it. The compounds below are all organic compounds and are important nutrient chemicals to the body:*

Compound	Elements present	Role in the body
Carbohydrates	Carbon, hydrogen, oxygen	Carbohydrates are the fuel of the body
Carbohydrates include:		
Monosaccharides (simple sugars)	Simple sugars are the building blocks of carbohydrates and a source of energy for chemical reactions Glucose is the main form in which sugar is used by your cells, fructose is found in fruits, and galactose is present in milk	
Some sugars also form parts of structural units; e.g., deoxyribose is a sugar that forms part of the DNA molecule, which carries hereditary information.		
Starch	This is a large molecule and is the main carbohydrate found in food	
Glycogen	Glycogen is an energy reserve and is stored in the liver and skeletal muscles	
Cellulose	This is a carbohydrate built by plants that we eat but cannot digest, and so it creates bulk that aids the movement of food and waste through our intestines; it is commonly referred to as fiber	

Compound	Elements present	Role in the body
Lipids (fats)	Carbon, hydrogen, oxygen	Lipids have over double the energy value of carbohydrates and proteins and are easily converted to body fat; they are composed of glycerol and fatty acids and most of them are *hydrophobic* (insoluble in water)
There are many different types of lipids with very diverse roles, the main ones being:		
Triglycerides (neutral fats)	These are the most plentiful fats in the body and in your diet and are solids (fats) or liquids (oils) at room temperature; they are found in fat deposits beneath the skin and around organs; they protect and insulate the organs and are also a major source of stored energy	
Phospholipids	These lipids form an integral part of the cell membrane and are also found in high concentrations in the nervous system	
Steroids	Steroids are a type of lipid, and many different types of steroids are found in the body; e.g., sex hormones and cholesterol (a steroid-alcohol or sterol)	

Other types of lipids include **eicosanoids**, which have diverse effects on inflammation, immunity, blood clotting, and other bodily responses; **fatty acids**, which are important energy-supplying molecules; **carotenes**, needed for the synthesis of vitamin A; **vitamin E**, which contributes to the functioning of the nervous system, wound healing, and is also an antioxidant; **vitamin K**, which is necessary for blood clotting; and **lipoproteins**, which help transport lipids in the body

MAJOR COMPOUNDS OF THE BODY

Compound	Elements present	Role in the body
Proteins	Carbon, hydrogen, oxygen, nitrogen; may contain sulfur	Proteins are the main family of molecules from which the body is built and are themselves built from amino acids; they are diverse in size, shape, and function
Proteins play the following roles in the body:		
Structural	Proteins are the building blocks of the body; e.g., bone is built from collagen and skin, hair and nails are built from keratin	
Regulatory	Hormones are made from proteins and they regulate the bodily functions; e.g., insulin helps regulate blood glucose levels	
Contractile	The proteins myosin and actin enable muscles to shorten, which allows for movement	
Immunity	Antibodies are proteins that protect against invading microbes	
Transport	Some carrier molecules are proteins; e.g., hemoglobin transports oxygen in the blood	
Catalytic	**Enzymes** are proteins that help speed up biochemical reactions	
Energy source	Proteins can also act as a source of energy in times of dietary inadequacy	

Proteins are the main family of molecules from which the body is built and are themselves built from amino acids; the standard genetic code encodes for 20 different amino acids, 9 of which are called **essential amino acids** because they cannot be made by the body and therefore must be obtained from proteins in the diet:

Compound	Elements present	Role in the body
Nucleic acids	Carbon, hydrogen, oxygen, nitrogen, phosphorus	Nucleic acids are very important molecules that are found inside cells
There are two types of nucleic acids:		
Deoxyribonucleic acid (DNA)	DNA is found inside the cell's nucleus and makes up chromosomes, which contain our genes	
	DNA is the inherited genetic material inside every cell; it provides instructions for building every protein in the body and it replicates itself before a cell develops to ensure that the genetic information inside every body cell is identical	
Ribonucleic acid (RNA)	RNA is the "molecular slave" to DNA (Marieb, 2003, p. 47); it transports the orders of DNA from the nucleus to ribosomes, where it is used to create specific proteins as per the genetic code	

Compound	Elements present	Role in the body
Adenosine triphosphate (ATP)	Carbon, hydrogen, oxygen, nitrogen, phosphorus	ATP is the main energy-transferring molecule in the body and provides a form of chemical energy that can be used by all body cells

Cellular Organization of the Body

Now that you understand the basic chemistry of the body, let us take a look at the next level up: the cellular level of organization. **Cytology** is the study of cells, which are the basic structural and functional units of the body. Cells vary greatly in size, shape, and structure, according to their function. For example, red blood cells are shaped like saucers. This biconcave shape serves two purposes: firstly it increases their surface area so that they can carry large amounts of oxygen, and, secondly, it enables red blood cells to squeeze through even the tiniest blood vessels. Nerve cells, on the other hand, have an entirely different shape: they have long, threadlike extensions for transmitting messages. In this chapter you will study a generalized animal cell.

Despite their differences, most cells are made up of a **nucleus, cytoplasm,** and a **plasma membrane**, and they are all bathed in **interstitial fluid,** a dilute saline solution derived from the blood.

Interstitial fluid is outside of the cell and is also known as extracellular fluid, intercellular fluid, or tissue fluid. The fluid inside the cells is called **intracellular fluid.** Both the interstitial fluid and the intracellular fluid are made up of oxygen, nutrients, waste, and other particles dissolved in water.

Figure 2.10 shows the structure of a generalized animal cell. The cell structures will be described on the pages following.

Did you know?

It is estimated that we are each made up of about 37.2 trillion cells. According to the writer Nicholas Bakalar (2015), "Even using the highest estimate for galaxies (200 billion) and the lowest estimate for human cells (1 trillion), there are at least 800 billion more cells in your body than there are galaxies in the known universe."

Infobox

Anatomy and physiology in perspective

Take a moment to put the chemistry you have just studied into perspective. A living cell is about 60% water and its structure is generally made up of the four elements carbon, oxygen, hydrogen, and nitrogen. A cell also contains small amounts of other elements that are essential to its functioning—for example, nerve cells need sodium and potassium in order to transmit messages.

Plasma membrane

Structure and function of the plasma membrane
The plasma membrane is a thin and flexible barrier that surrounds the cell and regulates the movement of all substances into and out of it. It is made up of lipids and proteins, which are organic compounds (see chart above, "Major Compounds of the Body," for further information on lipids and proteins).

Lipids
Three types of lipids are present in the plasma membrane:

Phospholipids: Approximately 75% of the lipids in the plasma membrane are phospholipids. Each phospholipid molecule has a head and a tail (like a tadpole). The head is **hydrophilic** (water-loving) while the tail is **hydrophobic** (water-hating), and the phospholipids lie tail to tail in two parallel layers. This is called a phospholipid bilayer and it forms the framework of the membrane. The hydrophilic heads are on the outside of the layers while the hydrophobic tails meet in the inside of the layers. Having the hydrophobic tails inside the membrane makes it impermeable to most water-soluble molecules.

Glycolipids: The functions of these lipids are still being discovered, but they do play a part in cell communication, growth, and development. They are cell identity markers and so enable the cell to

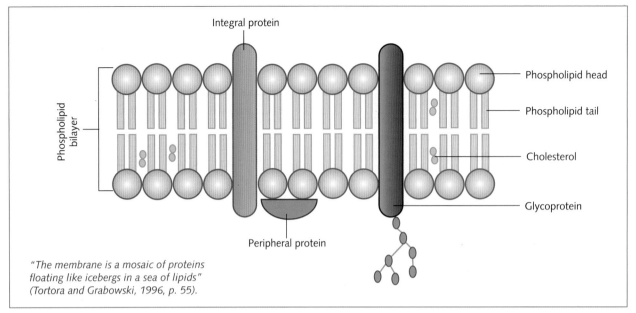

"The membrane is a mosaic of proteins floating like icebergs in a sea of lipids" (Tortora and Grabowski, 1996, p. 55).

Figure 2.4 *Structure of the plasma membrane*

recognize whether other cells are of its own type or if they are potentially harmful foreign cells. They are found in the phospholipid layer that faces the extracellular fluid.

Cholesterol: These lipids are found only in animal cells and help to strengthen the membrane.

Proteins

Two types of proteins are scattered in the phospholipid bilayer:

Integral proteins: These extend all the way through the membrane to create channels, which allow for the passage of materials in and out of the cell. Glycoproteins are proteins with attached sugar groups, and (like glycolipids) are cell identity markers.

Peripheral proteins: These are loosely attached to the surfaces of the membrane and they can separate easily from it.

The proteins in the cells determine the functions of the cell and they play a variety of roles. Proteins can act as:

- **Channels:** Some proteins have a pore (hole) in them through which other substances can move into and out of the cells.
- **Transporters:** Some proteins carry substances within the membrane.

- **Receptors:** Some proteins are able to identify and attach to specific molecules, such as hormones or nutrients, and thus guide them through the plasma membrane.

Other proteins act as enzymes or cytoskeleton anchors.

Transport across the plasma membrane

The life of a cell is dependent on the materials that are moved into and out of the cell: it needs energy and nutrition to function, and it also needs to get rid of waste products and harmful substances.

Materials are transported into and out of the cell via the plasma membrane, and there are two types of transport: **passive** processes and **active** processes.

Infobox

....

Anatomy and physiology in perspective

Next time you pour yourself a cup of coffee put some sugar in it but don't stir it. After a while, taste the coffee (without having stirred in the sugar). You will notice that it is sweet. Why? The particles of sugar will have diffused from an area of high concentration (the sugar) into an area of low concentration (the coffee). Diffusion is an example of passive transport.

Passive processes

In passive processes substances are moved without using cellular energy. These processes include:

Simple diffusion: The Latin word *diffus* means "spreading," and in diffusion substances move from areas of high concentration to areas of low concentration. Molecules that diffuse easily through the plasma membrane include oxygen, carbon dioxide, nitrogen, steroids, fat-soluble vitamins (A, D, E, and K), water, urea, and small alcohols.

Diffusion is a very simple process:

- All substances have **kinetic energy** and are continually moving about.
- If there are many particles of a substance in one area then it is termed an area of *high concentration.*
- An area with few particles of the substance will be called the area of *low concentration.*
- The difference between the two areas forms the *concentration gradient.*
- The particles from the area of high concentration will diffuse or spread into the area of low concentration until both areas have the same number of particles and **equilibrium** is reached.
- The rate of diffusion is determined by the temperature of the substance and the concentration gradient.

In the classroom

Demonstrate simple diffusion by putting a drop of food coloring into a glass of water and leaving it until all the water has changed color. This is diffusion.

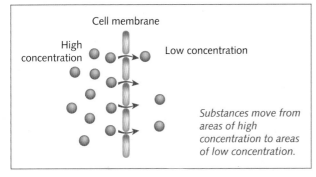

Figure 2.5 *Simple diffusion*

Osmosis: Osmosis is the diffusion of water through a selectively permeable membrane. A selectively permeable membrane allows only water molecules to move across it.

In osmosis, water molecules move from an area of higher water concentration to an area of lower water concentration. It must be remembered that where there is a high concentration of water molecules there will be a low concentration of solute molecules. Therefore, osmosis is also the movement of water molecules from an area of low solute concentration to an area of higher solute concentration.

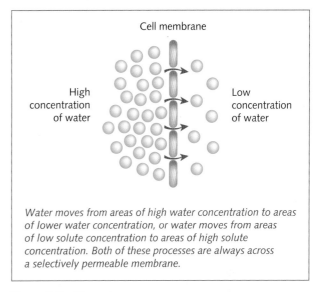

Water moves from areas of high water concentration to areas of lower water concentration, or water moves from areas of low solute concentration to areas of high solute concentration. Both of these processes are always across a selectively permeable membrane.

Figure 2.6 *Osmosis*

Facilitated diffusion: Molecules that are not lipid-soluble need help across the plasma membrane. These molecules include urea, glucose, fructose, galactose, and certain vitamins.

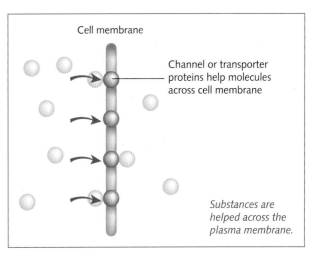

Figure 2.7 *Facilitated diffusion*

Channel or transporter proteins within the membrane help these molecules across the plasma membrane. The rate of facilitated diffusion is determined by the number of channels/transporters and the concentration difference on the two sides of the membrane.

Active processes

In active processes cells need to use some of their own energy gained from the splitting of ATP to transport materials across the plasma membrane. Active processes usually involve moving substances against a concentration gradient. These processes include:

Active transport: Integral membrane proteins act as pumps to push the molecules across the plasma membrane. These pumps are powered either directly or indirectly by ATP. Substances transported include ions, amino acids, and monosaccharides.

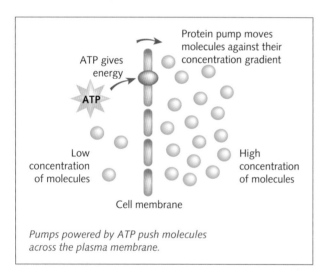

Pumps powered by ATP push molecules across the plasma membrane.

Figure 2.8   *Active transport*

Transport in a nutshell

Substances move across the plasma membrane through passive processes, which do not use cellular energy, and active processes, which do use cellular energy.

Vesicular transport: Vesicles are small, liquid-containing sacs, and in vesicular transport these sacs carry large particles such as bacteria, white blood cells, polysaccharides, and proteins across the cell membrane.

Substances enter the cells through **endocytosis,** a process in which a segment of the plasma membrane surrounds the substance, encloses it and brings it into the cell.

Substances exit the cells through **exocytosis,** a process in which the vesicles fuse with the plasma membrane to release their contents into the extracellular fluid.

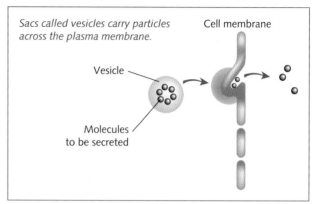

Figure 2.9   *Vesicular transport*

Cytoplasm and cell structures

The cytoplasm is all the cellular material inside the plasma membrane, excluding the nucleus. It is the site of most cellular activities and includes cytosol, organelles, and inclusions.

Cytosol

Cytosol is a thick, transparent, gel-like fluid made up of mainly water. It also contains solids and solutes, as well as spaces called **vacuoles,** which house cellular wastes and secretions.

Organelles

Organelles are the "little organs" of the cell and they play a specific role in maintaining the life of the cell. They are very specialized structures and differ according to the cell type and its functions. Some of the important organelles are:

- **Mitochondria:** These are the "powerhouses" of the cell and are where ATP is generated through the process of cellular respiration.

Did you know?

Mitochondria are fascinating organelles. There is a lot of compelling evidence that they were originally bacteria, and, unlike other organelles, mitochondria have their own DNA (mtDNA).

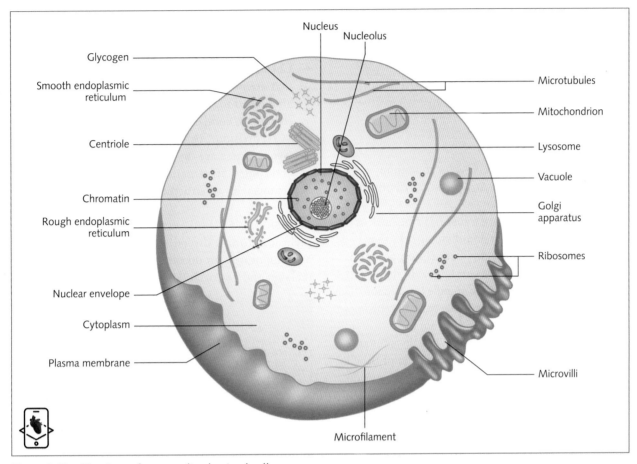

Figure 2.10 *Structure of a generalized animal cell*

Infobox

....

Anatomy and physiology in perspective

Active cells that need a lot of energy—for example, muscle cells—contain many mitochondria.

- **Ribosomes:** These tiny granules are the actual sites of protein synthesis in the cell—they are where proteins are made. Some ribosomes float freely in the cytoplasm and are called free ribosomes. Others are attached to the endoplasmic reticulum.
- **Endoplasmic reticulum (ER):** This is a network of fluid-filled **cisterns** (channels or tubules) that coils through the cytoplasm. It provides a large surface area for chemical reactions, and also transports molecules within the cell. There are two types of endoplasmic reticulum:
  - **Rough ER:** This has ribosomes attached to it and provides a site for protein synthesis. It also temporarily stores new protein molecules and participates in the formation of glycoproteins. In addition, the rough ER works together with the Golgi complex to make and package molecules that are to be secreted from the cell
  - **Smooth ER:** This has no ribosomes attached to it and therefore no proteins are made here. Instead, it provides a site for the synthesis of certain lipids (fatty acids, phospholipids, and steroids) and the detoxification of various chemicals such as alcohol, pesticides, and carcinogens
- **Golgi complex:** The Golgi complex, or Golgi apparatus, is located near the nucleus. It is made of flattened cisterns with tiny vesicles attached to their edges, and it processes, sorts, and packages proteins and lipids for delivery to the plasma membrane. It also forms lysosomes and secretory vesicles.
- **Lysosomes:** These vesicles are formed inside the Golgi complex. They contain powerful digestive enzymes and are able to break down and recycle many different molecules. They help recycle the cell's own worn-out structures as well as foreign substances.

Infobox
· ·
Anatomy and physiology in perspective

Lysosomal enzymes help digest any cellular debris at sites of injury, thus preparing the area for repair.

- **Peroxisomes:** These are vesicles containing enzymes that detoxify any potentially harmful substances in the cell.
- **Centrosomes:** These are found near the nucleus and have two roles. In non-dividing cells they organize the microtubules that help support and shape the cell and move substances. In dividing cells they form the mitotic spindle (see section "Cell division," below). Centrosomes contain centrioles.
- **Centrioles:** These are found within the centrosomes and play a role in cell division and also in the formation and regeneration of flagella and cilia. **Flagella** are projections on the outside of cells that enable them to move—a sperm cell, for example, has a flagellum. **Cilia** are hairlike projections that enable a cell to move substances across its surface—for example, ciliated cells of the respiratory tract move mucus.

Nucleus

The nucleus is the largest structure in the cell and controls all cellular structure and activities. It also contains most of the hereditary units, known as genes (mitochondria also contain a few genes). Almost all body cells except for red blood cells contain a nucleus, while some cells—such as skeletal muscle cells—contain several nuclei. The nucleus is constructed as follows:

- **Nuclear envelope:** The nucleus is surrounded by a double membrane of phospholipid bilayers (similar to the plasma membrane). This membrane contains nuclear pores (channels), which allow for the movement of molecules into and out of the nucleus.

- **Nucleolus:** Inside the nucleus is a spherical body made up of protein, some DNA, and RNA. This is where ribosomes are assembled.
- **Chromatin:** Chromatin is only present in cells that are not dividing. It is a mass of chromosomes all tangled together. During cell division the chromatin condenses and coils (see section "Cell division," below).
- **Genes:** These are the hereditary units of the cell and control its structure and activity. Genes are arranged along structures called chromosomes.

Inclusions

Inclusions form a diverse group of substances that are temporarily produced by some cells, for example, melanin and glycogen.

The cell in a nutshell
· ·

Imagine the cell as a bakery:

- The plasma membrane is the building's walls and doors.
- The cytoplasm is the bakery floor.
- The nucleus is the manager.
- Mitochondria are the generators.
- Ribosomes are the ovens.
- The endoplasmic reticulum is the production line.
- The Golgi complex is the packing and distribution department.
- Lysosomes are the recycling site.
- Peroxisomes are the cleaners.

Life Cycle of a Cell

A cell has two distinct periods in its life cycle—**interphase** and **cell division**.

Interphase and DNA replication

Interphase is the time in which a cell grows and carries out its usual metabolic activities. It is also the time in which the cell prepares itself for division through DNA replication.

The DNA molecule is the largest molecule in the cell and is the only type of molecule capable of independently forming a duplicate of itself. The DNA molecule is made up of two strands of repeating nucleotides. Nucleotides are molecules composed of a 5-carbon sugar, a phosphate group, and a nitrogen-containing base, and it is the unique order of these bases that determines an individual's characteristics. These bases are adenine, thymine, guanine, and cytosine, and genetic information is stored in DNA and RNA as sets of three nucleotides, referred to as a base triplet.

The chains of repeating nucleotides twist around each other into a double helix. This is a spiral curve that looks like a rubber ladder twisted around its axis.

In preparation for cell division, the DNA needs to be copied so that there is a copy for each resulting daughter cell. When DNA replicates, the molecule uncoils and separates into its two nucleotide strands. Each strand now serves as a template for building another nucleotide strand. This results in two identical double-stranded helices.

Study tip

Do not confuse DNA replication with gene expression. Both processes are very similar but they each serve a different function.

- DNA replication occurs within the nucleus of the cell and is necessary for cell division. It is a process that results in two identical DNA copies.
- Gene expression, on the other hand, is the process in which a gene's DNA is used as a template to synthesise a specific protein. It occurs in two phases:
  - Transcription—The information encoded in a specific region of DNA is copied (transcribed) to produce a specific molecule of ribonucleic acid (RNA)
  - Translation—The information now encoded into the RNA is translated into a corresponding sequence of amino acids. This process occurs when RNA attaches itself to a ribosome, and the result is a new protein molecule

Cell division

What happens if cells become damaged, diseased, or worn out and need to be replaced? They reproduce themselves through a process called cell division. There are two types of cell division:

- **Somatic cell division:** This occurs in all cells, except bacteria and some cells of the reproductive system, and it takes place when the body needs to replace dead and injured cells or produce new cells for growth. Through a process of nuclear division called **mitosis**, a single **diploid** parent cell duplicates itself to produce two identical daughter cells.
- **Reproductive cell division:** This occurs when a new organism is to be produced. Through a process of nuclear division called **meiosis, haploid** sperm and egg cells are produced, and these form a new organism.

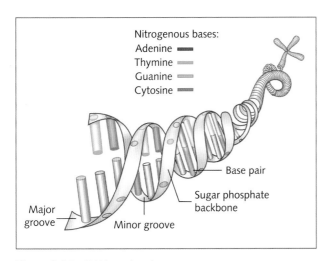

Nitrogenous bases:
Adenine
Thymine
Guanine
Cytosine

Base pair

Sugar phosphate backbone

Major groove

Minor groove

Figure 2.11 *DNA molecule*

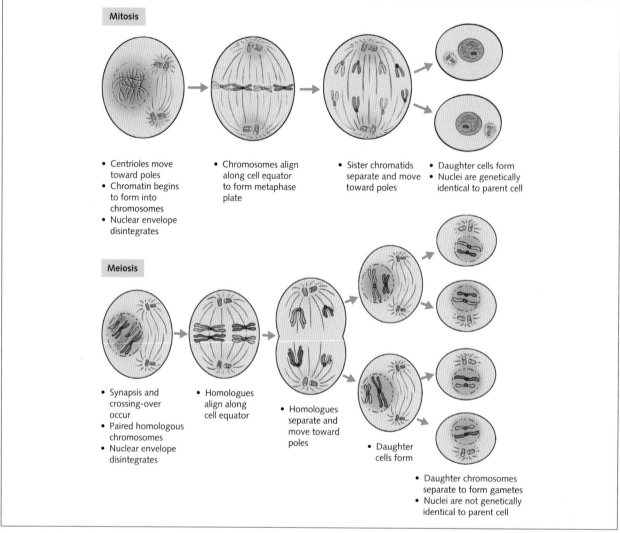

Figure 2.12 *Mitosis and meiosis*

TYPES OF CELL DIVISION	
Somatic cell division—Mitosis	**Reproductive cell division—Meiosis**
Cellular reproduction in which a mother cell divides into two daughter cells, each containing the same genes as the mother cell	Reproductive cell division in which four haploid daughter cells are produced
KEY DIFFERENCES TO REMEMBER	
Occurs in all cells, except bacteria and some cells of the reproductive system	Only occurs in reproductive cells
Takes place when the body needs to replace dead and injured cells or produce new cells for growth	Takes place when a new organism is to be produced
Two identical diploid daughter cells are produced. Diploid cells have two complete sets of chromosomes per cell	Four haploid daughter cells are produced. Haploid cells have only one set of chromosomes per cell. Human cells have 46 chromosomes. You inherit 23 chromosomes from your mother and 23 from your father

In this chapter we will only study somatic cell division in depth but, before we go any further, you need to know the following terms:

- **Somatic cell:** Any cell except the reproductive cells
- **Diploid:** Having two complete sets of chromosomes per cell
- **Haploid:** Having only one set of chromosomes per cell.

Human cells have 46 chromosomes. You inherit 23 chromosomes from your mother and 23 from your father.

Infobox

Anatomy and physiology in perspective

People with Down syndrome have 47 chromosomes instead of 46. They have an extra chromosome 21, which is why Down syndrome is also called trisomy 21.

Two processes take place during cell division: **mitosis** and **cytokinesis**.

Mitosis

Mitosis is the period in which a mother cell divides into two daughter cells, each containing the same genes as the mother cell. Although mitosis is a continuous process, it is easier to categorize it into the following four stages:

1. **Prophase:** In this stage:
   - *Chromatin fibers condense and shorten into chromosomes.* This condensing of fibers is thought to prevent the entangling of DNA strands as they move during mitosis.
   - *Centrosomes and centrioles form the mitotic spindle* through separating from each other and moving to opposite sides of the cell. The mitotic spindle is made of microtubules and is shaped like a football. It forms a site of attachment for the chromosomes and distributes them to opposite ends of the cell.

   - *Nuclear envelope and nucleus break down and are absorbed into the cytosol.*
2. **Metaphase:** This is a short phase in which the *centromeres line up at the center of the spindle.*
3. **Anaphase:** *The centromeres split and the chromatids/chromosomes move apart toward opposite ends of the cell.* Note that once they are separated the sister chromatids are now referred to as **daughter chromosomes.**
4. **Telophase:** This is prophase in reverse and is the period in which:
   - *Chromosomes go to the opposite ends of the cell, uncoil and become threadlike chromatin again.*
   - *Spindle breaks down and disappears.*
   - *Nuclear envelope forms around each chromatin mass.*
   - *Nucleoli appear in each of the daughter nuclei.*

Remember: pro = before, meta = after, ana = upward, telo = far/end

---

Study tip

Learning the life cycle of a cell can be challenging because there are so many new words that all sound similar! Take a moment to ensure you understand the differences between the following:

- **Chromosomes:** A chromosome is a threadlike structure composed of DNA coiled tightly around proteins called **histones**. Their function is to carry our genetic material.
- **Chromatin:** Chromatin is a substance made of DNA and proteins. During cell division it coils and condenses to form chromosomes. In other words, it is the substance in the nucleus that will form into chromosomes when the cell begins to replicate.
- **Chromatids:** During cell division the chromosome duplicates itself into two identical strands called chromatids. These chromatids are held together by a centromere and they later separate to become individual chromosomes.

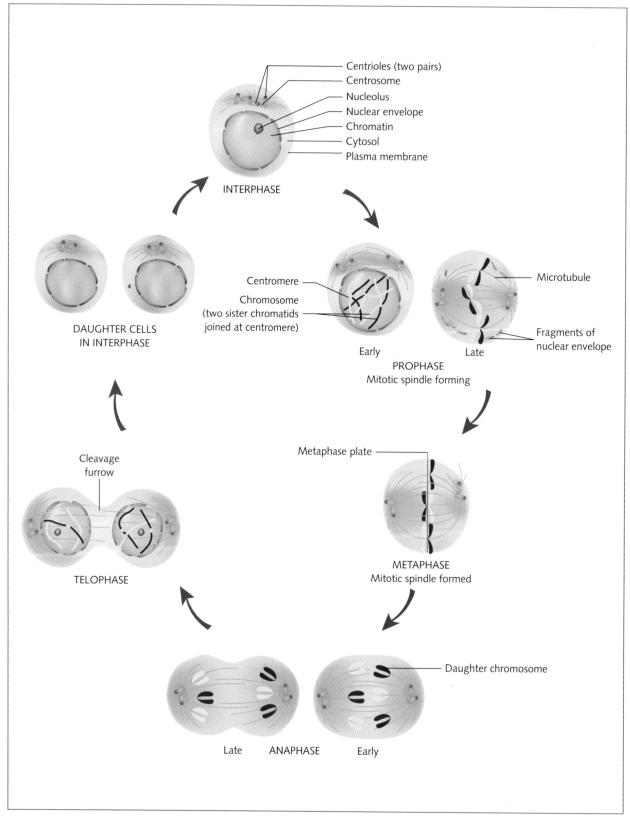

Figure 2.13 *Life cycle of a somatic cell—mitosis*

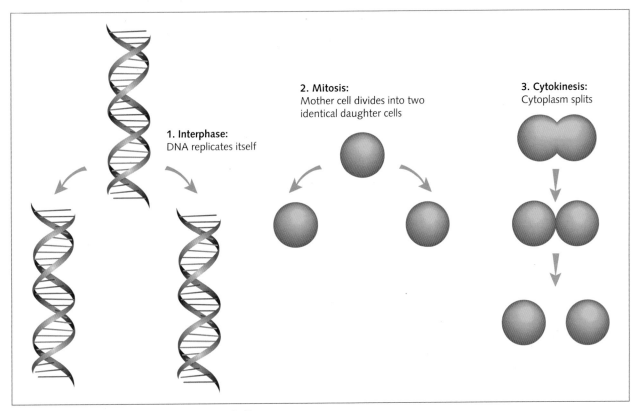

1. Interphase:
DNA replicates itself

2. Mitosis:
Mother cell divides into two identical daughter cells

3. Cytokinesis:
Cytoplasm splits

Figure 2.14 *Somatic cell division in a nutshell*

Cytokinesis (cytoplasmic division)

Cytokinesis actually happens during mitosis and is the process by which the cell splits into two new cells. During the late anaphase, a cleavage furrow forms in the plasma membrane. This is a slight indentation that extends around the center of the cell. The furrow deepens until the opposite surfaces of the cell make contact. The cell then splits into two daughter cells, each with its own separate portions of cytoplasm and organelles. The daughter cells are smaller than their mother cell, but genetically identical to it. They will soon grow and carry out normal cellular activities until it is their turn to divide—and so continues the cycle of life.

Infobox

Anatomy and physiology in perspective

Cancer is the uncontrolled division of body cells.

Tissue Level of Organization of the Body

Now that you know what a cell is, it is time to look at what happens when similar cells work together to perform a common function: they form groups called tissues. For example, nerve cells work together to form nervous tissue.

In this section you will learn about the different types of tissues, the study of which is known as **histology**.

Infobox

Anatomy and physiology in perspective

A biopsy is the removal of a sample of tissue for examination. It enables medical professionals to help diagnose diseases such as cancer.

There are four types of tissue in the body: epithelial, connective, muscle, and nervous. The table below gives a brief overview of them.

TYPES OF TISSUE IN THE BODY		
Name	**Function**	**Example**
Epithelial	Covers body surfaces and therefore functions in protection, absorption, and filtration Lines hollow organs, cavities, and ducts Forms glands and therefore functions in secretion	Skin
Connective	Protects and supports the body and its organs Binds organs together Stores energy reserves as fat Provides immunity	Blood, adipose tissue (fat), bone
Muscle	Provides movement and force	Skeletal muscle
Nervous	Initiates and transmits nerve impulses	Nerves

Epithelial tissue

Epithelial tissue, also called **epithelium**, forms body linings and glands. It is a large group of tissues that includes many different types, but they all generally share the same characteristics:

- Cells fit closely together with little extracellular material between them.
- Cells are arranged in continuous sheets.
- Cells always have:
  - A free surface, which is exposed to the body's exterior or a body cavity
  - An interior surface, which is attached to a basement membrane
- Cells are constantly being regenerated by mitosis.
- Tissues are firmly joined to connective tissue.
- Tissues are avascular, which means that they have no blood supply of their own. Therefore, they receive all nutrients and remove waste through the process of diffusion with the blood vessels located in the connective tissue below.

There are four different cell shapes that make up epithelial tissue:

1. **Squamous:** These cells are flat and thin, enabling substances to move through them rapidly for functions such as filtration, diffusion, osmosis, or secretion.
2. **Cuboidal:** Shaped like cubes, these cells can have microvilli on their surface and function in secretion and absorption.

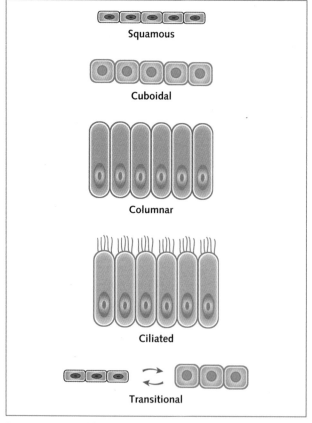

Figure 2.15 *Different types/shapes of epithelial cells*

3. **Columnar:** These cells are tall and rectangular in shape. They often have microvilli or cilia on their surface, they protect underlying tissues, and function in secretion and absorption.
4. **Transitional:** These cells change shape from squamous to cuboidal and back, enabling tissues to be stretched and return to their original size.

Epithelial tissue is classified according to the numbers of layers it has and the shape of its cells. The following chart details this classification.

CLASSIFICATION OF EPITHELIAL TISSUE

Simple epithelium: *Simple epithelium is a single layer of cells. It is usually very thin and functions in absorption, secretion, and filtration. It includes:*

	Simple squamous (pavement) epithelium	
	Description	A single layer of flat squamous cells
	Location example	Lines blood vessels, lymphatic vessels, and air sacs of lungs, and forms serous membranes
	Function	Filtration, diffusion, osmosis, and secretion
	Simple cuboidal epithelium	
	Description	A single layer of cube-shaped cells
	Location example	Covers the surface of the ovaries, lines kidney tubules, and forms the ducts of many glands
	Function	Secretion and absorption
	Simple columnar epithelium	
	Description	A single layer of rectangular cells; may contain goblet cells, which produce a lubricating mucus, and microvilli, which are fingerlike projections that increase the surface area of the plasma membrane
	Location example	Lines the gastrointestinal tract
	Function	Secretion and absorption
	Ciliated simple columnar epithelium	
	Description	A single layer of rectangular cells that contain hairlike projections called cilia, which help move substances
	Location example	Lines part of the upper respiratory tract, the fallopian tubes, and some of the sinuses
	Function	Moves fluids or particles along a passageway

Stratified epithelium: *Stratified epithelium consists of two or more layers of cells. It is durable and functions in protecting underlying tissues in areas of wear and tear. Some stratified epithelia also produce secretions. Stratified epithelium includes:*

	Stratified squamous epithelium	
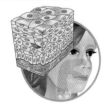	**Description**	Consists of several layers of cells, which are squamous in the superficial layer and cuboidal to columnar in the deep layers
		It exists in keratinized and non-keratinized forms; **keratin** is a tough, waterproof protein that is resistant to friction and helps repel bacteria
	Location example	The superficial layer of the skin is a keratinized form, while wet surfaces such as the mouth and tongue are non-keratinized
	Function	Protection

CLASSIFICATION OF EPITHELIAL TISSUE

	Transitional epithelium	
	Description	Consists of layers of cells that change shape when the tissue is stretched
	Location example	Organs of the urinary system, e.g., the bladder
	Function	Allows for distension

Connective tissue

Connective tissue is the most abundant and widely distributed tissue in the body and takes many forms. For example, fat, blood, and bone are all types of connective tissue.

The characteristics common to all types of connective tissue are:

- Cells are surrounded and separated by a matrix made of protein fibers and a fluid, gel, or solid ground substance. This ground substance is usually produced by the connective tissue cells and deposited in the space between the cells.
- The tissue has a rich blood supply, except for cartilage and tendons.
- The tissue has a nerve supply, except for cartilage.

CLASSIFICATION OF CONNECTIVE TISSUE

Loose connective tissue: Loose connective tissue has loosely woven fibers and many cells. It is a softer connective tissue and includes:

	Areolar tissue	
	Description	This is a loose, soft, pliable, semifluid tissue and is the most widely distributed type of connective tissue in the body
		It contains collagen, elastic, and reticular fibers, which give areolar tissue its elasticity and extensibility (see chapter 3 for more information on these fibers)
	Location example	Surrounds body organs and is found in the subcutaneous layer of the skin
	Function	Strength, elasticity, and support (it is often the glue that holds the internal organs in their positions)
	Adipose tissue	
	Description	This is an areolar tissue that contains mainly fat cells
	Location example	Subcutaneous layer of the skin, surrounding organs such as the kidneys and heart, and found in the mammary glands
	Function	Insulation, energy reserve, support, and protection
	Lymphoid (reticular) tissue	
	Description	Contains thin fibers that form branching networks to form the **stroma** (a support framework for many soft organs)
	Location example	Lymph nodes, the spleen, red bone marrow
	Function	Support

CLASSIFICATION OF CONNECTIVE TISSUE

Dense connective (fibrous) tissue: Dense connective tissue contains thick, densely packed fibers and fewer cells than loose connective tissue. It forms strong structures and there are different types of dense connective tissue, including the following:

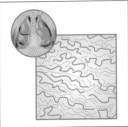

Elastic connective tissue (yellow elastic tissue)	
Description	Consists of many freely branching elastic fibers, few cells, and little matrix; the elastic fibers give the tissue a yellowish color
Location example	Lung tissue, walls of arteries, trachea, bronchial tubes
Function	Elasticity for stretching and strength

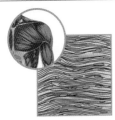

Dense regular connective tissue (white fibrous tissue)	
Description	Consists mainly of collagen fibers arranged in parallel bundles with cells in between the bundles; the matrix is a shiny white color
Location example	Tendons, ligaments, aponeuroses
Function	Attachment

*Bone (osseous tissue): Bone is an exceptionally hard connective tissue that protects and supports other organs of the body. It consists of bone cells sitting in **lacunae** (cavities) surrounded by layers of a very hard matrix that has been strengthened by inorganic salts such as calcium and phosphate. It includes compact and cancellous bone:*

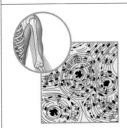

Description	**Compact bone** is the hard, more dense, outer type of bone, while **cancellous bone** lies internally to the compact bone and is spongy
Location example	Bones
Function	Support, protection, movement, and storage

Cartilage: Cartilage is a resilient, strong connective tissue that is less hard and more flexible than bone. It consists of a dense network of collagen and elastic fibers embedded in a rubbery ground substance. Cartilage has no blood vessels or nerves and includes:

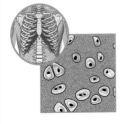

Hyaline cartilage	
Description	This is the most abundant cartilage in the body but is also the weakest It consists of a resilient, gel-like ground substance, fine collagen fibers, and cells
Location example	Ends of long bones, ends of ribs, nose
Function	Movement, flexibility, and support

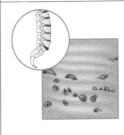

Fibrocartilage	
Description	This is the strongest of the three types of cartilage and consists of cells scattered between bundles of collagen fibers; it is a strong and rigid cartilage
Location example	Intervertebral discs
Function	Support and strength

CLASSIFICATION OF CONNECTIVE TISSUE

Elastic cartilage	
Description	This is a strong and elastic cartilage consisting of cells in a threadlike network of elastic fibers within the matrix
Location example	Eustachian tubes, supports external ear and epiglottis
Function	Supports and maintains shape

Blood (vascular tissue): Blood is an unusual type of connective tissue whose matrix is a fluid called blood **plasma***. Plasma consists mainly of water, with a variety of dissolved substances such as nutrients, wastes, enzymes, gases, and hormones. Blood also contains:*

Red blood cells (erythrocytes): These transport oxygen to body cells and remove carbon dioxide from them

White blood cells (leucocytes): These are involved in phagocytosis (the destruction of microbes, cell debris, and foreign matter), immunity and allergic reactions

Platelets: These function in blood clotting

Muscle tissue

The fibers of muscle tissue are actually elongated cells that provide a long axis for contraction. Thus, muscle tissue is able to shorten (contract) to produce movement. Muscle tissue also maintains posture and generates heat. Muscle tissue is characterized according to its location and function. There are three types: **skeletal, cardiac,** and **smooth (visceral).**

CLASSIFICATION OF MUSCLE TISSUE

Skeletal muscle tissue	
Description	Skeletal muscle tissue is attached to bones and composed of long, cylindrical fibers with multiple nuclei
	The fibers are striated, which means that when looked at under a microscope alternating light and dark bands are seen
	Skeletal muscles are under conscious control and are therefore called voluntary muscles
Location example	Attached to bones by tendons
Function	Motion, posture, and heat production
Cardiac muscle tissue	
Description	Cardiac muscle tissue forms most of the wall of the heart and consists of branched, striated fibers
	Cardiac tissue is not under conscious control; it is regulated by its own pacemaker and the **autonomic nervous system** and is therefore an involuntary muscle
Location example	Heart wall
Function	Pumps blood

CLASSIFICATION OF MUSCLE TISSUE

	Smooth (visceral) muscle tissue	
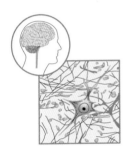	Description	Smooth muscle tissue is so called because it contains non-striated (smooth) fibers
		It is not under conscious control; it is regulated by the autonomic nervous system and is therefore an involuntary muscle
	Location example	Walls of hollow structures, such as blood vessels and intestines
	Function	Constricts and dilates structures to move substances within the body (e.g., blood in blood vessels, foods through gastrointestinal tract)

Nervous tissue

Nervous tissue is made up of **neurons** and **neuroglia** and it is found in the brain, spinal cord, and nerves. Its function is that of communication—of being sensitive to stimuli, generating and conducting impulses. Neurons are composed of a cell body, whose cytoplasm is drawn out into a long extension. These extensions are called **dendrites** or **axons** and they receive and conduct electrochemical impulses. Neuroglia are the supporting cells that insulate, support, and protect the neurons. They do not generate or conduct nerve impulses.

Membranes

Membranes are thin, flexible sheets made up of different tissue layers. They cover surfaces, line body cavities, and form protective sheets around organs. They are categorized as epithelial and connective tissue (**synovial**) membranes.

CLASSIFICATION OF MEMBRANES

*Epithelial membranes: Epithelial membranes consist of an epithelial layer and an underlying connective tissue layer, and include **mucous**, **serous**, and **cutaneous** membranes:*

	Mucous membranes	
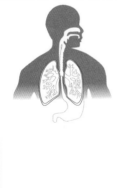	Description	Mucous membranes line body cavities that open directly to the exterior
		They are "wet" membranes whose cells secrete mucus, which prevents cavities from drying out, lubricates food as it moves in the gastrointestinal tract, and traps particles in the respiratory tract (**note:** urine, not mucus, moistens the urinary tract)
		Mucous membranes also act as a barrier that is difficult for pathogens to penetrate
	Location example	The hollow organs of the digestive, respiratory, urinary, and reproductive systems
	Function	Lubrication, movement, and protection

CLASSIFICATION OF MEMBRANES

Serous membranes

Description	Serous membranes line body cavities that do not open directly to the exterior, and they cover the organs that lie within those cavities
	They are composed of two layers: the **parietal layer** is attached to the cavity wall and the **visceral layer** is attached to the organs inside the cavity; between these two layers is a watery lubricating fluid called the **serous fluid**, which enables the organs to move and glide against each other easily
	The layers of a serous membrane consist of thin layers of areolar connective tissue covered by a layer of simple squamous epithelium
Location example	There are three serous membranes in the body:
	Pleura lines the thoracic cavity and covers the lungs
	Pericardium lines the cardiac cavity and covers the heart
	Peritoneum lines the abdominal cavity and covers the abdominal organs and some of the pelvic organs
Function	Lubrication and protection

Cutaneous membrane

Description	This is the skin, and it is composed of a superficial keratinizing stratified squamous epithelium and an underlying dense connective tissue layer; it will be discussed in more detail in the following chapter

Connective tissue membranes (synovial membranes): *Connective tissue membranes are known as synovial membranes and are composed of areolar connective tissue with elastic fibers and fat. They line:*

The cavities of freely movable joints, and secrete **synovial fluid**, which lubricates the joints

Bursae and tendon sheaths, which provide cushioning

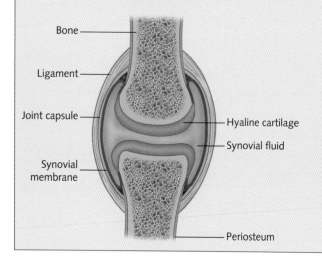

Bone
Ligament
Joint capsule
Hyaline cartilage
Synovial fluid
Synovial membrane
Periosteum

Tissues in a nutshell

- Epithelial tissue lines and protects.
- Connective tissue connects.
- Muscle tissue moves.
- Nervous tissue communicates.
- Membranes cover.

System Level of Organization of the Body

You have studied the body at the chemical, cellular, and tissue levels and now it is time to briefly look at the system level of organization. You will learn more about the systems and their organs in the following chapters, but for now they are illustrated for you on pp. 50–51.

There are certain things you need to do in order to survive. For example, you need to be able to do such things as eat, breathe, and move. The systems of our body carry out these crucial life processes, and each system is composed of several related organs that share a common function. These systems are the:

- Integumentary system (the skin, hair, and nails)
- Skeletal system
- Muscular system
- Nervous system
- Endocrine system
- Respiratory system
- Cardiovascular system
- Lymphatic and immune system
- Digestive system
- Urinary system
- Reproductive system.

These systems work together to ensure that the body maintains a stable internal environment despite any changes in its external environment. This process is known as **homeostasis**.

Pathology Basics

This book covers many different diseases and in order to learn them it helps to be aware of their underlying pathophysiology. Whenever you encounter a new disease, always ask yourself the following questions:

1. What is happening on a cellular level? What is injuring the cell?
   - **Lack of oxygen:** Oxygen is vital to the life and functioning of a cell. If blood supply to an area is reduced or inadequate this is called **ischemia**. Ischemia results in **hypoxia**, which is a reduced oxygen supply, or **anoxia**, which is the absence of oxygen. Cells cannot survive without oxygen.
   - **Physical injury:** Cells can be injured by mechanical trauma (such as occurs in a fall or car accident), temperature extremes, radiation, electric shocks, or sudden changes in atmospheric pressure.
   - **Chemical injury:** Many chemicals are known to injure our cells. Examples include medications, poisons, and pesticides.
   - **Infection:** Cells can be injured by biological agents such as parasites, bacteria, viruses, and fungi.
   - **Injury as a result of an immune response:** Although the function of our immune system is to protect us, the immune system can sometimes damage our own cells. Autoimmune disease is one example.
   - **Injury as a result of a genetic defect.**
   - **Injury as a result of nutritional imbalances:** Many diseases are caused by either a lack of nutrients or an excess intake of them.
2. What is happening on a tissue level? What is the underlying process, the pathophysiology? Ideas include edema, jaundice, inflammation, infection, and cell death.
3. What organs are affected? What will be the consequences of that particular organ being affected?
4. What is the systemic effect? How is this disease affecting the body system involved? Are other systems affected?
5. How does this condition affect the person's quality of life and their mental health? For example, acne vulgaris involves inflammation and can also involve infection. Although signs are localized, symptoms can include itchiness and pain and an important consequence can be how it affects the person's self-confidence.

Cancer

Cancer is the uncontrolled division of cells and it can affect any system in the body. Tumors are swellings, lumps, or growths in the body and they can be cancerous (**malignant**), non-cancerous (**benign**), or pre-cancerous. Although most cancers present as tumors, which either grow into nearby tissue or have cells that break away and travel to other parts of the body (**metastasis**), some cancers, such as those of the blood, do not take the form of tumors.

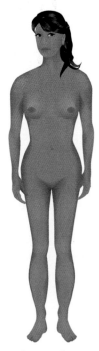

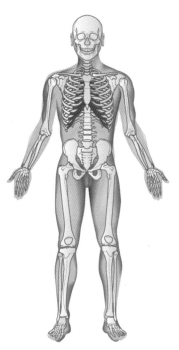

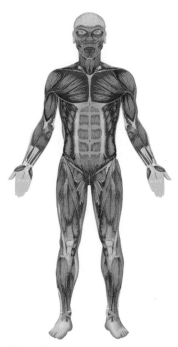

Integumentary system—*protects the body; regulates body temperature; eliminates waste; helps produce vitamin D; contains nerve endings sensitive to pain, temperature, and touch*

Skeletal system—*provides movement, support, and protection; stores minerals; houses the cells that create blood cells*

Muscular system—*powers movement; maintains posture; generates heat*

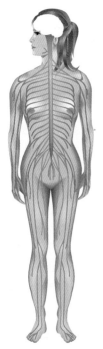

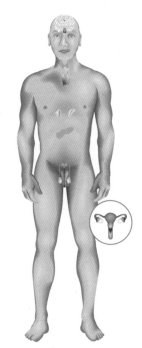

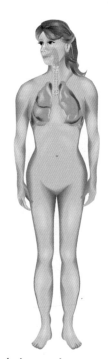

Nervous system—*regulates body activities through detecting, processing, and responding to change in both the external and internal environments*

Endocrine system—*regulates body activities through hormones*

Respiratory system—*supplies oxygen and removes carbon dioxide; helps produce vocal sounds*

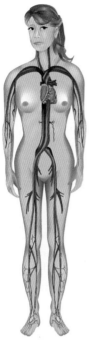

Cardiovascular system—transports blood, which carries oxygen, carbon dioxide, nutrients, and waste to and from cells; regulates body temperature

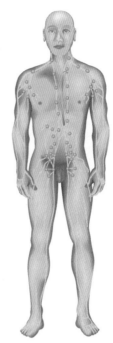

Lymphatic and immune system—functions in immunity, protection, and waste removal; returns proteins and plasma to the cardiovascular system; transports fats

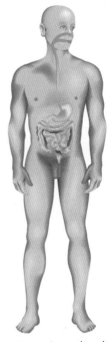

Digestive system—breaks down food and absorbs nutrients; eliminates waste

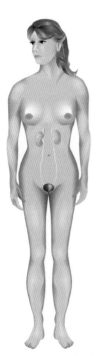

Urinary system—eliminates waste; regulates water, electrolyte, and acid–base balance of blood

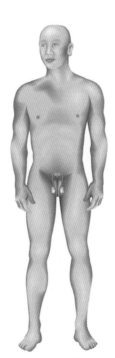

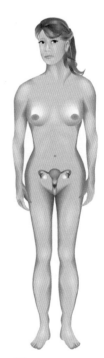

Reproductive system—reproduces life

Generalized effects of cancer include:

- Nausea
- Vomiting
- Diarrhea
- Fever
- Weight loss.

These signs and symptoms in a patient should always be a red flag to further investigation.

Asking yourself the following questions will help you understand the effects (and therefore signs and symptoms) of a particular cancer:

- Where in the body is the cancer? What tissues and types of cells are affected? What is the normal function of those cells?
- Is the tumor putting pressure on, growing into, or obstructing neighboring organs? How is that affecting the functioning of that organ? For example, cancer of the prostate can make urination difficult.
- Is there ulceration, bleeding, or secondary infection involved? How does this affect the patient?
- Is the patient in a lot of pain?
- How is the patient coping emotionally? Does he or she have support from family and friends?
- How is the cancer and treatment affecting the patient's everyday life/job/family and relationships?

As a therapist it is important to have a basic understanding of the different treatments available for cancer. This will help you decide whether or not it is safe for you to work on a client. Although there are many different types of cancer, most of them are treated with either one or a combination of the following:

Surgery is usually used to treat tumors that have not spread beyond their original site of growth. However, surgery cannot always be used if the ttumor is in an inaccessible area or if the surgery would involve the removal of an entire vital organ.

Radiation therapy involves the focusing of radiation (an emission of energy in the form of X-rays or similar rays) on a specific area or organ of the body. It can be given via an external beam focused on the body or via radioactive substances that are introduced into the body. Radiation kills cells, such as cancer cells, that divide rapidly. However, it can also

damage non-cancerous cells that divide rapidly, e.g. those of the skin; hair follicles; or the lining of the mouth, esophagus, and intestines. Possible side effects of radiation therapy can include tiredness, changes in appetite, weight loss, skin reactions similar to sunburn, and skin sensitivity to the sun or to cold winds. Unfortunately, some types of cancer cells are resistant to radiation.

Chemotherapy involves the use of drugs to destroy cancer cells by interfering with their ability to divide. The drugs often affect non-cancerous cells as well, especially those of the skin, the lining of the mouth, the bone marrow, the hair follicles, and the digestive system (these are all cells that divide rapidly). However, damage to these cells is temporary. Chemotherapy drugs can be given via injections, as tablets, or as creams.

There are many possible side effects to chemotherapy, including a reduction in the number of blood cells produced by the bone marrow; fatigue, nausea and vomiting; loss of appetite, diarrhea and/or constipation; mouth ulcers and changes in taste; hair loss; skin changes such as rashes, dryness, discoloration and an increased skin sensitivity to sunlight; brittle or flaky nails, slow nail growth, and the appearance of white lines across the nails; tingling or numbness in the hands or feet; anxiety, restlessness, dizziness, and sleeplessness; headaches and changes in hearing. Please note, this is an extensive list of the side effects of chemotherapy and someone receiving it will not necessarily have all of the above.

Immunotherapy involves stimulating the body's immune system against the cancer. Substances such as vaccines, antibodies, and biologic response modifiers are used to encourage the immune system to destroy the cancer cells.

Certain cancers—such as breast and prostate cancers—use hormones to grow. **Hormone, or endocrine, therapy** is usually used in conjunction with other types of cancer treatment and either blocks the body's ability to produce specific hormones or interferes with how those hormones behave in the body. Side effects from hormone therapy depend greatly on the hormones involved and may range from hot flushes and mood swings to diarrhea, nausea, and fatigue.

Unlike chemotherapy, which acts on cell division, **targeted therapies** are designed to act only on specific molecules (targets), without harming other cells. Targets may be genes that need to be switched on or off, or specific proteins within cancer cells that need to be destroyed. Certain immunotherapies can be classified as targeted therapy. Targeted therapy is usually used together with other cancer treatments and side effects depend on the type of targeted treatment used.

NEW WORDS	
Anoxia	The absence of oxygen in an area
Autonomic nervous system	Part of the nervous system responsible for the control of functions that are not under conscious control, e.g., the beating of the heart
Benign	Not harmful, non-cancerous
Cistern	A channel or tubule in the cell
Cytology	The study of cells
Diploid	Having two complete sets of chromosomes per cell
Enzyme	A protein that speeds up the rate of a reaction without itself being used in the reaction
Equilibrium	Balance
Gene	The basic unit of genetic material
Haploid	Having one complete set of chromosomes per cell
Histology	The study of tissues
Homeostasis	The process by which the body maintains a stable internal environment
Hydrophilic	Water-loving
Hydrophobic	Water-hating
Hypoxia	A lack, or deficiency, of oxygen in an area
Ischemia	A reduced or inadequate blood supply to an area
Kinetic energy	The energy of motion
Malignant	Cells are dividing abnormally and uncontrollably, cancerous
Metabolism	The changes that take place within the body to enable its growth and function
Metastasis	The spread of cancer cells
Phagocytosis	The engulfment and destruction of microbes, cell debris, and foreign matter by phagocytes, which are a type of white blood cell
Solvent	A liquid in which a solid is dissolved
Somatic	Any cell except the reproductive cells
Vacuole	A space within the cytoplasm of a cell that contains material taken in by the cell
Vesicle	A small, fluid-filled sac

Study Outline

Levels of structural organization of the body

The body can be divided into six levels of structural organization. From the simplest to the most complex level, they are: chemical, cellular, tissue, organ, system, and organismic.

Chemical organization of the body

1. Atoms are the basic unit of matter.
2. Elements consist of uniquely structured atoms.
3. The 4 major elements in the body are carbon, hydrogen, oxygen, and nitrogen.
4. The 9 lesser elements in the body are calcium, phosphorus, potassium, sulfur, sodium, chlorine, magnesium, iodine, and iron.
5. The 13 trace elements in the body are aluminum, boron, chromium, cobalt, copper, fluorine, manganese, molybdenum, selenium, silicon, tin, vanadium, and zinc.
6. Chemical reactions occur when atoms combine with or break apart from other atoms to form new products.
7. Molecules are the combination of two or more atoms.
8. Compounds are molecules of different types of atoms.
9. Water is the most abundant substance in the body. It functions in maintaining body temperature, acting as a lubricant, providing cushioning, and being a solvent.
10. Carbohydrates are the fuel of the body and are made up of simple sugars (monosaccharides).
11. Lipids (fats) insulate and protect the body, are a source of stored energy, and form an integral part of many structures and functions of the body. They are made up of glycerol and fatty acids.
12. Proteins are the building blocks of the body and are made up of amino acids.
13. Nucleic acids are found inside our cells. Deoxyribonucleic acid (DNA) makes up chromosomes, which contain our genes. Ribonucleic acid (RNA) is used to create specific proteins as per the genetic code.
14. Adenosine triphosphate (ATP) is the main energy-transferring molecule in the body.
15. Nutrients are essential for the growth, maintenance, and repair of the body. Macronutrients are carbohydrates, proteins, fats, essential minerals, and water. Micronutrients are vitamins and trace minerals.
16. Vitamins are organic compounds required in minute amounts for the normal functioning of the body.
17. Minerals play a role in body growth and maintenance.
18. Essential fatty acids are fats that cannot be made by the body and therefore need to be supplied by the diet.
19. Free radicals are highly unstable, reactive molecules that can damage cells.
20. Antioxidants are substances that combat or neutralize free radicals.

Cellular organization of the body

1. Cytology is the study of cells.
2. Cells are the basic structural and functional units of the body.
3. Cells are made up of a nucleus, cytoplasm, plasma membrane, and various organelles.
4. The plasma membrane is a barrier that surrounds the cells and regulates the movements of substances into and out of it. It consists of lipids and proteins.
5. Lipids make up the structure of the membrane, which is a phospholipid bilayer that also contains glycolipids and cholesterol.
6. Proteins are scattered in the phospholipid bilayer and act as channels, transporters, and receptors.
7. Materials are moved in and out of the cell through two types of transport: passive processes and active processes. Passive processes are simple diffusion, osmosis, and facilitated diffusion. Active processes are active transport and vesicular transport.
8. Simple diffusion is the movement of substances from areas of high concentration to areas of low concentration.
9. Osmosis is the movement of water from areas of high water concentration to areas of lower water concentration across a selectively permeable membrane.
10. In facilitated diffusion, substances are helped across the plasma membrane by channel or transporter proteins.
11. In active transport, pumps powered by ATP push molecules across the plasma membrane.
12. In vesicular transport, vesicles carry particles across the plasma membrane. Substances enter

cells through endocytosis and leave cells through exocytosis.

> Enter = endo
> Exit = exo

13. The cytoplasm is all the cellular material inside the plasma membrane excluding the nucleus. Cytoplasm contains cytosol, organelles, and inclusions.
14. Organelles are mitochondria, ribosomes, endoplasmic reticulum, Golgi complex, lysosomes, peroxisomes, centrosomes, and centrioles.
15. Mitochondria are the powerhouses of the cells.
16. Ribosomes are where proteins are made.
17. Endoplasmic reticulum (ER) transports molecules and rough ER contains ribosomes, which are the site for protein synthesis. Smooth ER has no ribosomes and is the site for lipid synthesis and detoxification.
18. The Golgi complex processes, sorts, and packages proteins and lipids.
19. Lysosomes break down and recycle molecules.
20. Peroxisomes detoxify harmful substances.
21. Centrosomes contain centrioles and function in cell division.
22. Centrioles function in cell division and play a role in the formation of flagella and cilia.
23. The nucleus is the control center of the cell. It is surrounded by a membrane called the nuclear envelope/membrane and it contains a nucleolus and chromatin.
24. The nucleolus is where ribosomes are made.
25. Chromatin is the material of which chromosomes are composed. Chromosomes are made up of DNA, which carries the genetic material of the cell.
26. Cells reproduce themselves through the process of cell division.
27. In somatic cell division, a single parent cell duplicates itself into two identical daughter cells. This process is called mitosis and it happens in four stages: prophase, metaphase, anaphase, and telophase.

> **P-MAT**
> Prophase—Metaphase—Anaphase—Telophase

28. In reproductive cell division, sperm and egg cells are produced. This process is called meiosis.

Tissue level of organization

1. Tissues are groups of cells that share a common function.
2. Histology is the study of tissues.
3. There are four types of tissue in the body: epithelial, connective, muscle, and nervous.

> Emergencies Create Nervous Muscles
> Epithelial, Connective, Nervous, Muscle

4. Epithelial tissue forms body linings and glands and functions in protection, absorption, and filtration.
5. There are four types of cells that make up epithelial tissue: squamous (thin and flat), cuboidal (cube-shaped), columnar (column-shaped), and transitional (changing shapes).
6. Simple epithelium is a single layer of cells. There are four types: squamous, cuboidal, columnar, and ciliated. It is very thin and functions in absorption, secretion, and filtration. It lines vessels such as blood and lymph vessels, and the respiratory and gastrointestinal tracts.
7. Stratified epithelium consists of two or more layers of cells. There are two types: stratified squamous and transitional. It is durable and functions in protecting underlying tissues in areas of wear and tear. Some also produces secretions. Examples include the skin and the organs of the urinary system.
8. Connective tissue is the most abundant and widely distributed tissue in the body. Cells are surrounded and separated by a matrix made of protein fibers and a fluid, gel, or solid ground substance. There are many different types of connective tissue, including loose connective tissue (areolar, adipose, lymphoid), dense connective tissue (yellow elastic, white fibrous), bone, cartilage (hyaline, fibrocartilage, elastic), and blood.

> Lucy Always Ate Lizards Despite
> their Yellow and White Blood
> Carl Hated the Fibers Enveloped in their Bones
> Loose (Areolar, Adipose, Lymphoid),
> Dense (Yellow elastic, White fibrous), Blood,
> Cartilage (Hyaline, Fibrocartilage, Elastic), Bone

9. Loose connective tissue has loosely woven fibers and many cells. It is a softer connective tissue that includes areolar tissue, adipose tissue, and lymphoid tissue. Examples include the tissue that surrounds the organs of the body and lymph nodes.

10. Dense connective tissue contains thick, densely packed fibers and fewer cells than loose connective tissue. It forms strong structures and includes elastic connective tissue and dense regular connective tissue. Examples include lung tissue, tendons, and ligaments.

11. Bone tissue consists of a very hard matrix that has been strengthened by inorganic salts. It includes compact and cancellous bone and it functions in protection and support.

12. Cartilage consists of a dense network of collagen and elastic fibers embedded in a rubbery ground substance. It has no blood vessels or nerves and it functions in movement, flexibility and support. It includes hyaline cartilage, fibrocartilage and elastic cartilage.

13. Blood consists of a fluid matrix called plasma and red blood cells, white blood cells, and platelets.

14. Muscle tissue is made of elongated cells and is able to contract and produce movement. It also helps maintain posture and generates heat. There are three types of muscle tissue: skeletal, cardiac, and smooth (visceral).

15. Skeletal muscle is attached to bones and composed of long, cylindrical, striated fibers with multiple nuclei. These are voluntary muscles.

16. Cardiac muscle forms most of the wall of the heart and consists of branched, striated fibers. It is involuntary muscle tissue.

17. Smooth muscle moves substances within the body and consists of non-striated, or smooth, fibers. It is an involuntary tissue.

18. Nervous tissue is made up of neurons and neuroglia and functions in communication. It is found in the brain, spinal cord, and nerves.

Membranes

1. Membranes are thin, flexible sheets made up of different tissue layers. They cover surfaces, line body cavities, and form protective sheets. There are two groups of membranes: epithelial and connective tissue.

2. Epithelial membranes consist of epithelial tissue and an underlying layer of connective tissue. They include mucous membranes, which line body cavities that open directly to the exterior (for example, the hollow organs of the respiratory system), and serous membranes, which line body cavities that do not open directly to the exterior (for example, the pleura).

3. Connective tissue membranes are synovial membranes and are composed of areolar connective tissue with elastic fibers and fat. They line joints, bursae, and tendon sheaths.

System level of organization

1. Systems are groups of organs that share a common function.

2. The systems of the body are the integumentary system, skeletal system, muscular system, nervous system, endocrine system, respiratory system, cardiovascular system, lymphatic and immune system, digestive system, urinary system, and the reproductive system.

3. Homeostasis is the process by which the body maintains internal equilibrium despite changes in its external environment.

Review

1. Name the six levels of organization of the body.
2. Define the following:
   - Atom
   - Element
   - Molecule
   - Compound.
3. Name the four major elements that make up the body.
4. Describe the importance of water in the body.
5. Describe the term carbohydrate. List the functions of carbohydrates.
6. Describe the term lipid. List the functions of lipids.
7. Describe the term protein. List the functions of proteins.
8. Explain what a cell is.
9. List the functions of the following:
   - Nucleus
   - Mitochondria
   - Ribosomes
   - Golgi complex
   - Lysosomes
   - Peroxisomes.
10. Describe how somatic cells reproduce.
11. Put the following processes into their chronological order: telophase, metaphase, anaphase, prophase.
12. Describe cytokinesis.
13. Describe the term "tissue."
14. Name the four major types of tissues in the body. For each one give an example.
15. Name the major systems of the body and briefly describe their functions.

Multiple-Choice Questions

1. Which of the following statements is correct?
   a. Oxygen, carbon, cholesterol, and nitrogen are major elements in the body
   b. Selenium, lipids, chromium, and nitrogen are major elements in the body
   c. Oxygen, carbon, hydrogen, and nitrogen are major elements in the body
   d. Ergosterol, carbon, hydrogen, and chromium are major elements in the body

2. Water is the:
   a. Solvent in body fluids
   b. Solute in body fluids
   c. Solution in body fluids
   d. None of the above

3. Carbohydrates are:
   a. Atoms
   b. Elements
   c. Compounds
   d. Matter

4. Glycogen and cellulose are:
   a. Proteins
   b. Lipids
   c. Carbohydrates
   d. None of the above

5. Triglycerides are:
   a. Proteins
   b. Lipids
   c. Carbohydrates
   d. None of the above

6. The building blocks of the body are:
   a. Proteins
   b. Lipids
   c. Carbohydrates
   d. None of the above

7. Which of the following statements is false?
   a. Nucleic acids are found inside cells
   b. Nucleic acids make up our genes
   c. DNA and RNA are nucleic acids
   d. Nucleic acids are vitamins

8. The fat-soluble vitamins are:
   a. B, C
   b. A, D, E, K
   c. B, C, D, K
   d. A, D, C

9. Cytology is the study of:
   a. Tissues
   b. Plants

c. Cells

d. Chemicals

10. The plasma membrane:
    a. Surrounds the cell
    b. Surrounds the nucleus
    c. Surrounds the organ
    d. Surrounds the mitochondria

11. Which of the following are passive forms of transport across the cell membrane?
    a. Simple diffusion and vesicular transport
    b. Osmosis and facilitated diffusion
    c. Active transport and simple diffusion
    d. Facilitated transport and vesicular transport

12. Which of the following is an organelle?
    a. Plasma membrane
    b. Cytosol
    c. Cytoplasm
    d. Ribosome

13. The process by which a parent cell duplicates itself into two identical daughter cells is called:
    a. Meiosis
    b. Mitosis
    c. Somosis
    d. Somotosis

14. What happens during interphase?
    a. A cell grows and DNA replicates itself
    b. A cell grows and divides itself
    c. A cell grows and dies
    d. A cell grows and DNA does not replicate itself

15. Which of the following is a type of connective tissue?
    a. Smooth muscle tissue
    b. Stratified squamous epithelium

c. Nerves

d. Bone

16. Which type of tissue initiates and transmits impulses?
    a. Muscle
    b. Connective
    c. Epithelial
    d. Nervous

17. Simple squamous epithelium consists of:
    a. Two or more layers of flat cells
    b. A single layer of flat cells
    c. Two or more layers of rectangular cells
    d. A single layer of rectangular cells

18. Which of the following statements is correct?
    a. Bone tissue has a rubbery ground substance
    b. Cartilage has a very hard matrix that has been strengthened by inorganic salts
    c. Blood has a matrix called plasma
    d. None of the above

19. Cardiac muscle is:
    a. Striated and involuntary
    b. Striated and voluntary
    c. Non-striated and involuntary
    d. Non-striated and voluntary

20. Membranes are:
    a. Sheets made up of neurons and neuroglia
    b. Sheets made up of the same tissue layers
    c. Sheets made up of different tissue layers
    d. Sheets made up of fibers

3

The Skin, Hair, and Nails

Introduction

Which is the largest organ in your body?

Here is a clue—in an average adult it can weigh almost 11 lb (5 kg) and cover an area about the size of a large dining-room table. Although it is so large, it can be as thin as ½ mm, and yet it is the only solid protection we have against the environment (Tortora and Derrickson, 2009). In addition, it reflects the state of our health and emotions.

You guessed it … the skin!

In this chapter you will discover the intricacies that make up the skin, hair, and nails, and you will see how they combine to form the **integumentary system.**

Student objectives

By the end of this chapter you will be able to:

*   Explain the functions of the skin
*   Describe the anatomy of the skin
*   Describe the structure and function of the hair
*   Describe the structure and function of the nail
*   Describe the structure and function of the cutaneous glands
*   Identify common pathologies of the skin, hair, and nails.

Did you know?

It is normal to lose about 500 ml of sweat per day—that's about one and a half cans of coke.

Skin

Functions of the skin

The skin is the ultimate overcoat. It keeps us warm when it is cold and cool when it is hot; it protects us from sunlight, rain, and injury; it secretes substances to keep itself in good condition; and, in addition to all of this, it even repairs itself when cut or torn.

Heat regulation

The body works hard at keeping its normal internal temperature at around 98.6°F (37°C). It does this by adapting to environmental changes in temperature by either cooling itself down in a warm environment or warming itself up in a cool environment. The body also needs to adapt to internal changes in temperature in times of fever or exercise. It regulates its temperature by:

*   Cooling itself down through:
    *   **Sweating:** Tiny glands release sweat on to the skin's surface; from here the sweat evaporates, drawing heat from the body and cooling it down
    *   **Vasodilation:** Blood vessels dilate and this causes blood to rush to the capillaries in the surface of the skin. From here the heat in the blood is lost through radiation. The skin also appears pinker and warmer
*   Warming itself up through:
    *   **Decreased sweat production**
    *   **Vasoconstriction:** Blood vessels constrict and this reduces the flow of blood through the capillaries. Thus the heat in the blood is conserved. The the skin also appears whiter and cooler
    *   **Goosebumps:** The arrector pili muscles contract and cause the hairs to stand on end in what is known as goosebumps. This this traps a layer of warm air close to the surface of the body
    *   **Shivering:** Our muscles contract more frequently to create heat within the body

Sensation

The dermis of the skin contains nerve endings that are known as **cutaneous sensory receptors.** They are sensitive to:

*   Touch
*   Temperature
*   Pressure
*   Pain.

Some areas have more receptors than others and are therefore more sensitive. For example, the lips and fingertips are extremely sensitive areas of the body.

Protection

What would happen to you if your skin was only a membrane that held your insides in? You would go swimming, absorb all the water in the pool, and become waterlogged. Millions of bacteria from the environment would enter your body and make you ill. The moment you went outdoors into the sun you would burn. As you can see, the skin is a unique barrier that protects you from a range of things, including:

- **Physical trauma and abrasion:** The skin insulates and cushions the organs and structures of the body.
- **Bacterial invasion:** The skin secretes acidic substances, which form an **acid mantle**. This inhibits the growth of bacteria. The skin also contains phagocytes, which ingest foreign substances and pathogens.
- **Dehydration:** Keratin in the skin forms a waterproof barrier, which prevents water from passing into and out of the body. This prevents us from literally drying out.
- **Ultraviolet radiation:** Melanin helps to protect us from the sun's damaging ultraviolet radiation.
- **Chemical damage:** The skin acts as a physical barrier to many potentially harmful substances.
- **Thermal damage:** The skin acts as a barrier that can help protect us from burns and scalds.

It is also important to remember that one of the main functions of the skin is that of sensation. The skin is sensitive to touch, pressure, pain, and temperature. This gives it further protective properties in that it enables the body to react to stimuli and so protect itself from further injury.

Absorption

Although the skin is a waterproof protective barrier, certain substances can still be absorbed through the skin. These substances include:

- Fat-soluble substances such as vitamins A, D, E, and K

- Topical steroids used to treat skin conditions such as eczema
- Drugs used in transdermal patches, e.g. hormones used in hormone replacement therapy (HRT) and nicotine used in nicotine patches
- Some toxic chemicals, such as mercury
- Essential oils used in aromatherapy.

Excretion

The skin excretes wastes from the body. These include:

- Urea
- Salts
- Water
- Aromatic substances, e.g., garlic.

Secretion

Sebaceous glands found in the skin secrete sebum, which is a fatty substance that keeps the skin supple and waterproof.

Synthesis of vitamin D

Despite being called a vitamin, vitamin D is actually a prohormone that helps regulate calcium levels in the body and is necessary for the growth and maintenance of bones. Exposure to the sun can meet 90% of our vitamin D needs. The skin contains a compound called 7-dehydrocholesterol, which, in the presence of sunlight, is converted to previtamin D3. Previtamin D3 is then metabolized by the liver and the kidneys into the active form of vitamin D, the steroid hormone called calcitriol.

Did you know?

The more we understand about vitamin D, the more we realize how vital it is we get out into the sunshine. Vitamin D helps metabolize calcium, improves the absorption of many vitamins, strengthens immunity, and influences gene expression. A lack of vitamin D is now known to play a role in conditions as diverse as depression, cardiac disease, and certain cancers.

Minor functions of the skin

The functions discussed previously are the major functions of the skin; however, the skin also functions in:

- **Immunity:** The skin is a strong physical barrier against invading microbes and also contains specific immune cells, such as Langerhans cells. Langerhans cells recognize and bind to foreign molecules that stimulate an immune response (known as **antigens**) and then transport these antigens to regional lymph nodes.
- **Blood reservoir:** In a resting adult, 8–10% of the body's total blood flow is in the dermis. In times of moderate exercise the dermal capillaries dilate and blood flow to the area increases to help cool the body. However, in times of strenuous exercise, dermal blood vessels actually constrict so that more blood can circulate to the muscles.
- **Communication:** Our skin communicates information about both our health and our emotions.

Anatomy of the skin

Dermatology is the study of the skin, which is a cutaneous membrane made of two distinct layers:

- The **epidermis** is a tough, waterproof outer layer that is continuously being worn away.
- The **dermis** lies beneath it and is a thicker layer that contains nerves, blood vessels, sweat glands, and hair roots.

The dermis is attached to the **subcutaneous layer**, which anchors the skin to the other organs in the body.

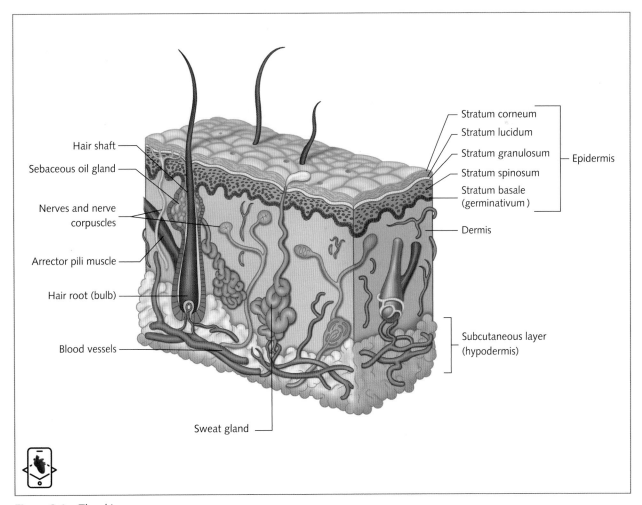

Figure 3.1 *The skin*

TISSUES THAT MAKE UP THE SKIN		
Name	**Tissue type**	**General description**
Epidermis	Keratinized stratified squamous epithelium	A thin layer of flat, dead cells that are continually being shed; this is a waterproof and protective layer
Dermis	Connective tissue containing collagen and elastic fibers	A thicker layer that supports the epidermis above it by enabling the passage of nutrients and oxygen; it also allows the skin to move, absorbs shocks, and cools and warms the body
Subcutaneous layer (also called subcutis, superficial fascia, or hypodermis)	Areolar and adipose tissue	This is not considered part of the skin but it anchors the skin to other organs and provides shock absorption and insulation

Did you know?

A blister from a burn or excess friction is simply an area where the epidermis and dermis have separated.

Epidermis

The epidermis is composed of five layers of stratified squamous epithelial tissue, which becomes tough and hard through a process called **keratinization.**

Before looking at the different layers of the epidermis it helps to know a little about the four types of cells that are found in these layers.

- **Keratinocytes:** These make up about 90% of epidermal cells and they produce a protein called **keratin.** Keratin helps waterproof and protect the skin. Its name comes from the Greek word *kerato*, meaning "horny."
- **Melanocytes:** The Greek word *melan* means "black," and melanocytes produce a brown-black pigment called **melanin.** Melanin contributes to skin color and absorbs ultraviolet light. Melanin granules actually form a protective layer over the nuclei of cells. This layer is only over the side of the nuclei that faces the surface of the skin, and the melanin is like a sun hat, protecting the nuclei from ultraviolet light.
- **Langerhans cells:** These arise from bone marrow and move to the epidermis. They respond to foreign bodies and thus play a role in skin immunity.

- **Merkel cells:** These are only found in the stratum basale of hairless skin and are attached to keratinocytes. They make contact with nerve cells to form Merkel discs, which function in the sensation of touch.

We will now look at the five layers of the epidermis and the meanings of their names. This will give you an idea of the appearance of each layer.

Infobox

Anatomy and physiology in perspective

The thickness of the skin varies depending on the area of the body. For example, the skin on the soles of the feet and the palms of the hands is thickest. This is because these areas are subject to a great deal of pressure and friction. On the other hand, the skin on the eyelids is very thin as it needs to be flexible and move quickly.

From the deepest to the most superficial layer, they are the:

- **Stratum basale:** *Basale* means "base" (this layer is also called the **stratum germinativum,** which means "to sprout"). This is the deepest layer of the epidermis and is the base from where new cells germinate or "sprout."
- **Stratum spinosum:** *Spinosum* means "thorn-like," or "prickly." This layer consists of prickly cells that are beginning to go through the process of keratinization.

- **Stratum granulosum:** *Granulosum* means "little grains." This layer is made up of degenerating cells that are becoming increasingly filled with little grains or granules of keratin.
- **Stratum lucidum:** *Lucidum* means "clear." This is a waterproof layer of dead, clear cells.
- **Stratum corneum:** *Corneum* means "horny." This is the outermost layer of the skin. Its cells are dead and now completely filled with keratin. Thus they are tough, durable and horny.

The epidermis can also be divided into two major layers:

- **The inner layer (Malpighian layer):** This layer of epidermis contains only dividing, non-keratinized cells. It includes the stratum basale, where new cells are constantly being produced, and the stratum spinosum, where some cells are only beginning to go through the process of keratinization.

Did you know?

···

When you shave the hairs off your skin, you are also cutting off many layers of dead skin, yet you don't bleed. This is because the epidermis is **avascular**. That means it contains no blood vessels.

- **The outer layer:** This layer is composed of keratinized, non-dividing cells. It includes the strata granulosum, lucidum, and corneum.

Stratum basale (stratum germinativum)—basal-cell layer

The stratum basale forms the deepest layer of the epidermis and is the layer closest to the dermis. Because it is close to the dermis it can receive nutrients and oxygen from it through the process of diffusion. This nourishment enables the stratum basale to produce millions of new cells each day.

The stratum basale has the following characteristics:

- It is composed of a single layer of cuboidal or columnar cells that have nuclei.
- It is constantly producing new cells through cell division. This is the reason it is sometimes called the stratum germinativum.
- The cells are pushed upward toward the superficial layers of the skin by newly produced cells below.
- The different cells present in the stratum basale are:
  – Stem cells for reproduction
  – Keratinocytes
  – Melanocytes
  – Merkel discs

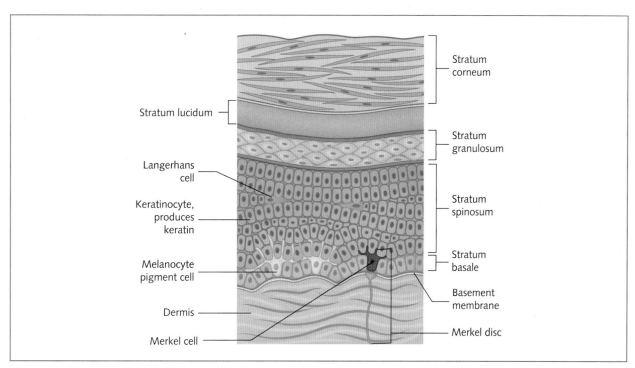

Figure 3.2 *The skin, showing the main layers of the epidermis*

Stratum spinosum—prickle-cell layer

The stratum spinosum consists of eight to ten layers of many-sided, irregular cells that appear to be covered with prickly thorns or spines. These spines join the cells tightly to one another. This is a transitional layer between the stratum basale and the stratum granulosum and it contains some dividing cells as well as cells that are beginning to go through the process of keratinization.

Stratum granulosum—granular-cell layer

The stratum granulosum consists of three to five layers of flattened cells whose nuclei are beginning to degenerate and die. This is because the cells are now far away from the nutrient-supplying dermis and they are becoming increasingly keratinized.

Stratum lucidum—clear-cell layer

The stratum lucidum is composed of three to five layers of clear, flat, dead cells that have no nuclei and contain eleidin, the precursor to keratin. This layer is waterproof and most apparent in the thick skin on the palms of the hands and soles of the feet.

Stratum corneum—horny-cell layer

The uppermost layer of the skin is the one that is exposed to all the harsh changes of the external environment as well as ultraviolet radiation, countless pathogens, and chemicals. It is the layer that needs to protect the skin from the external environment and so it must be the strongest and toughest of all the layers. This layer is made of 25–30 layers of flat, dead cells that are completely filled with keratin. This durable layer makes up about three-quarters of the total thickness of the epidermis and it has the following characteristics:

- All cells are non-nucleated (i.e., they are dead).
- The cytoplasm of the cells has been replaced by the fibrous protein keratin.
- Cells are constantly shed through a process called **desquamation.**
- Cells are constantly replaced from beneath.

Dermis

The dermis is the supportive layer beneath the epidermis and it is composed of connective tissue that contains both collagen and elastic fibers. It contains many different cells and structures, including:

- **Fibroblasts:** These are large, flat cells that synthesize the following fibers:
  - **Collagen fibers:** These are very tough yet flexible fibers that are resistant to pulling force and give skin its **extensibility** (ability to stretch). Collagen fibers also attract and bind water and are thus responsible for keeping skin hydrated. They contain the protein collagen
  - **Elastic fibers:** These are strong, thin fibers that give skin its **elasticity** (ability to return to its original shape after stretching). They can be stretched up to 150% of their relaxed length without breaking, and contain the protein elastin
  - **Reticular fibers:** These are thin fibers that form a branching network around other cells and give support and strength. They contain the protein collagen, coated with glycoprotein
- **Macrophages:** These are cells that engulf and destroy bacteria and cell debris by a process called **phagocytosis.**
- **Adipocytes:** These are fat cells.
- **Mast cells:** These cells produce histamine, which dilates small blood vessels during inflammation.
- **Blood and lymphatic vessels.**
- **Nerves.**
- **Glands.**
- **Hair follicles.**

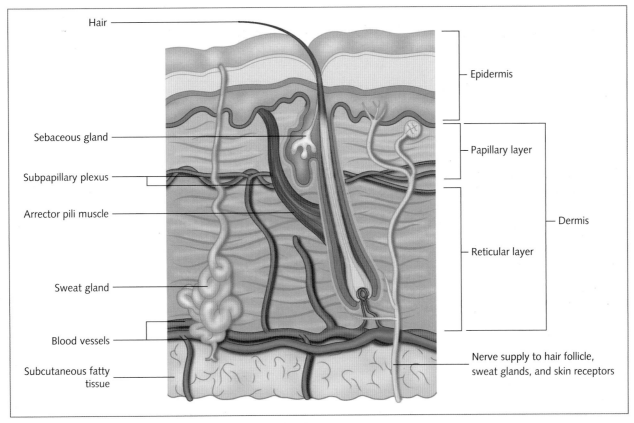

Figure 3.3 *The skin, showing the main structures in the dermis*

Did you know?

··

When the skin stretches beyond its ability, for example in pregnancy, small tears can occur in the dermis. These tears are stretch marks.

The dermis can be divided into two layers:

- **The papillary layer:** So named because of its nipple-shaped projections that go into the epidermis (papilla means "nipple").
- **The reticular layer:** Due to its nature, contributes to the varying thickness of the skin.

Papillary layer

The papillary layer is an undulating membrane that makes up approximately one-fifth of the thickness of the dermis. It is composed of areolar connective tissue and fine elastic fibers and has nipple-shaped, fingerlike projections called papillae. These papillae go into the epidermis and:

- Greatly increase the surface area of the papillary layer
- Contain loops of capillaries so that diffusion of nutrients and oxygen can take place between the dermis and epidermis
- May contain Meissner's corpuscles, which are nerve endings that are sensitive to touch.

Infobox

··

Anatomy and physiology in perspective

On the thick skin of the hand, the dermal papillae cause ridges in the overlying epidermis. These ridges are arranged in whorled and looped patterns that increase friction and act as suction cups so that you can pick up and grip objects. Sweat secretions into these ridges leave fingerprints on objects. Fingerprints are unique to each person and genetically determined. They develop in the embryo and do not change as a person grows—they only enlarge. Because of their uniqueness they are used to identify individuals.

Reticular layer

The reticular layer is deep to the papillary layer and is composed of dense, irregular connective tissue containing bundles of collagen and elastic fibers. These fibers give skin its extensibility, elasticity, and strength. The reticular layer is the main support structure of the skin, and it also contains:

- Hair follicles
- Nerves
- Oil glands
- Ducts of sweat glands
- Adipose tissue.

Subcutaneous layer

Although it is not part of the skin, it is important to learn about the subcutaneous layer as it is the tissue that attaches the reticular layer to the underlying organs. The subcutaneous layer contains:

- Areolar connective tissue
- Adipose tissue
- Lamellated corpuscles (Pacinian corpuscles): These are nerve endings that are sensitive to pressure.

Did you know?

All races have approximately the same number of melanocytes in their skin, yet differing amounts of pigments. It is these pigments that make a difference to skin color. The three pigments in your skin that are responsible for your color are:

- **Melanin**, which varies in color from pale yellow to black
- **Carotene**, which is a yellowish-orange pigment
- **Hemoglobin**, which is the pigment that carries oxygen in the red blood cells.

Types of skin

Now that you know the structure and functions of the skin, it is time to take a look at what you really see on a person and what distinguishes one person's skin from another. The common skin types are:

- **Normal (balanced) skin:** Normal skin is a balanced skin in which there are no signs of oily or dry areas. It is actually a "perfect" skin and is, of course, quite rare in adults. Normal skin:
  - Has an even texture
  - Has good elasticity
  - Has small pores
  - Feels soft and firm to the touch
  - Is usually blemish-free
- **Oily skin:** In an oily skin there is an overproduction of sebum by the sebaceous glands. This can be caused by hormones, e.g., in puberty. Oily skin:
  - Has an uneven texture
  - Has normal elasticity
  - Has large pores
  - Feels thick and greasy to touch
  - Often has blemishes such as comedones, papules, pustules, and scars
  - Appears sallow (unhealthy yellow or pale brown in color) and has a characteristic shine
  - Ages slowly
- **Dry skin:** In dry skin there is either an underproduction of sebum or a lack of moisture, or both together. Dry skin:
  - Has flaky, dry patches and a thin, coarse texture
  - Has poor elasticity
  - Feels dry, coarse, and papery to touch
  - Looks like parchment and often has dilated capillaries around the cheek and nose areas
  - May also be sensitive
  - Ages prematurely, especially around the eyes, mouth and neck
- **Combination skin:** Combination skin is a mixture of dry, normal, and greasy skin and is the most common type of skin. Combination skin:
  - Has an oily T-zone (forehead, nose, and chin), which feels thick and greasy and is often blemished
  - Has dry cheeks and neck, which feel flaky and coarse and may have dilated capillaries
  - Has varying tone and elasticity
  - May also have sensitive areas
- **Sensitive skin:** Sensitive skin often accompanies dry skin and is easily irritated. Sensitive skin:
  - Is hypersensitive and reactions can include reddening, itching, and chafing
  - Often has dilated capillaries
  - Is often dry and transparent
  - Is usually warm to touch

- **Mature skin:** As a person ages, both sun exposure and hormonal changes affect the skin, causing it to age. Mature skin:
  - Is dry, thin, less elastic, and bruises easily
  - Can become sensitive and irritated and take longer to heal
  - Can have pigmentation, deep wrinkles, and dilated capillaries

Infobox

Anatomy and physiology in perspective

As we age, our skin changes. We are born with soft, smooth skin that has a thick layer of fat and only a thin layer of protective keratin. It is not a very effective barrier against harmful substances.

As we grow our skin thickens and strengthens, and by adulthood we have strong, supple skin that functions effectively in protecting us and regulating our body temperature.

Then, as we age, the skin begins to thin. In old age both the dermis and epidermis are thinner and a lot of the underlying fat layer that usually insulates us has disappeared. The number of sweat glands and blood vessels in our skin also decreases and this lowers our skin's ability to regulate our body temperature. Therefore, we become more susceptible to both the cold and the heat. The skin also loses its elasticity with old age and begins to wrinkle and sag, and there is a decrease in melanocytes which causes an increase in sensitivity to the sun. Finally, a decrease in the number of nerve endings results in less sensitivity to external stimuli.

Hair

Hairs (or pili) grow over most of the body, except the palms of the hands, the soles of the feet, the eyelids, lips and nipples. They come in different types:

- **Lanugo hair:** This is a soft hair that begins to cover a fetus from the third month of pregnancy. It is usually shed by the eighth month of pregnancy.

- **Vellus hair:** This is a soft and downy hair and it is found all over the body, except the palms of the hands, soles of the feet, eyelids, lips and nipples.
- **Terminal hair:** This is a longer, coarser hair that is found on the head, eyebrows, eyelashes, under the arms and in the pubic area.

Structure of the hair

Hairs are columns of keratinized dead cells. When looked at longitudinally, they are made up of two parts:

- **Hair shaft:** The superficial end of the hair that projects from the surface of the skin; what we often call the hair "strand."
- **Hair root:** Penetrates into the dermis.

Infobox

Anatomy and physiology in perspective

It is the shape of the shaft that determines what type of hair you will have. For example, a round shaft produces straight hair, an oval shaft produces wavy hair and a flat shaft produces curly hair.

Did you know?

It is normal to lose 70–100 hairs per day. We don't usually notice this because adjacent hairs grow in different phases. However, these growth phases can be synchronized by a shock or stress to the body, such as illness or childbirth. This causes alarmingly large amounts of hair to be lost at the same time and is called **telogen effluvium**. Poor diet, illness, drugs, emotional stress, and hormonal changes also accelerate hair loss.

A cross-section of a hair shows that it consists of three concentric layers:

- **Inner medulla:** This consists of two to three rows of polyhedral cells and contains pigment granules and air spaces.

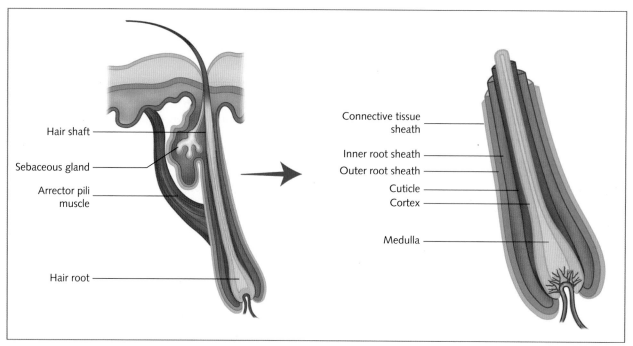

Figure 3.4 *Structure of a hair and hair follicle*

- **Middle cortex:** This is made up of elongated cells containing pigment granules in dark hair and air in white hair.
- **Outer cuticle:** This is a single layer of keratinized, flat, dead cells. These cells provide strength and help keep the inner layers of the hair tightly compacted.

Infobox

Anatomy and physiology in perspective

Cuticle cells overlap one another like tiles on a roof. This overlapping of the cells keeps the hairs apart and prevents them from matting.

Did you know?

Humans are born with all the hair follicles they will ever have, and hair is one of the fastest growing tissues in the body.

Hairs grow out of hair follicles that surround the root of the hair. At the base of the follicle is the bulb, which houses a nipple-shaped projection called the hair papilla. The papilla contains:

- Areolar and connective tissue
- Blood vessels that provide nourishment to the cells
- The matrix—a ring of cells that divide to create the hair.

Associated with hairs are:

- **Sebaceous oil glands:** These secrete sebum, which lubricates the hair.
- **Arrector pili muscles:** These are bands of smooth muscle cells that attach the side of the hair to the dermis. They contract to pull the hairs into a vertical position as a response to cold, fright, or differing emotions.

Life cycle of a hair

The life cycle of a hair includes growing, transitional, and resting stages. The growth stage is called **anagen**, and in this stage a follicle reforms and the matrix divides to create a new hair. As with the skin, the older cells are pushed upward as new cells develop below. The transitional stage is known as **catagen** and usually lasts one to two weeks. During this stage the hair separates from the base of the follicle as the dermal papilla breaks down. Finally, in the resting stage, or **telogen,** the follicle is no longer attached to the dermal papilla and the hair moves up the follicle and is naturally shed.

Functions of the hair

Hair has two main functions:

- It helps to keep the body warm.
- It protects the body. For example:
  - Hair on the head guards the scalp against the harmful rays of the sun
  - The eyebrows and eyelashes protect the eyes from foreign particles
  - Nostril hairs prevent the inhalation of insects and other foreign bodies
  - The hairs in the external ear canal protect the ears from insects and foreign particles

Hair in a nutshell

Living cells in the matrix divide constantly and push the hair upward. As the cells move upward they fill with keratin and die, forming the hair shaft, which warms and protects us.

Infobox

Anatomy and physiology in perspective

It is the pigments in your hair that determine its color. For example, people with dark hair have mainly true melanin in their hair; blondes and redheads have melanin and varying amounts of the minerals iron and sulfur; and those with gray hair have a decreased amount of the enzyme needed for the synthesis of melanin.

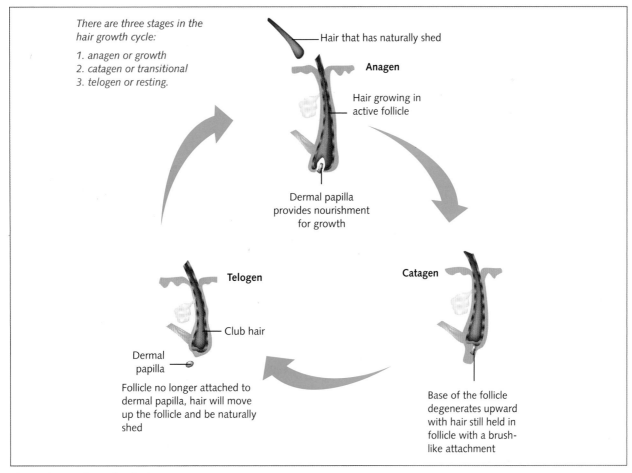

There are three stages in the hair growth cycle:

1. anagen or growth
2. catagen or transitional
3. telogen or resting.

Hair that has naturally shed

Anagen

Hair growing in active follicle

Dermal papilla provides nourishment for growth

Catagen

Base of the follicle degenerates upward with hair still held in follicle with a brush-like attachment

Telogen

Club hair

Dermal papilla

Follicle no longer attached to dermal papilla, hair will move up the follicle and be naturally shed

Figure 3.5 *Life cycle of a hair*

Nails

....

Nails are hard plates that cover and protect the ends of the fingers and toes and enable us to pick up small objects easily. *Onyx* is a Latin word meaning "nail," and another term for a nail is *unguis*.

Anatomy of the nail

For ease of learning, we will look at the nail in two parts. To begin with, we will look at the area beneath the nail plate. Starting at the proximal end is the:

- **Germinal matrix:** This area is rich in nerves and blood vessels and is the region where cell division takes place and growth occurs. Cells in this area are pushed upward toward the lunula.
- **Nail groove:** Grooves on the sides of the nail guide it up the fingers and toes.
- **Nail bed:** This area lies directly beneath the nail plate and secures the nail to the finger or toe. It contains blood vessels for nourishment and sensory nerve endings.

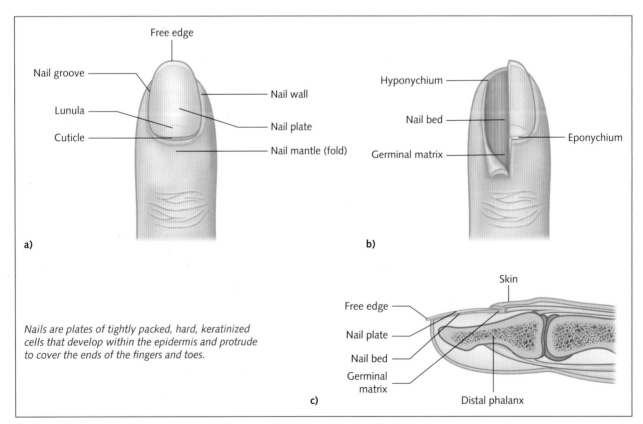

Nails are plates of tightly packed, hard, keratinized cells that develop within the epidermis and protrude to cover the ends of the fingers and toes.

Figure 3.6 *Structure of the nail*

Nails in a nutshell

Living cells at the matrix divide constantly and push the nail forward. As the cells move toward the fingertips they fill with tough keratin and die, forming the nail plate, which helps protect our fingers and toes.

We will now look at the top of the nail, again starting from its proximal end:

- **Nail mantle:** This is the skin that lies directly above the germinal matrix; it is sometimes referred to as the **nail fold.**
- **Cuticle:** This is an extension of the horny layer of the epidermis from the nail mantle (fold) that overlaps the base of the nail plate. Its function is to protect the germinal matrix from infection.
- **Lunula:** This is the crescent-shaped white area at the proximal end of the nail.
- **Eponychium:** This is an extension of the cuticle from the base of the nail fold. Its function is to protect the matrix from infection.
- **Hyponychium:** This is located under the nail plate, where the free edge forms. It protects the nail bed from infection.
- **Nail plate:** This is the visible body of the nail. It does not contain any blood vessels or nerves and it functions in protecting the nail bed beneath it.
- **Nail wall:** This is the skin that covers the sides of the nail plate and it protects the nail grooves.
- **Free edge:** This is also called the **distal edge** and is the part of the nail that extends past the end of the finger or toe.

Functions of the nail

The key functions of the nail are:

- The nails protect the ends of the toes and fingers from physical trauma
- The nails help us to grasp and pick up small objects
- The nails enable us to scratch parts of the body.

Cutaneous Glands

Glands are groups of specialized cells that secrete beneficial substances and also excrete waste products. There are several kinds of glands associated with the skin, the main ones being sebaceous and sweat glands. These glands are generally found in the dermis of the skin.

Sebaceous glands

The word *sebaceous* means "oily" and sebaceous glands are oil glands that usually empty into hair follicles, although some do open directly on to the surface of the skin. Sebaceous glands secrete **sebum**, which is an oily substance composed of fats, cholesterol, protein, and inorganic salts. Sebum acts as a lubricant that:

- Prevents hair from drying out and becoming brittle
- Prevents excessive evaporation of moisture from the skin, thus keeping it soft and moist
- Inhibits the growth of certain bacteria.

Cutaneous glands in a nutshell

Cutaneous glands are groups of specialized cells that secrete substances such as sebum and excrete waste products such as sweat.

composed of water, ions, urea, uric acid, amino acids,
ammonia, glucose, lactic acid, and ascorbic acid.
It aids heat regulation of the body and also helps
eliminate small amounts of waste. Sweat is acidic and
therefore helps to inhibit the growth of bacteria on
the skin's surface.

Sudoriferous glands are divided into two types,
depending on their location, structure, secretion,
and function: **eccrine** and **apocrine**. The table below
highlights the differences between eccrine and
apocrine glands.

Sudoriferous (sweat) glands

Sudoriferous glands excrete sweat on to the
surface of the skin. Sweat, or perspiration, is

	Eccrine glands	Apocrine glands
Location	These are very common sweat glands found all over the body except for on the lips, nail beds, some of the reproductive organs, and the eardrums; they are most numerous on the palms of the hands and the soles of the feet	These are found in the axilla (armpits), pubic region, and the areolae of the breasts
Structure	Their secretory portion is located in the subcutaneous layer and their duct extends outward through the skin, opening as a pore on the surface of the skin	Their secretory portion is located in the dermis or subcutaneous layer and their duct opens into hair follicles
Excretion	Sweat	Sweat, fatty acids, and proteins
Function	They excrete waste and help to regulate the body's temperature by keeping it cool	Their exact function is not yet known, but they are activated by pain, stress, and sexual foreplay

In the classroom

....

Diseases and disorders of the skin are surprisingly
common. Have a class discussion and see who has had
which of the following skin conditions. Question your
classmates on what the condition looked like, how it
felt, how they got it, etc. It is always easier to remember
conditions if you can learn from someone who has
experienced them.

Common Pathologies of the Skin

The condition of a person's skin and hair reflects their general health and emotional well-being. It is positively influenced by:

- Healthy nutrition
- Exercise
- Adequate water intake
- Sufficient sleep
- Rest and relaxation
- Hygiene and care.

Factors that have a negative effect on one's skin and hair include:

- Poor nutrition and minimal water intake
- Insufficient exercise
- Lack of sleep, rest, or relaxation
- Emotional stress and tension
- Excess alcohol and caffeine consumption
- Smoking
- Medication (some drugs have negative side effects on the skin)
- Excess exposure to ultraviolet radiation
- Use of harsh chemicals in detergents and soaps
- Environmental pollution
- Hormonal changes
- Aging.

Red flags

- Any rash accompanied by fever, nausea, and/or headache
- Widespread, generalized erythema (reddening) of the skin
- Widespread, generalized pruritus (itching) of the skin
- Skin conditions that are infected, blistering, painful, or rapidly worsening
- Severe sunburn
- Severe jaundice (yellowing) of the skin
- Moles that are changing, itchy, or bleeding.

Infobox

Anatomy and physiology in perspective

Remember that although some skin disorders have no medical consequences, they can have a traumatic effect on a person's confidence and self-image.

Study tip

Make sure you learn both the clinical term and the common name of the following diseases and disorders. You may find that you know a lot of them already. For example, *herpes simplex* is simply a cold sore—something you may already know all about.

Terms for marks and growths on the skin

Although you may not need to learn the following terms, they will help you to visualize and thus learn some of the diseases described later.

Abrasion	A damaged area of the skin caused by the skin being scraped or worn away
Bruise	A discoloration of the skin caused by the escape of blood from underlying vessels
Bulla	A large, fluid-filled spot
Callus	A thick, protective layer of skin caused by repeated pressure or friction; common on the fingers and feet
Chilblains (perniosis)	Red, itchy swellings occurring on the extremities or legs due to exposure to the cold; they can occasionally blister
Corn (clavus)	A small cone of compacted cells found either on the toes or between the toes; caused by continual pressure and often accompanied by pain and inflammation
Crust (scab)	An accumulation of dried blood, pus, or skin fluids on the surface of the skin; forms wherever the skin has been damaged
Cyst	A semi-solid or fluid-filled lump above and below the skin
Excoriation	The removal of the skin caused by scratching or scraping
Fissure	A crack in the skin that penetrates into the dermis
Macule	A small, flat, discolored spot of any shape, e.g., freckles

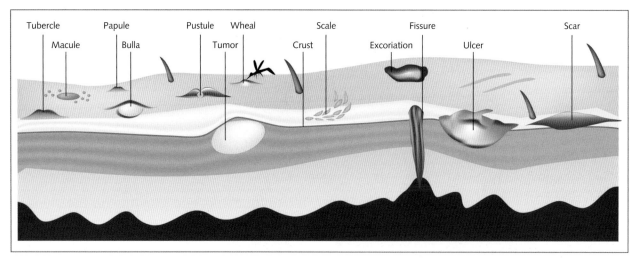

Figure 3.7 *Marks and growths on the skin*

Mole	A small and dark skin growth; it is a concentrated area of melanin
Nodule	A solid bump that may be raised
Papule	A small, solid bump that does not contain fluid; for example, warts, insect bites, and skin tags
Plaque	A large, flat, raised bump or group of bumps
Pustule	A lump containing pus
Scales	Areas of dried, flaky cells; for example, in psoriasis or dandruff
Scar	An area where normal skin has been replaced by fibrous tissue; forms after an injury
Stretch marks	Small tears in the dermis caused by the skin stretching beyond its ability
Telangiectasia	A localized collection of blood vessels in the skin; it is characterized by a red spot that can sometimes be spidery in appearance and that blanches under pressure
Tubercle	A solid lump that is larger than a papule
Tumor	An abnormal growth of tissue
Ulcer	A deep, open lesion on the skin; ulcers penetrate the dermis
Vesicle	A small, fluid-filled spot; for example, chickenpox and burns
Wheal (hive)	A common allergic reaction in which there is swelling with an elevated, soft area

Abnormal growth disorders

Acrochordon (skin tags)

Harmless soft, small, flesh-colored or dark growths that generally appear on the neck, in the armpits, or in the genital area.

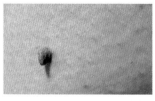

Acrochordon (skin tags)

Alopecia

Absence of hair growth where it is expected to grow. Forms of alopecia include:

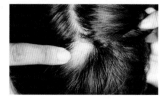

Alopecia areata

- **Alopecia areata**—loss of patches of hair
- **Alopecia totalis**—complete loss of scalp hair
- **Alopecia universalis**—complete loss of all hair
- **Androgenetic alopecia**—male-pattern baldness associated with hormonal changes.

Keloids

Form over healed wounds and are an overgrowth of scar tissue that appear as smooth, shiny, flesh-colored growths of fibrous tissue. Although they

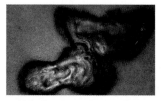

Keloids

are not painful, they can itch or be sensitive to touch, and can form in any scar, even acne scars.

Psoriasis

Chronic disorder characterized by raised, red patches that have silvery scales. These patches are caused by unusually rapid cell growth, but the reason for this rapid

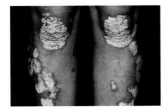

Psoriasis

cell growth is unknown. Some people with psoriasis will also have deformed, thickened nails. Psoriasis often runs in families and can be aggravated by sunburn, injuries, or stress. It is sometimes improved through gentle exposure to the sun. Psoriasis can be accompanied by psoriatic arthritis.

Seborrheic keratoses (senile warts)

Common in middle-aged to elderly people and are harmless darkish brown or black growths. They are common on the torso and temples, but can appear anywhere on the skin. Usually

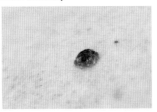

Seborrheic keratoses (senile warts)

round, although can be oval in shape.

Xanthoma

Fatty deposit beneath the skin that usually appear on joints such as the elbows or knees or around the eyes. Xanthomas appearing on the eyelids are called xanthelasma.

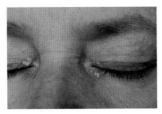

Xanthoma

Xanthomas can be suggestive of hyperlipidemia.

Allergies

When a person has an allergic reaction to a substance, it is usually an inappropriate immune response to what is normally a harmless substance. When the skin is involved in an allergic reaction, the most obvious sign is inflammation. Inflammation is a localized, protective response involving redness, swelling, and pain.

Dermatitis and eczema

Dermatitis is a broad term for inflammation of the upper layers of the skin and it includes a variety of signs and symptoms that usually involve itching, blistering, redness, and swelling. Severe signs are oozing, scabbing, and scaling. Dermatitis can be caused by allergens, irritants, dryness, scratching, or fungi.

- **Contact dermatitis:** This is an itchy rash that is confined to a specific area and the result of direct contact with a substance. It can be caused by cosmetics,

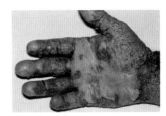

Contact dermatitis

metals such as nickel, certain plants such as poison ivy, drugs in some creams, and certain chemicals used in clothing manufacturing.

- **Eczema:** This is a form of dermatitis that can be caused by either internal or external factors. It is characterized by itchiness, redness, and blistering. It can

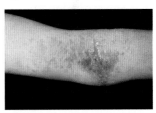

Eczema

be either dry or weeping, and can cause scaly and thickened skin.

Urticaria (nettle rash, or hives)

Commonly called hives, this is an allergic reaction triggered by certain foods, drugs, or insect stings. It is identified by itchy wheals, which are pale, slightly elevated

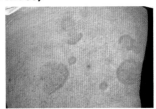

Urticaria (nettle rash, or hives)

swellings surrounded by an area of redness.

Bacterial infections of the skin

We come into contact with bacteria every day, but most of the time our skin forms a barrier that prevents infection. However, some bacterial infections do occur. These are usually in people with a weakened immune system or with damaged skin (from sunburn, scratching, or trauma). Many types of bacteria can affect the skin and the most common are **staphylococcus** and **streptococcus**.

Carbuncles

Collection of small, shallow abscesses that are connected to one another under the skin. If a person has carbuncles, they will usually also have a fever and feel ill and tired.

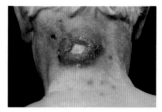

Carbuncle

Cellulitis

Spreading bacterial infection of the skin that begins as redness, pain, and tenderness over an area and then develops into hot, swollen areas that appear slightly pitted. Cellulitis is caused by bacteria and can occur after being bitten by humans or animals or injuring oneself in water or dirt.

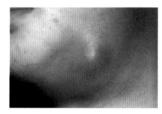

Cellulitis

Conjunctivitis

This is described in chapter 6 under the heading "Eye disorders."

Folliculitis

Bacterial infection of a hair follicle and appears as a small white pimple at the base of a hair. One or many follicles can be infected.

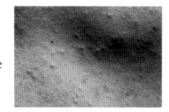

Folliculitis

Furuncles (boils)

Also known as boils or skin abscesses, these are pus-filled pockets of infection beneath the skin. They are bacterial infections that are more common in people with poor hygiene or weakened immune systems.

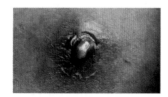

Furuncle (boil)

Hordeolum (stye)

This is described in chapter 6 under the heading "Eye disorders."

Impetigo

Very contagious bacterial infection that is common in children. Signs and symptoms include itchiness; pain; and scabby, yellow-crusted sores or fluid-filled blisters. It most commonly occurs on the face, arms, and legs and is easily spread through scratching.

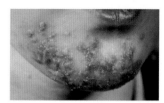

Impetigo

Burns

Injuries to the skin that can be caused by heat, sunlight, chemicals, electricity, or radiation. Burns differ according to their cause and the degree of the burn. For example, a first-degree burn is a shallow, superficial burn in which only the epidermis has been affected; a second-degree burn extends into the dermis; and a third-degree burn involves injury to all layers of the skin, including the subcutaneous layer. Symptoms of burns also vary according to the degree of the burn, from simple redness and swelling to blistering and even blackening and scarring of the skin.

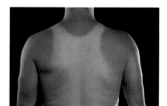

Sunburn

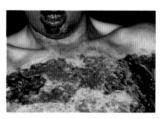

Second- and third-degree burns

Cancers

There are three main types of skin cancer: squamous cell carcinoma, basal cell carcinoma, and melanoma. Long-term sun exposure generally plays a role in the development of skin cancer, and fair-skinned people, who produce less melanin, are more susceptible to developing it.

Most skin cancers are curable if treated early enough, and so it is vitally important that any unusual, persistent skin growth be examined by a doctor as soon as possible.

Basal cell carcinoma (rodent ulcers)

This is the most common form of skin cancer. Although it is called "basal cell," it does not necessarily originate in the basal cells of the epidermis. Basal cell carcinoma

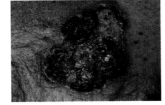

Basal cell carcinoma

can appear in many forms. For example, it may appear as raised bumps that break open and form scabs; or as a flat, pale or red patch; or it may be an enlarged papule with a thickened, pearly border. Basal cell carcinomas may also be mistaken for sores that constantly bleed, scab, and heal. These carcinomas rarely metastasize (spread to distant parts of the body). However, they can invade surrounding tissues and this can be serious if the carcinomas are located close to the brain, eyes, or mouth.

Melanoma

Originates in the melanocytes of the skin and can develop in sun-exposed areas or on moles and can metastasize. Melanomas vary in appearance and signs to

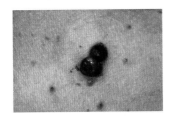

Melanoma

watch for include moles or freckles that are growing, changing in color, or changing in shape; moles that bleed or break open; or irregular black or gray lumps that appear on the skin.

Squamous cell carcinoma (prickle-cell cancer)

Originates in the stratum spinosum (prickle-cell layer) of the epidermis and usually occurs on sun-exposed areas in fair-skinned people. Occasionally, it may develop in areas that

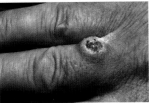

Squamous cell carcinoma

are not exposed to the sun, e.g., the mouth. It is characterized by a thick, scaly, warty appearance, and if left untreated it can develop into an open sore that grows into the underlying tissue. In addition to prolonged sun exposure, causes of squamous cell carcinoma include certain chemicals, chronic sores, burns, and scars. Squamous cell carcinomas do occasionally metastasize.

Red flags

When examining a person's skin, take note of any moles or pigmented lesions. Ask if the lesion is new, changing, growing, itchy, or bleeding. Also ask if there is a family history of skin cancers and check the rest of the body for other suspicious lesions. Refer the patient if you are at all concerned, especially if the answer is yes to any of the following ABCDE questions:

- **A = Asymmetry**
  - Is it irregular in shape?
- **B = Bleeding and border**
  - Does it bleed or have an irregular or rough border?
- **C = Color**
  - Is the color uneven or changing?
- **D = Diameter**
  - Is the mole or lesion growing, or >6 mm in diameter?
- **E = Evolving**
  - Is it changing or evolving?

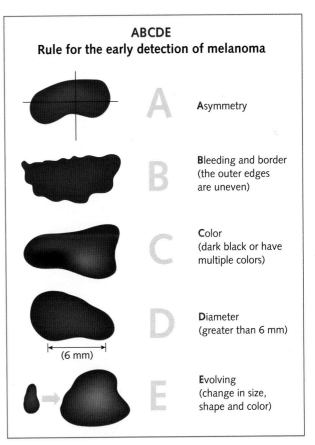

ABCDE
Rule for the early detection of melanoma

Asymmetry

Bleeding and border (the outer edges are uneven)

Color (dark black or have multiple colors)

Diameter (greater than 6 mm)

(6 mm)

Evolving (change in size, shape and color)

Fungal infections of the skin

Fungi are organisms that often make their homes in moist areas of the skin, e.g., between the toes or in folds of skin.

Candidiasis (thrush or yeast infection)

Also called **candidosis**, this is an infection by the yeast candida. This yeast is normally found in the mouth, digestive tract, and vagina, but it can infect other areas of the body if it is allowed to grow unchecked.

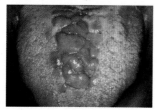

Candidiasis (thrush or yeast infection)

Pregnant women, obese people, and people with diabetes are more prone to candidiasis. So are those taking antibiotics. Different forms of candidiasis include:

- **Infections in skin folds:** These are characterized by a bright red rash with a softening and sometimes breaking down of the skin. The rash may itch or burn and small pustules may appear. Areas that are sometimes infected by candidiasis include the navel, the anus, and the diaper (nappy) area of a baby.
- **Vaginal candidiasis:** This is characterized by burning, itching, and redness around the vagina that is accompanied by a white or yellow discharge.
- **Penile candidiasis:** This characterized by a red, raw, painful rash on the penis.
- **Thrush:** This is candidiasis of the mouth, and it is characterized by white, painful patches on the tongue and sides of the mouth.
- **Candidal paronychia:** This is candidiasis of the nail bed, and it is characterized by redness and swelling that may lead to the nail turning white or yellow and separating from the nail bed.

Tinea (ringworm)

Contagious fungal infection that is identified by ring-shaped patches on the skin. It is generally classified by its location on the body, and includes:

- **Tinea capitis (scalp ringworm):** This is an itchy, scaly, pink rash on the scalp that can cause patches of hair loss.

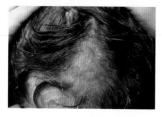

Tinea capitis (scalp ringworm)

- **Tinea corporis (body ringworm):** This appears as round patches that have pink, scaly borders and clear centers. It can be very itchy.
- **Tinea pedis (athlete's foot):** This is a common infection found between the toes. Its signs and symptoms include scaling with, or without, redness and itching. It is easily spread in moist areas where people walk barefoot, e.g., communal showers.

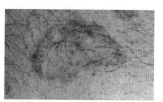

Tinea corporis (body ringworm)

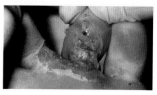

Tinea pedis (athlete's foot)

Infestations of the skin

Most skin infestations are caused by skin parasites, which are tiny insects or worms that burrow into the skin and live there.

Pediculosis (lice)

Lice are tiny, wingless insects, which spread easily from person to person by physical contact. Although lice are difficult to find, their eggs (nits) are easily seen as shiny, grayish eggs that are firmly attached to hair shafts. Lice can occur on different parts of the body and generally cause severe itching.

A lice infestation needs to be treated as soon as possible as intense scratching can lead to bacterial infections.

- **Pediculosis capitis (head lice):** These infect scalp hair and are common in young children. They are spread through sharing personal items such as hair brushes and hats.

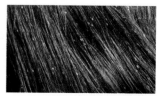

Pediculosis capitis (head lice)

- **Pediculosis corporis (body lice):** These are usually only found in people with poor hygiene or who live in overcrowded housing. The lice generally inhabit the seams of clothing.

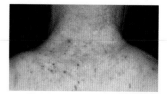

Pediculosis corporis (body lice)

- **Pediculosis pubis (pubic lice):** These are sometimes called crabs. These lice infest the genital hair and are spread through sexual contact.

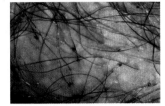
Pediculosis pubis (pubic lice)

Scabies (itch mites)

Highly contagious infestation caused by the female itch mite, who burrows her way into the horny layer of the skin. Here she lays her eggs and within a few days young mites have hatched. Tiny, itchy bumps develop, which are usually worse at night.

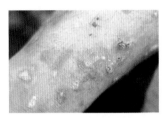
Scabies (itch mites)

Pigmentation disorders

Most pigmentation disorders are related to either an overproduction or an underproduction of the pigment melanin. Melanin is produced by cells called melanocytes, and it is the pigment responsible for the color of a person's skin. A few pigment disorders can be related to other pigments—for example, jaundice is a buildup of the pigment bilirubin.

Albinism

Hereditary disorder caused by a lack of melanin in the body and can occur in people of all races. It is characterized by white hair, pale skin, and pink or pale blue eyes.

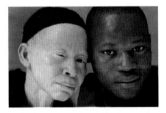
Albinism

Albinism also results in abnormal vision, involuntary eye movements, and extreme sensitivity to sunlight.

Chloasma

Also known as **melasma**, this is a blotchy, brownish patch caused by the overproduction of melanin. It is more common in women and usually affects the

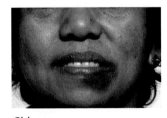
Chloasma

forehead, cheeks, and around the lips. Chloasma can be triggered by hormonal changes in pregnancy or when taking the contraceptive pill. It can occasionally be caused by excessive sun exposure or as a reaction to some skin cosmetics, and it usually fades with time.

Dilated capillaries

Capillaries are the tiny blood vessels found in the dermis of the skin. When they dilate, more blood rushes to them and this appears as erythema.

Ephelides (freckles)

Flat, irregular patches of melanin produced in response to sunlight. They are harmless, and common in fair-skinned people.

Erythema

Term used to describe inflammation or redness of the skin. It is caused by the engorgement of skin capillaries.

Lentigines

Lentigines (singular *lentigo*) are small, pigmented patches that can be flat or slightly raised. They can occur anywhere on the body and vary in color from tan-brown to black. They can appear at birth or in early childhood or can

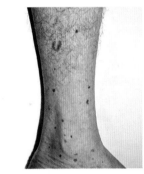
Lentigines

be due to sun exposure. In older people they are sometimes called "liver spots" or "sun spots."

Leucoderma (leukoderma) and vitiligo

Leucoderma is the name given to depigmented, white patches on the skin that has many causes, including genetics, immunological problems, inflammatory conditions, infections, medications, or exposure to certain chemicals.

Vitiligo is a pigmentary disorder characterized by smooth, white patches of skin where there is a lack of melanocytes. Due to this lack of melanocytes, it is important to protect

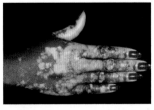
Vitiligo

the skin from the sun with sunscreen and clothing. The exact cause of vitiligo is unknown but it is currently thought to be a hereditary immunological disorder precipitated by stress, trauma, or illness, and it is associated with autoimmune diseases such as diabetes, pernicious anemia, and thyroid and adrenal disorders. Although it has no medical consequences, it can be very distressing for an individual.

Vascular naevi

Naevi (singular *naevus*) are malformed, dilated blood vessels in the skin. They appear as red or purple blotches and can occur anywhere on the body. Birthmarks are a common type of naevus. There are different types of naevi, including:

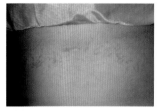

Vascular naevi

- **Port-wine stains:** These are flat, red to purplish discolorations, which are present at birth.
- **Spider naevi:** These are small, red spots surrounded by slender, dilated capillaries that look like spider's legs. They are common in fair-skinned people and are sometimes associated with sun exposure.
- **Strawberry naevi:** These are birthmarks that usually disappear during childhood. They are red and raised above the surface of the skin.

Pressure sores (decubitus ulcers)

Also called bed sores, these are caused by constant pressure to an area. This pressure prevents the flow of blood to the area and results in the death of the skin. The dead skin then breaks down and forms sores or ulcers. Pressure sores are common in people who are bedridden, and are characterized by redness and inflammation.

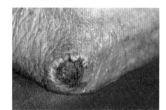

Pressure sores

Sebaceous gland disorders

Acne rosacea

Sometimes called "adult acne" and usually affects the central area of the face. It is characterized by redness, noticeable blood vessels, and tiny pimples. Its cause is unknown, but it is aggravated by alcohol, spicy foods, menopause, and stress.

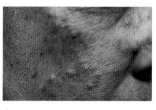

Acne rosacea

Acne vulgaris

An inflammatory disorder of the sebaceous glands that is thought to be caused by an interaction between hormones, skin oils, and bacteria. It can range from mild to severe.

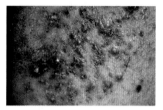

Acne vulgaris

Acne vulgaris occurs mainly on the face, chest, shoulders, and back and signs include comedones, papules, pustules, cysts, and sometimes abscesses.

Comedones (blackheads)

Enlarged sebaceous glands can become blocked by accumulated sebum; this is known as a whitehead. When the sebum oxidizes and dries, it darkens and forms blackheads.

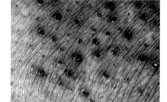

Comedones (blackheads)

Milia

Commonly found around the eyes and over the cheek area, appearing as white, hard nodules under the skin. They are small, harmless, keratin-filled cysts found just beneath the epidermis and are common in newborn babies.

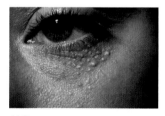

Milia

Seborrhea

Characterized by an oily skin with enlarged, blocked pores, comedones, and pustules and is due to an excessive secretion of sebum by the sebaceous glands.

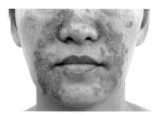

Seborrhea

Steatomas (sebaceous cysts, or wens)

Usually found on the face, neck, scalp, and back, these are round lesions that have a smooth and shiny surface.

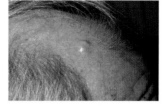

Steatoma (sebaceous cyst)

Sudoriferous (sweat) gland disorders

Anhidrosis

Also called **hypohidrosis**, this is a lack of sweating in the presence of an appropriate stimulus, such as heat. It can be congenital or due to an illness.

Bromhidrosis (body odor)

Also called **bromidrosis** or **osmidrosis**, this is caused by the breakdown of sweat by bacteria and yeasts that normally live on the skin. It can also be influenced by one's diet, genetics, and general health.

Hyperhidrosis

Also called **hyperidrosis**, this is excessive or almost constant sweating. It can affect the entire surface of the skin but is usually limited to the armpits, genitals, palms, and soles. It can be caused by an illness or a medical condition such as hyperthyroidism, or may occur after the use of certain drugs.

Miliaria rubra (prickly heat)

Common in warm, humid climates and is caused by sweat that is trapped in the narrow ducts that carry it to the surface. This trapped sweat causes inflammation and a prickling, itching sensation. It can appear as an itchy rash of very tiny blisters or as large, reddened areas of the skin.

Viral infections of the skin

Viruses are tiny organisms that invade living cells and then multiply within them. They cause many common infections, such as cold sores and warts. Diseases caused by viruses are often accompanied by rashes, spots or sores on the skin.

Herpes simplex (cold sore)

Small, fluid-filled blisters that can keep recurring and are normally found on the face and around the mouth. Cold sores usually begin with a tingling sensation at the site, followed by redness, swelling, and the development of blisters. These blisters then break open, leaving sores and scabs. This condition is passed through direct contact with the sores.

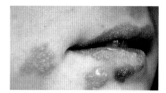

Herpes simplex (cold sore)

Herpes zoster (shingles)

Re-emergence of the chickenpox virus and usually occurs when a person's immune system is weakened. It develops as a painful eruption of blisters

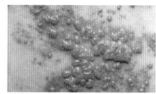

Herpes zoster (shingles)

limited to an area served by infected nerves. If the trigeminal (V) nerve is affected the rash can affect the eye, leading to long-term complications and possible loss of sight. The infected person may feel unwell and feverish and/or may experience pain, tingling, and itching.

Rubella (German measles)

Contagious infection that begins with mild flu-like signs, such as a runny nose and cough. Painless, rose-colored spots appear on the roof of the mouth

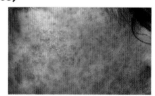

Rubella (German measles)

and then merge and extend over the back of the throat. The lymph glands swell in the neck and a characteristic rash then appears, which begins on the face and neck and spreads down the body. This rash is often accompanied by a reddening or flushing of the skin. Joint pain can also accompany rubella. Rubella is spread by airborne droplets of moisture. Rubella in pregnancy (congenital rubella) can cause birth defects in the unborn child.

Rubeola (measles)

Highly contagious infection that begins with flu-like signs, such as a fever, runny nose, sore throat, cough, and red eyes. Two to four days later small white spots appear inside

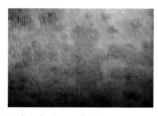

Rubeola (measles)

the mouth, and then a few days later an itchy rash appears. This rash usually begins on the neck and then spreads to the rest of the body. Measles is spread by airborne droplets of moisture.

Varicella (chickenpox)

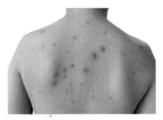

Varicella (chickenpox)

Very contagious infection characterized by a mild fever that is followed by an itchy rash of small, raised spots that can blister, crust, and scab. These scabs drop off after about 12 days. Chickenpox is spread by airborne droplets of moisture, and after the infection the virus can remain dormant in the body and reactivate as shingles in later life.

Warts

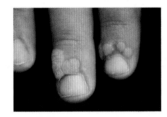

Warts

Small, firm growths that have a rough surface and are usually caused by the human papillomavirus (HPV). They can grow in clusters or as an isolated growth. Warts on the body are generally painless, and are common on areas that are frequently injured, e.g., the knees, face, fingers, and around the nails. Warts include:

- **Filiform warts (verrucae filiformis):** These are small, pedunculated warts that occur on the margins of the eyes and mouth. They are also referred to as digitate or facial warts.
- **Genital warts (condylomata acuminata):** These occur on the skin of the genital and perianal areas and are often sexually transmitted. They can be itchy and uncomfortable.
- **Palmar warts:** These occur on the palms of the hands.
- **Plantar warts (verrucae):** These occur on the feet and can be painful owing to the pressure of the weight of the body on them.

Common Pathologies of the Nails

The nails can be affected by many skin conditions and they can also be indicators of internal imbalances, neglect, or stress and anxiety. It is important to be able to recognize diseases and disorders of the nail, as some can lead to **cross-infection**.

Factors that affect nail growth positively include:

- Good nutrition
- A good supply of blood to the nails.

Factors that have negative effects on nail growth include:

- Poor health
- Poor nutrition
- Overexposure to chemicals such as detergents
- Poor manicure and pedicure techniques
- Injuries to the nail bed
- Aging.

Agnail (hang nail)

Characterized by dry, split cuticles and is often caused by poor treatment techniques, the use of detergents, or soaking the hands in water for long periods. Although it is a harmless disorder, it can become infected.

Anonychia

Congenital absence of a nail.

Beau's lines

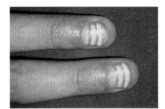

Beau's lines

Transverse (horizontal) ridges or grooves on the nail plate that can reflect a temporary retardation of growth due to ill health, a very high fever, or a zinc deficiency in the body.

Egg-shell nails (soft, thin nails)

Unusually soft, thin, white nails that are curved over the free edge that can be the result of poor diet, ill health, medication, or some nervous disorders.

Koilonychia (spoon nails)

Term given to spoon-shaped, concave nails resulting from abnormal growth. Spoon nails can be congenital, due to a lack of minerals such as iron or a result of illness. The nails are also thin, soft, and hollowed.

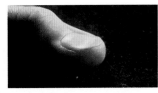

Koilonychia (spoon nails)

Leuconychia (white nails or white spots)

Term given to white spots or streaks on the nail, or to nails that are white or colorless. Leuconychia is often the result of trauma to the nail or air bubbles but can also be an indication of poor health. The white spots will grow out with the nail.

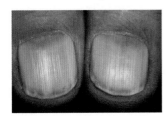

Leuconychia (white nails)

Longitudinal furrows

Longitudinal (vertical) ridges can occur in the nail as a result of uneven nail-tissue growth. To an extent, they are normal in adults and increase with age. However, severe ridges can result from injury to the nail matrix through poor treatment techniques or from the excessive use of detergents and other harsh chemicals. They can also be caused by conditions such as psoriasis and poor circulation.

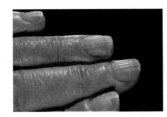

Longitudinal furrows

Onychauxis (thick nails) and onychogryposis (ram's horn nail)

Unusual thickness of the nail caused by trauma to the nail matrix, fungal infection, or neglect that can also be hereditary. Chronic thickening of the nail can lead to onychogryposis, a condition in which the nail thickens and curves into a hooked nail. It usually results from damage to the nail bed and can cause pain and injury to adjoining toes.

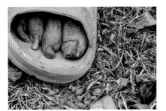

Onychauxis (thick nails) and onychogryposis (ram's horn nail)

Onychocryptosis (ingrowing nail)

Condition in which the sides of the nail penetrate the skin. It is characterized by red, shiny skin around the nail and can be very sensitive and painful if touched. Ingrowing nails are most common on the large toe, and can be caused by ill-fitting shoes or improper nail cutting.

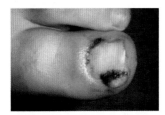

Onychocryptosis (ingrowing nail)

Onycholysis (separation of the nail from the nail bed)

Condition where the nail usually begins to loosen at the free edge and this continues up to the lunula, but the nail does not fall off. It can be caused by illness, trauma, infection, certain drugs, or abuse of the nails.

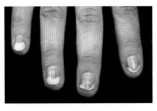

Onycholysis (separation of the nail from the nail bed)

Onychophagy (nail biting)

Common in people who suffer from stress or anxiety. It can result in an exposed nail bed that is inflamed and sore. Onychophagy is the term given to nails that have become deformed through excess nail biting.

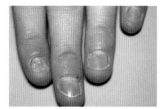

Onychophagy (nail biting)

Onychoptosis (nail shedding)

Condition in which parts of the nail shed and usually occurs during ill health or as a reaction to some drugs. It can also be caused by trauma to the nail.

Onychorrhexis (brittle nails)

Term given to dry, brittle, splitting nails that also have longitudinal ridges and is common in old age and in people with arthritis or anemia. It can also be caused by poor treatment techniques and excessive soaking of the hands in water or detergents.

Paronychia (bacterial infection of the cuticle)

Bacterial infection of the skin surrounding the nails where the tissues become red, swollen, and painful. It is a common infection that can be the result of injury, nail biting, or poor manicure techniques.

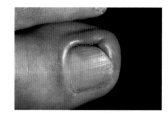

Paronychia (bacterial infection of the cuticle)

Pterygium inversum unguis (pterygium)

Often appears as an overgrown cuticle but is actually scar tissue attaching to the nail plate and growing over the nail as it grows out. It is caused by damage to the nail matrix. Don't confuse pterygium inversum unguis with pterygium conjunctiva, which occurs in the eye!

Severely bruised nail

Usually as a result of physical damage or trauma to the nail bed. A clot of blood forms under the nail plate and, in some cases, a severely bruised nail can fall off.

Tinea unguium (onychomycosis)

Ringworm—fungal infection—of the nail that is characterized by thickened and deformed nails. Infected nails may separate from the nail bed, crumble, or flake off.

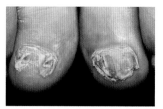

Tinea unguium

NEW WORDS	
Acid mantle	A film of sebum and sweat on the surface of the skin that protects against bacteria
Avascular	Lacking in blood vessels
Cross-infection	The transfer of infection from one person to another
Cutaneous	Relating to the skin
Dermatology	The study of the skin
Desquamation	The process through which the skin is shed
Elasticity	The ability to return to the original shape after stretching
Extensibility	The ability to stretch
Integumentary system	The system of the skin and its derivatives (hair, nails, and cutaneous glands)
Keratinization	The process through which cells die and become full of the protein keratin
Phagocytosis	The ingestion of bacteria
Vasoconstriction	The constriction of blood vessels
Vasodilation	The dilation of blood vessels

Study Outline

Skin

Functions of the skin

1. **Sensation:** The skin contains cutaneous sensory receptors that are sensitive to touch, temperature, pressure, and pain.
2. **Absorption:** The skin absorbs certain substances.
3. **Protection:** The skin protects against trauma, bacteria, dehydration, ultraviolet radiation, chemical damage, and thermal damage.
4. **Heat regulation:** It cools the body through sweating and vasodilation. It warms the body through decreased sweat production, vasoconstriction, contraction of the arrector pili muscles, and shivering.
5. **Excretion:** The skin excretes wastes.
6. **Secretion:** The skin secretes sebum, which keeps the skin supple and waterproof.
7. **Vitamin D synthesis:** The skin functions in the synthesis of vitamin D, which helps regulate the calcium levels of the body and is necessary for the growth and maintenance of bones.

> Skin Always Protects Humans, Every Single Day
> Sensation, Absorption, Protection, Heat regulation, Excretion, Secretion, vitamin D

Anatomy of the skin—main layers

1. The skin is a cutaneous membrane made of two distinct layers: the epidermis and the dermis.
2. The epidermis is the tough, waterproof outer layer that is continuously being worn away. It is made of keratinized stratified squamous epithelium.
3. The dermis is the thicker layer that contains nerves, blood vessels, sweat glands, and hair roots. It is made of areolar connective tissue containing collagen and elastic fibers. It lies beneath the epidermis.
4. The dermis is attached to the subcutaneous layer, which is made of areolar and adipose connective tissue.

Epidermis

1. The epidermis is made up of five layers: the stratum basale (basal-cell layer), stratum spinosum (prickle-cell layer), stratum granulosum (granular-cell layer), stratum lucidum (clear-cell layer) and stratum corneum (horny-cell layer).

> Bad Skin Grafts Look Comical
> Basale, Spinosum, Granulosum, Lucidum, Corneum

2. The basal-cell layer constantly produces new cells that are pushed upward.
3. The prickle-cell layer is a transitional layer where some cells are dividing but others are starting to become keratinized.
4. In the granular-cell layer cells begin to die as they become increasingly keratinized.
5. The clear-cell layer is a waterproof layer of dead cells.
6. The horny-cell layer is the outermost layer and consists of strong, tough, dead cells that are completely full of keratin. The cells are constantly being shed through the process of desquamation.
7. Keratinocytes produce keratin, which is a waterproof protein.
8. Melanocytes produce melanin, which is a pigment that contributes to skin color and absorbs ultraviolet light.

> Your body dresses itself for all seasons.
> It puts on a **raincoat made of keratin**
> and a **sun hat made of melanin.**

9. Skin is thickest on the palms of the hands and soles of the feet and thinnest on the eyelids.

Dermis

1. The dermis is the supportive layer beneath the epidermis and it is composed of two layers: the superficial papillary layer and the deeper reticular layer.
2. The papillary layer has fingerlike projections that go into the epidermis. These projections contain loops of capillaries and nerve endings sensitive to touch.
3. The reticular layer houses hair follicles, nerves, oil glands, ducts of sweat glands, and adipose tissue.

Subcutaneous layer

The subcutaneous layer attaches the reticular layer to the underlying organs and it contains areolar and adipose connective tissue and nerve endings that are sensitive to pressure.

Skin types

1. There are six basic skin types: normal, oily, dry, combination, sensitive, and mature.
2. Normal skin is a balanced skin in which there are no signs of oily or dry areas.
3. Oily skin has an overproduction of sebum by the sebaceous glands.
4. Dry skin has an underproduction of sebum or a lack of moisture, or both together.
5. Combination skin is a mixture of dry, normal, and greasy skin and is the most common type of skin.
6. Sensitive skin often accompanies dry skin and is easily irritated.
7. Mature skin is often dry, thin, lacks elasticity, and is easily damaged.

Hair

1. There are three types of hair: lanugo, vellus, and terminal.
2. Lanugo hair is a soft hair only found in a fetus.
3. Vellus hair is a soft hair found all over the body except the palms, soles, eyelids, lips, and nipples.
4. Terminal hair is a long, coarse hair found on the head, eyebrows, eyelashes, under the arms, and in the pubic area.

Structure of a hair

1. Hairs are columns of keratinized dead cells.
2. Hairs grow out of hair follicles.
3. Hairs are made up of a superficial end called the "shaft" and a "root" that penetrates into the dermis.
4. Arrector pili muscles pull the hair up to a vertical position as a response to cold, fright, or differing emotions.

Functions of hair

Hair provides warmth and protection.

Life cycle of a hair

1. There are three distinct phases in the life cycle of a hair: anagen, catagen, and telogen.
2. Anagen is the growing or active phase in which a new hair develops at the matrix.
3. Catagen is the transitional or changing stage in which a now fully grown hair detaches from the matrix.

4. Telogen is the resting or "tired" phase in which a fully grown hair sits high up in the follicle and the hair bulb beneath it is inactive.

> ACT
> Anagen = Active
> Catagen = Changing
> Telogen = Tired

Nails

Structure of a nail

1. The nail covers the ends of the fingers and toes.
2. The nail plate is the visible body of the nail. Its sides are covered by the nail wall and at its proximal end is the lunula, which is a crescent-shaped white area.
3. The nail mantle, or proximal nail fold, is skin that lies above the matrix.
4. The cuticle is an extension of the horny layer of the epidermis from the nail mantle (fold). It protects the germinal matrix from infection.
5. The distal edge of the nail is called the free edge.
6. Beneath the nail mantle is the germinal matrix, where cell division and nail growth occur.
7. The nail bed is beneath the nail plate and attaches it to the finger or toe.

Functions of a nail

Functions of the nail include protection, helping us pick up small objects, and enabling us to scratch.

Cutaneous glands

1. Glands are specialized cells that secrete substances.
2. Cutaneous glands are usually found in the dermis of the skin.
3. Sebaceous glands secrete sebum.
4. Sebum is a lubricant that helps condition and protect the skin and hair.
5. Sudoriferous glands are sweat glands.
6. Sweat functions in heat regulation and in the elimination of waste.
7. There are two types of sudoriferous glands: eccrine and apocrine.
8. Eccrine glands are found almost all over the body and open as pores on the surface of the skin. They

secrete sweat and function in regulating the body's temperature and excreting waste.

9. Apocrine glands are found only in the armpits, pubic region, and the areolae of the breasts. They open into hair follicles and secrete sweat, fatty acids, and proteins. They are activated by pain, stress, and sexual foreplay.

Review

1. What type of membrane is the skin?
2. Name the two layers that make up the skin.
3. Name the tissue type that makes up the epidermis.
4. Name the tissue type that makes up the dermis.
5. Name the skin layer that contains the nerves, blood vessels, and sweat glands.
6. Put the following layers of the epidermis into their correct order, starting from the deepest and ending with the most superficial layer: stratum spinosum, stratum granulosum, stratum basale, stratum corneum, stratum lucidum.
7. Identify the layer of the epidermis in which cells divide.
8. Identify the layer of the epidermis that consists of dead cells that are completely filled with keratin.
9. Name the process through which cells are constantly shed from the skin.
10. Name two types of fibers that are found in the dermis.
11. Name the two layers that make up the dermis.
12. Identify which layer of the dermis has fingerlike projections that protrude into the epidermis.
13. Name the tissue type that makes up the subcutaneous layer.
14. Describe the main functions of the skin.
15. Explain how the body cools itself when it is too hot.
16. Explain how the body warms itself when it is too cold.
17. Name the type of cells found in hair.
18. Name the superficial end of the hair.
19. Name the end of the hair that penetrates the dermis.
20. Describe the two main functions of the hair.
21. Name the type of cells found in the nail.
22. Identify where in the nail the cells divide.
23. Give the name of the visible body of the nail.
24. Give the name of the white, crescent-shaped area on the nail.
25. Describe three functions of the nail.
26. Explain what a gland is.
27. Identify where cutaneous glands are found.
28. What do sebaceous glands secrete?
29. What do sudoriferous glands excrete?
30. Name the two types of sudoriferous glands.
31. Identify the type of sudoriferous gland found in the axilla.

Multiple-Choice Questions

1. Which of the following statements is correct?
   a. The skin is one of the smallest organs of the body
   b. The skin is one of the largest organs of the body
   c. The skin is not an organ of the body
   d. The skin is the smallest organ of the body

2. Keratinized stratified squamous epithelium tissue is found in the:
   a. Reticular layer
   b. Dermis
   c. Epidermis
   d. Subcutaneous layer

3. Functions of the hair include:
   a. Excretion
   b. Protection
   c. Sensation
   d. Absorption

4. In the nail, cell division takes place in:
   a. The nail mantle
   b. The lunula
   c. The matrix
   d. The nail plate

5. Sebaceous glands secrete:
   a. Sweat
   b. Sebum
   c. Uric acid
   d. Glucose

6. Which of the following statements is true?
   a. Keratin helps waterproof and protect the skin
   b. Keratin contributes to skin color
   c. Keratin absorbs ultraviolet light
   d. Keratin functions in the sensation of touch

7. Which is the correct order of the layers of the epidermis, from the most superficial to the deepest layer?
   a. Stratum spinosum, stratum basale, stratum lucidum, stratum granulosum, stratum corneum
   b. Stratum basale, stratum spinosum, stratum granulosum, stratum lucidum, stratum corneum
   c. Stratum corneum, stratum lucidum, stratum spinosum, stratum granulosum, stratum basale
   d. Stratum corneum, stratum lucidum, stratum granulosum, stratum spinosum, stratum basale

8. Herpes simplex is a:
   a. Fungal infection of the nail
   b. Viral infection of the nail
   c. Fungal infection of the skin
   d. Viral infection of the skin

9. The skin functions in warming the body through which of the following processes:
   a. Sweating
   b. Shivering
   c. Vasodilation
   d. None of the above

10. Which of the following is responsible for the color of your skin?
    a. Melanin
    b. Keratin
    c. Elastin
    d. Collagen

11. Tinea corporis is ringworm of the:
    a. Feet
    b. Body
    c. Scalp
    d. Nails

12. New skin cells are constantly produced in the:
    a. Stratum spinosum
    b. Stratum basale
    c. Stratum corneum
    d. Stratum granulosum

13. Where on the body are eccrine glands located?
    a. In the axilla only
    b. In the axilla, pubic region and areolae
    c. Everywhere except the lips, nail beds, eardrums, and on some of the reproductive organs
    d. Everywhere

14. Keloids are:
    a. Harmless, soft, flesh-colored growths
    b. Thickened nails
    c. Senile warts
    d. An overgrowth of scar tissue

15. The clinical term for nail biting is:
    a. Koilonychia
    b. Onychophagy
    c. Onycholysis
    d. Leuconychia

The Skeletal System

Introduction

Imagine what we might look like with no bones. How would we move? How would we stand up straight? We would be a mass of soft tissues lying on the floor unable to move or sit up.

In this chapter you will learn about the skeletal system and discover what a unique and vital system it is.

Student objectives

By the end of this chapter you will be able to:

- Describe the functions of the skeletal system
- Describe bone tissue and identify the different types of bones found in the body
- Explain the structure of a long bone
- Identify the organization of the skeleton and name the bones of the body
- Describe the joints of the body
- Identify the common pathologies of the skeletal system.

Did you know?

- Weight for weight, bone is approximately five times stronger than steel.
- Bones are hard, yet flexible—your ribs are strong enough to protect your heart but flexible enough to allow movement for breathing.
- Bones are hard, yet light, and account for only approximately 14% of the body's total weight.

Functions of the Skeletal System

Bones are not dead materials that simply support your body. They are living structures that are constantly changing by reshaping, rebuilding, and repairing themselves, and they play vital roles in both the structure and functioning of the body. Bones support and protect the body, allow for movement and mineral homeostasis, and are a site of blood-cell production as well as energy storage.

Support

Bones are the scaffolding of the body and provide a framework that supports and anchors soft tissues and organs.

Shape

Acting as a framework, bones form the basic shape of the body.

Protection

Bones are extremely hard and able to protect the body's vital organs. For example, the cranial bones protect the brain and the vertebrae protect the spinal cord.

Movement

Without bones we would not be able to stand, walk, run, or even chew. Our bones are sites of attachment for skeletal muscles. When the muscles contract or shorten they pull on the bones and this generates movement.

Mineral homeostasis

Bones store most of the calcium present in our bodies. In addition to forming bones, calcium is vital for nerve transmission, muscular contraction, blood clotting, and the functioning of many enzymes in the body. Depending on the blood calcium levels, bones either release calcium into or absorb it from the blood to ensure there is always the correct amount of calcium present in the blood. Bones also store other minerals such as phosphorus. Mineral homeostasis in bones is controlled by hormones.

Site of blood-cell production

Some bones in the body contain red bone marrow, which, through the process of **hemopoiesis**, produces red blood cells, white blood cells, and platelets.

Storage of energy

The yellow bone marrow found in some bones stores lipids, which are an important energy reserve in the body.

Anatomy of Bones

Bone tissue

Osteology is the study of bone. **Osseous tissue** (bone tissue) is a connective tissue whose matrix is composed of water, protein, fibers, and mineral salts. The fibers are made of a protein called **collagen**, which enables bone to resist being stretched or torn apart. This is known as "tensile strength," and without collagen bones would be hard and brittle. The mineral salts are mainly calcium carbonate and a crystallized compound called **hydroxyapatite**. These salts give bone its hardness.

Before learning about the different types of bones, it helps to know the cells that make up bone tissue:

- **Osteoprogenitor cells:** These are stem cells derived from mesenchyme (the connective tissue found in an embryo). They have the ability to become osteoblasts.
- **Osteoblasts:** These cells secrete collagen and other organic components to form bone.
- **Osteocytes:** These are mature bone cells that maintain the daily activities of bone tissue. They are derived from osteoblasts and are the main cells found in bone tissue.
- **Osteoclasts:** These cells are found on the surface of bones and they destroy or resorb bone tissue.

Two types of bone tissue exist: **compact** and **spongy**.

- **Compact (dense) bone tissue:** This is a very hard, compact tissue that has few spaces within it. It is composed of a basic structural unit called an **osteon**, or **Haversian system**, which consists of concentric rings called **lamellae** made of a hard, calcified matrix. Between the lamellae are small spaces called **lacunae** where osteocytes are housed. Through the center of the lamellae run **Haversian canals**, in which nerves and blood and lymph vessels are found. These Haversian canals are connected to one another and the periosteum

through perforating channels called **Volkmann's canals**. **Canaliculi** are tiny canals that radiate outward from the central canals to other lacunae. The main functions of compact bone tissue are protection and support. It forms the external layer of all bones.

- **Spongy (cancellous) bone tissue:** This is a light tissue with many spaces within it, and it has a sponge-like appearance. It does not contain osteons. Instead, it is made up of lamellae arranged in an irregular latticework of thin plates of bone called **trabeculae**. Within the trabeculae are lacunae containing osteocytes. Spongy bone tissue contains red bone marrow, which is the site of blood-cell production. It is found in the hip bones, ribs, sternum, vertebrae, skull, and the ends of some long bones.

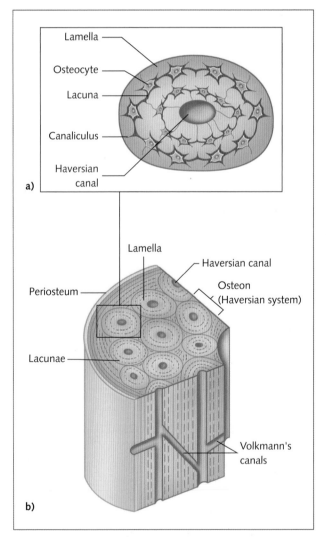

Figure 4.1 *Compact bone tissue*

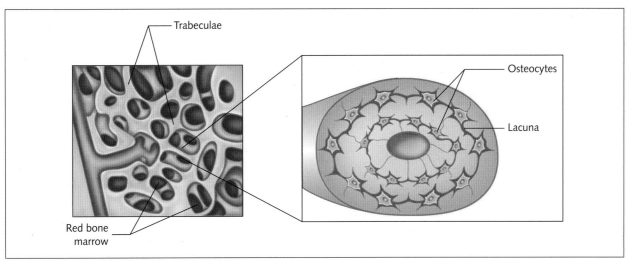

Figure 4.2 *Spongy bone tissue*

Did you know?

Every bone in your body is completely reformed approximately every ten years, and the distal portion of your thigh bone is replaced approximately every four months (Tortora and Grabowski, 1996).

Bone formation and remodeling

Bone is a dynamic, living tissue that is constantly changing, repairing, and reshaping itself. Most bones are formed through **ossification**, a process that begins somewhere between the sixth and seventh week of embryonic life and continues throughout adulthood. There are two types of ossification:

- **Intramembranous ossification**: Bone forms on or within loose, fibrous connective-tissue membranes without first going through a **cartilage** stage.
- **Endochondral ossification**: Bone forms on **hyaline cartilage,** which has been produced by cells called **chondroblasts.**

New bone tissue constantly replaces old, worn-out or injured bone tissue through the process of **remodeling**. Mechanical stress, in the form of the pull of gravity and the pull of skeletal muscles, is integral to the process of remodeling. If these stresses are absent the bones weaken, or if they are excessive the bones thicken abnormally. For example, the bones of people who are bedridden diminish, while those of some athletes are found to be thicker than usual.

Infobox

Anatomy and physiology in perspective

X-ray studies of the astronauts of the Gemini and Apollo space missions revealed that the heel bones of two of the three crewmen had decreased in density. This is thought to be because of their weightless experience in space leading to a lack of the mechanical stress necessary for bone remodeling (Barnard, 1981). Horse riders, on the other hand, are known to develop small new bones in their thighs (called rider's bones, or heterotopic bones) owing to chronic muscle strain (Colledge et al., 2010).

What does aging do to our bones?

Why do people often get shorter and smaller as they age? Why do their bones seem so brittle and easily broken? Why do they take so long to repair? Aging has two specific effects on our bones. Firstly, aging causes **demineralization** of the bones. This is a loss of calcium and other minerals from the bone matrix and this process is especially evident in women after the age of 30. By the age of 70, a woman can easily have lost almost 30% of the calcium in her bones. Secondly, aging decreases the body's ability to produce collagen, which gives bones their tensile strength. Thus, bones become more brittle and susceptible to fracture.

In the classroom

Having now learned about bone remodeling, have a discussion around why *weight-bearing* exercises are so important in the prevention of osteoporosis.

Types of Bones

The body contains many bones, which are generally classified into the following types: **long, short, flat, irregular,** and **sesamoid**.

- **Long bones:** These have a greater length than width and usually contain a longer shaft with two ends (see section "Structure of a Long Bone" for further details). Long bones are slightly curved

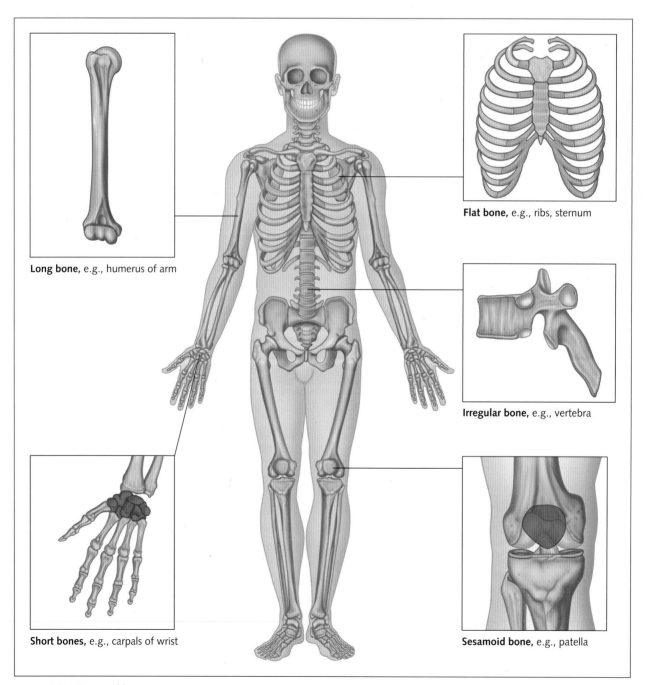

Long bone, e.g., humerus of arm

Flat bone, e.g., ribs, sternum

Irregular bone, e.g., vertebra

Short bones, e.g., carpals of wrist

Sesamoid bone, e.g., patella

Figure 4.3 *Types of bone*

to provide strength and are composed of mainly compact bone tissue with some spongy bone tissue. Examples of long bones include the femur, tibia, fibula, phalanges, humerus, ulna, and radius.

- **Short bones:** These are cube-shaped and nearly equal in length and width. They are made up of mainly spongy bone with a thin surface of compact bone. Examples of short bones include the carpals and tarsals.
- **Flat bones:** These are very thin bones consisting of a layer of spongy bone enclosed by layers of compact bone. Flat bones act as areas of attachment for skeletal muscles and also provide protection. Examples of flat bones include the cranial bones, sternum, ribs, and scapulae.
- **Irregular bones:** Most bones that cannot be classified as long, short, or flat bones fall into the category of irregular bones. They have complex shapes and varying amounts of compact and spongy tissues. An example of an irregular bone is a vertebra.
- **Sesamoid bones:** These are oval bones that develop in tendons where there is considerable pressure. An example is the patella (kneecap).

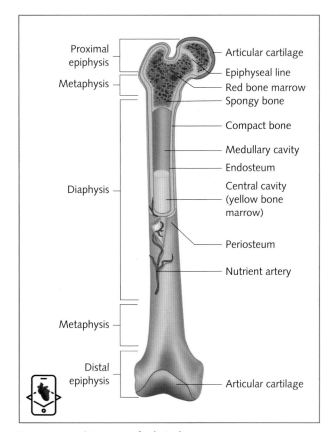

Figure 4.4 *Structure of a long bone*

Structure of a long bone

To help you understand the structure of a bone, we will look at the structure of the femur. This is the long bone in your thigh.

A long bone has a main, central shaft called a **diaphysis**. The diaphysis is covered by a membrane known as the **periosteum**. The periosteum provides attachment for muscles, tendons, and ligaments and is also essential for nutrition, repair, and growth in diameter of bone. The periosteum consists of two layers:

- **Outer fibrous layer:** Made of dense, irregular connective tissue that contains blood vessels, lymph vessels, and nerves that pass into the bone.
- **Inner osteogenic layer:** Made of elastic fibers and containing blood vessels and bone cells.

Each end of the diaphysis is called an **epiphysis**. Each epiphysis is covered by a thin layer of hyaline cartilage called **articular cartilage**. This cartilage reduces friction and absorbs shock at the area where the bone forms an articulation (joint) with the surface of another bone. The epiphysis is made of mainly spongy bone tissue and contains red bone marrow. This is where blood cells are produced.

The region where the diaphysis joins the epiphysis is the **metaphysis**. In a growing bone the metaphysis has a layer of hyaline cartilage that allows the diaphysis to grow in length. This is called the **epiphyseal plate**. In a mature bone that is no longer growing in length, the epiphyseal plate is replaced by the **epiphyseal line**.

Inside the diaphysis is a space known as the **medullary** or **marrow cavity**. The medullary cavity is lined by a membrane called the **endosteum**. This contains cells necessary for bone formation. In adults this cavity contains fatty yellow bone marrow, which stores lipids.

Infobox

Anatomy and physiology in perspective

If a child fractures a bone and damages the epiphyseal plate, then the bone will always be shorter than it should be. However, if the epiphyseal plate has not been damaged, then the bone will be able to grow to its normal length.

Organization of the Skeleton

There are approximately 206 bones in the human body. This number can differ slightly depending on age and sex; for example, a baby has between 270 and 300 bones at birth.

The skeleton is made up of a central **axial skeleton**, which supports and protects the major organs of the head, neck, and trunk, and an **appendicular skeleton**, which forms the upper and lower extremities and their girdles.

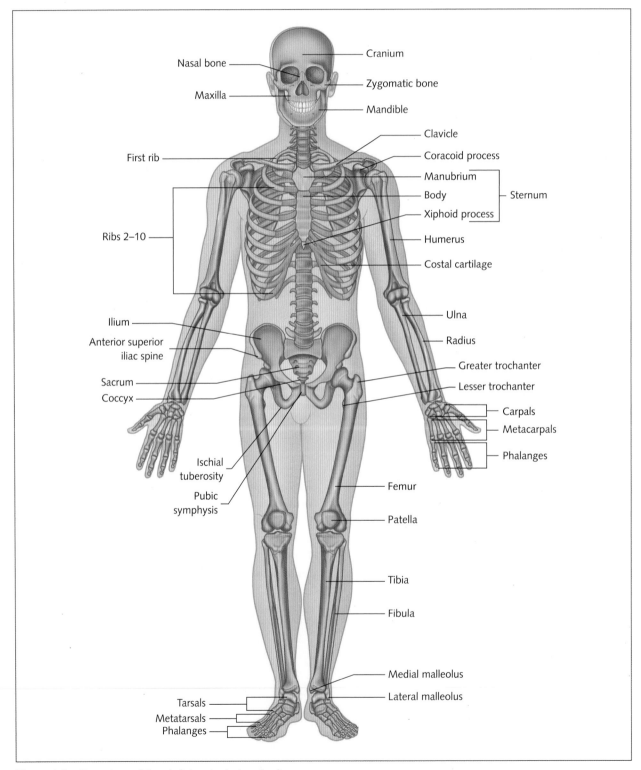

Figure 4.5 *Overview of the skeleton (anterior view)*

- **The axial skeleton:** This consists of the 80 bones that are found in the center of the body; namely, the skull, hyoid, ribs, sternum, and vertebrae. The auditory ossicles are also usually included in the axial skeleton (these are discussed in chapter 6).

- **The appendicular skeleton:** This consists of the 126 bones of the upper and lower limbs and their girdles, which connect the limbs to the axial skeleton.

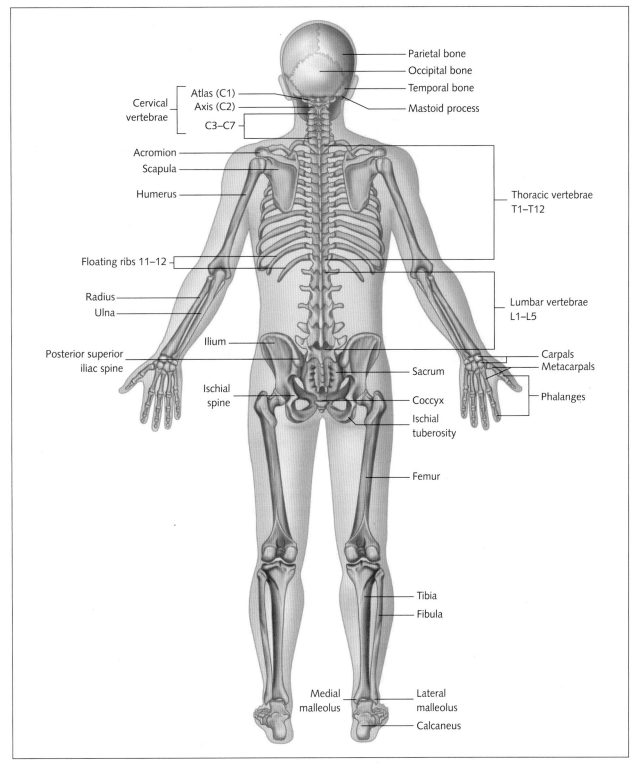

Figure 4.6 *Overview of the skeleton (posterior view)*

The bones of the skeleton are attached to one another by **ligaments**. Ligaments are tough, fibrous cords of connective tissue that contain both collagen and elastic fibers. They surround joints and bind them together.

Study tip

Learn the names of the bones well and you will be relieved later that you did so. Many of the muscles, blood vessels, and nerves that you also need to learn are named after the bones along which they run. For example, the tibialis anterior is a muscle located on the anterior surface of the tibia bone, the radial artery is located near the radius bone, and the ulnar nerve is found near the ulna bone. The time you spend learning the bones will not be wasted!

In the classroom

One of the most fun ways to learn the bones of the body is to draw them on another person. Be sure to use a non-toxic, non-permanent marker! Alternatively, spend some time drawing stick figures of the skeleton. Repeat these again and again, and as you draw each bone say the name aloud.

Please note

The charts below mention joint types and movements. You may want to read the section "Joints" that comes afterward before reading the following information.

Axial Skeleton

Bones of the skull

The skull consists of 22 bones, excluding the ossicles of the ear. Except for the mandible, which forms the lower jaw, the bones of the skull are attached to each other by sutures, are immobile, and form the cranium (from Greek *kranion* = "the upper part of the head"). The skull, or cranium, can be divided into the **neurocranium**, which forms the protective casing of the brain, and the **viscerocranium**, which forms the skeleton of the face.

Bones of the neurocranium

The neurocranium has a domed roof called the **calvaria** (skullcap) and a floor called the cranial base (**basicranium**). Together the calvaria and cranial base are composed of eight bones: two parietals, two temporals, one frontal, one occipital, one sphenoid, and one ethmoid bone.

Parietal bones
Form most of the superior and lateral walls of the cranium. They meet in the midline at the sagittal suture, and meet with the frontal bone at the coronal suture.

Temporal bones
Lie inferior to the parietal bones. There are three important markings on the temporal bones: (1) the **styloid process**, which is just in front of the mastoid process, a sharp needle-like projection to which many of the neck muscles attach; (2) the **zygomatic process**, a thin bridge of bone that joins with the zygomatic bone, just above the mandible; and (3) the **mastoid process**, a rough projection posterior and inferior to the styloid process (just behind the lobe of the ear).

Frontal bone
Forms the forehead, the bony projections under the eyebrows, and the superior part of each eye orbit.

Occipital bone
The most posterior bone of the cranium. It forms the floor and back wall of the skull, and joins the parietal bones anteriorly at the lambdoid suture. In the base of the occipital bone is a large opening, the **foramen magnum**, through which the spinal cord passes to connect with the brain. To each side of the foramen magnum are the **occipital condyles**, which rest on the first vertebra of the spinal column (the **atlas**).

Sphenoid
Butterfly-shaped bone that spans the width of the skull and forms part of the floor of the cranial cavity.

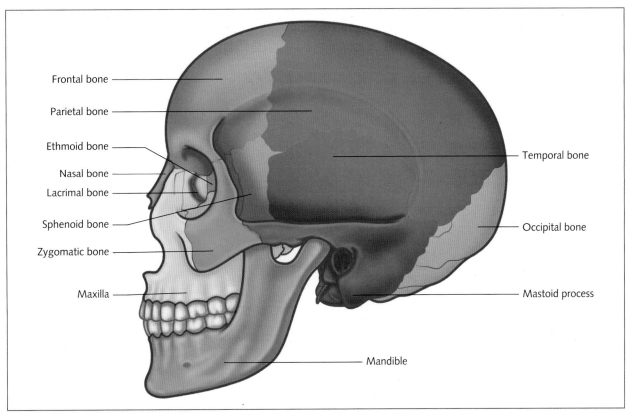

Figure 4.7 *Bones of the skull (lateral view)*

Parts of the sphenoid can be seen forming part of the eye orbits, and the lateral part of the skull.

Ethmoid bone
Single bone in front of the sphenoid bone and below the frontal bone. It forms part of the nasal septum and superior and medial conchae.

BONES OF THE NEUROCRANIUM	
Parietal	Two parietal bones form the sides and roof of the cranium
Temporal	Beneath the parietal bones are two temporal bones; they form the inferior lateral sides of the cranium and part of the cranial floor
Frontal	Forms the forehead and the roofs of the orbits (eye sockets)
Occipital	Forms the back of the cranium and most of the base of the cranium

BONES OF THE NEUROCRANIUM	
Sphenoid	This butterfly-shaped bone articulates with all the other cranial bones and holds them together; it lies at the middle part of the base of the skull and forms part of the floor of the cranium, the sides of the cranium, and parts of the eye orbits
Ethmoid	This is the major supporting structure of the nasal cavity; it forms the roof of the nasal cavity and part of the medial walls of the eye orbits

Bones of the viscerocranium

The viscerocranium, the skeleton of the face, consists of fourteen bones: six pairs of bones and two single bones. The paired bones are the nasal, palatine, zygomatic, lacrimal, maxillae, and inferior nasal conchae. The single bones are the vomer and the

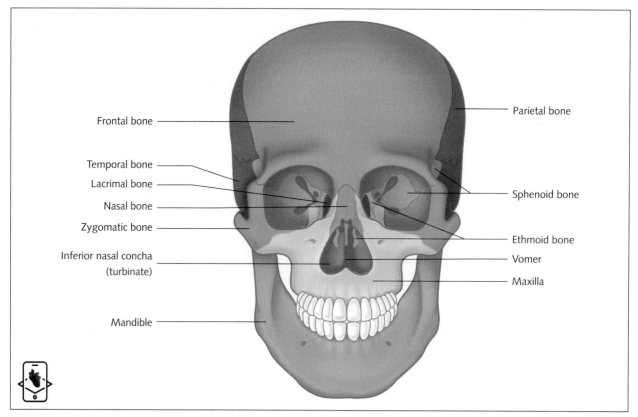

Figure 4.8 *Bones of the skull (anterior view)*

mandible. (The ethmoid bone can be classified with either the neurocranium or the viscerocranium. In this book it has been classified as part of the neurocranium.)

Nasal bones
Small rectangular bones that form the bridge of the nose (the lower part of the nose is made up of cartilage).

Palatine bones
These L-shaped bones are situated at the back of the nasal cavity between the maxilla and the pterygoid process of the sphenoid bone.

Zygomatic bones
More commonly known as the **cheekbones**, they also form a large portion of the lateral walls of the eye orbits.

Lacrimal bones
The smallest of the facial skeleton, these bones sit inside the bony orbit, and have two surfaces and four borders.

Maxillae
These bones fuse to form the upper jaw into which the upper teeth are embedded.

Inferior nasal concha (turbinate)
These bones (pl. conchae) sit on the nasal septum, separating the nasal cavity into two bilateral and symmetrical anatomical caves.

Vomer
Runs vertically within the nasal cavity, separating the left and right sides. It is part of the nasal septum.

Mandible (lower jawbone)
The strongest bone in the skull; it joins the temporal bones on each side of the face at the temporomandibular joints, forming the only freely movable joints in the skull. The horizontal part of the mandible, or the body, forms the chin. Two upright bars of bone, or **rami**, extend from the body to connect the mandible with the temporal bone. The lower teeth are embedded in the mandible.

BONES OF THE VISCEROCRANIUM	
Nasal	These two bones form the bridge of the nose
Maxilla	These two bones unite to form the upper jawbone, part of the floors of the orbits, part of the lateral walls and floor of the nasal cavity, and most of the roof of the mouth; the maxillae articulate with every bone in the face except the mandible
Zygomatic	These two bones are the cheekbones and form part of the lateral wall and floor of the orbits
Lacrimal	These tiny bones form part of the medial wall of the eye orbit; they are about the same size and shape as a fingernail and are the smallest bones in the face
Palatine	These two bones form part of the palate (roof of the mouth), part of the floor and lateral wall of the nasal cavity, and part of the floors of the orbits
Inferior nasal concha (turbinate)	These two bones form part of the lateral wall of the nasal cavity and help to circulate, filter, and warm air before it passes into the lungs
Vomer	This bone forms part of the nasal septum, which divides the nose into left and right sides
Mandible	This is the lower jaw; it is the only moveable bone in the skull and is also the largest and strongest facial bone

Bones of the neck and spine

Bones of the neck
The neck comprises the cervical vertebrae (to be discussed shortly), as well as a unique bone that does not articulate with any other bone in the body. This is the **hyoid bone** and it is suspended from the temporal bones by ligaments and muscles.

The hyoid supports the tongue and provides attachment for some of the muscles of the neck and pharynx.

Bones of the spine (vertebral column)
The spine is a strong, flexible structure that is able to bend and rotate in most directions. It supports the head, encloses and protects the spinal cord, and is also a site of attachment for the ribs and the muscles of the back.

The spine is composed of 33 vertebrae, as follows: 7 cervical, 12 thoracic, 5 lumbar, 5 sacral and 4 coccygeal. The sacral vertebrae fuse to form the sacrum, and the coccygeal vertebrae fuse to form the coccyx. Thus, there are 26 separate bones that make up the spine.

Cervical vertebrae (7)
The word *cervix* means "neck," and seven cervical vertebrae form the neck. The first cervical vertebra (C1) is called the **atlas**, and it supports the head, just as the mythological figure Atlas supported the world on his shoulders. The second (C2) is called the **axis**, and it literally acts as an axis on which the atlas and head can rotate in a side-to-side movement. The third to sixth cervical vertebrae are quite normal, but the seventh (C7) is called the **vertebra prominens**, and is the large prominence that can be seen and felt at the back of the neck.

Thoracic vertebrae (12)
The word *thorax* means "chest," and there are 12 thoracic vertebrae, 10 of which articulate with the ribs. These vertebrae are larger and stronger than the cervical vertebrae.

Lumbar vertebrae (5)
Five lumbar vertebrae support the lower back. They are the largest, strongest vertebrae and provide attachment for the large muscles of the back that support the weight of the upper body.

Sacral vertebrae (5)
Five sacral vertebrae fuse to form a triangular bone called the **sacrum**, which is the strong foundation of the pelvic girdle.

Coccygeal vertebrae (4)

Four coccygeal vertebrae fuse to form a triangular shape called the **coccyx**, or tailbone.

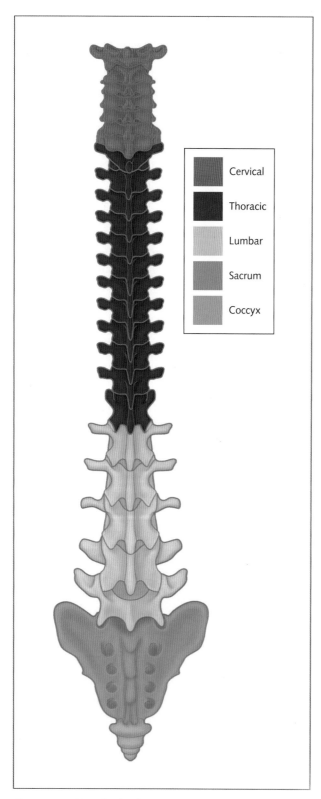

Cervical

Thoracic

Lumbar

Sacrum

Coccyx

Figure 4.9 *Vertebral column (posterior view)*

A closer look at the spine

The spine is a simple yet invaluable structure that needs to not only protect the spinal cord but also be able to move in a number of directions, withstand pressure, hold the weight of the upper body, and maintain the body in an upright position. It is able to perform all these functions because it is made up of so many small, strong bones and joints.

Structure of a vertebra

Although vertebrae do differ in size and shape according to where in the spine they are found, they all share a similar structural pattern.

- **A vertebral body:** This is a thick, disc-shaped anterior portion that is weight bearing. (Except the atlas, the body of which is represented by the dens.)
- **A vertebral arch:** This is formed by two thick posterior **processes** (projections) called the **pedicles** and the **laminae**. The body and arches form a space called the **vertebral foramen**.
- **The vertebral foramen:** This is the space formed by the body and arches. It contains the spinal cord, adipose and areolar connective tissues, and blood vessels. The vertebral foramina of all vertebrae join together to form the **spinal canal**.
- **Transverse processes:** These are two prominences that project laterally from either side of the vertebral arch, where the pedicles and lamina join. These processes serve as points of attachment for muscles and articulations with the ribs.
- **Spinous process:** This is a single prominence that projects posteriorly from the vertebral arch where the laminae meet. It is also called the spine of a vertebra and serves as a point of attachment for muscles.
- **Superior and inferior articular processes:** These four processes form joints with the vertebrae above and below.

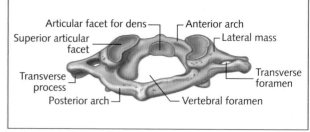

Figure 4.10 *Atlas (C1), posterosuperior view*

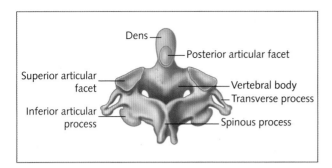

Figure 4.11 *Axis (C2), posterosuperior view*

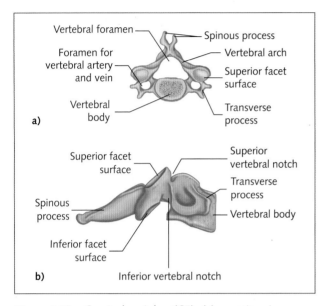

Figure 4.12 *Cervical vertebra (C5), (a) superior view; (b) lateral view*

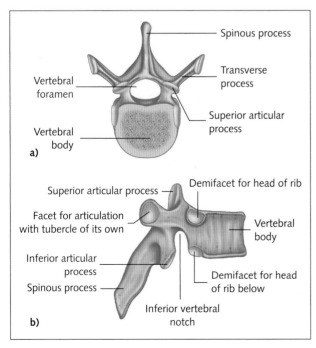

Figure 4.13 *Thoracic vertebra (T6), (a) superior view; (b) lateral view*

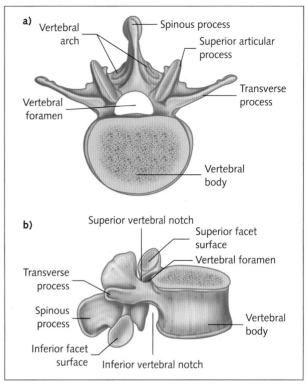

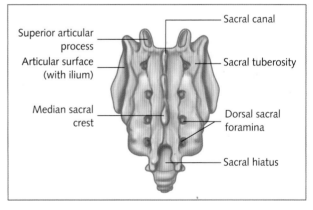

Figure 4.14 *Lumbar vertebra (L5), (a) superior view; (b) lateral view*

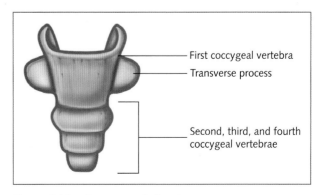

Figure 4.15 *Sacrum, posterior view*

Figure 4.16 *Coccyx, posterior view*

Intervertebral discs

Intervertebral discs are found between the vertebrae. They are composed of an outer ring of fibrocartilage called the **anulus fibrosus** and a soft, elastic inner core called the **nucleus pulposus**. Intervertebral discs form strong joints that allow the spinal column to move in many directions, and they also provide a cushioning that can flatten and absorb vertical shock when under compression.

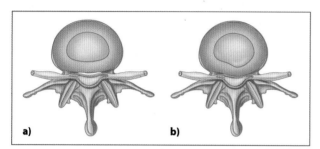

Figure 4.17 *(a) A normal intervertebral disc; (b) a compressed intervertebral disc (superior view)*

Infobox

Anatomy and physiology in perspective

A slipped disc is not a disc that has slipped out of the spinal column. It is actually a herniated disc, and is often called a **prolapsed intervertebral disc** (PID). This means that the disc's outer ring of fibrocartilage has ruptured and its inner nucleus pulposus is protruding. This usually occurs when the ligaments surrounding the discs are injured or weakened and the discs are put under excess pressure.

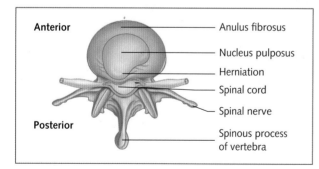

Figure 4.18 *Herniated (slipped) disc (superior view)*

Curves of the spine

When viewed from the side, the spine has four natural curves that increase its strength and flexibility,

help maintain balance, and absorb shock. They are named after the vertebrae that form them:

- Cervical curve
- Thoracic curve
- Lumbar curve
- Sacral curve.

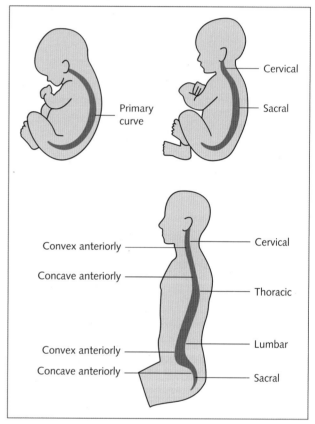

Figure 4.19 *Curves of the spine*

Infobox

Anatomy and physiology in perspective

A fetus curled up inside the womb has only a single, concave curve. When it is a baby and it starts to hold its head erect, a second curve, the cervical curve, then develops. When the baby starts to sit up straight, stand, and walk, the lumbar curve develops. This curve separates the thoracic and sacral curves, which are known as the primary curves. The cervical and lumbar curves are the secondary curves.

Bones of the thorax

The thorax, or thoracic cage, is a bony cage formed posteriorly by 12 thoracic vertebrae and their intervertebral discs, latero-anteriorly by 12 pairs of ribs and their associated costal cartilages, and anteriorly by the sternum.

The **sternum** is commonly known as the breastbone and is actually the fusion of three bones: the manubrium, the body, and the xiphoid process. The sternum is attached to the first seven pairs of ribs by costal cartilage.

The **ribs** consist of 12 pairs in total, and comprise true, false, and floating.

The thorax encloses and protects the heart and lungs and supports the bones of the shoulder girdle and upper limbs.

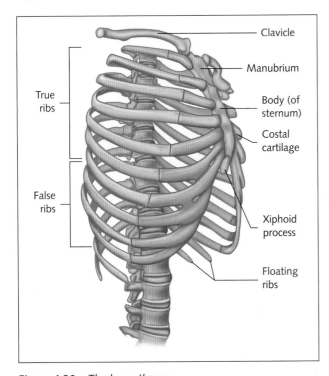

True ribs

False ribs

Clavicle

Manubrium

Body (of sternum)

Costal cartilage

Xiphoid process

Floating ribs

Figure 4.20   *The bony thorax*

BONES OF THE THORAX	
Sternum	This is the breastbone; it is a flat, narrow, long bone that is found in the middle of the anterior thoracic wall The sternum is composed of three parts: • The superior **manubrium**, which articulates with the clavicle and the costal cartilages of the first two ribs • The long, middle **body**, which articulates with the costal cartilages of the second through seventh ribs • The inferior **xiphoid process**, which provides attachment for some abdominal muscles
Ribs	There are 12 pairs of ribs: • The first 7 pairs of ribs are attached to the sternum by a type of hyaline cartilage called **costal cartilage**; these 7 pairs are known as **true ribs** because they are directly attached to the sternum
	• The remaining 5 pairs of ribs are **false ribs** because they are not directly attached to the sternum • The 8th, 9th, and 10th pairs are attached to each other by their cartilages and then to the cartilages of the 7th pair of ribs • The 11th and 12th pairs of ribs are **floating ribs** that are only attached to abdominal muscles
Thoracic vertebrae	See section "Bones of the neck and spine" above for more information on the thoracic vertebrae

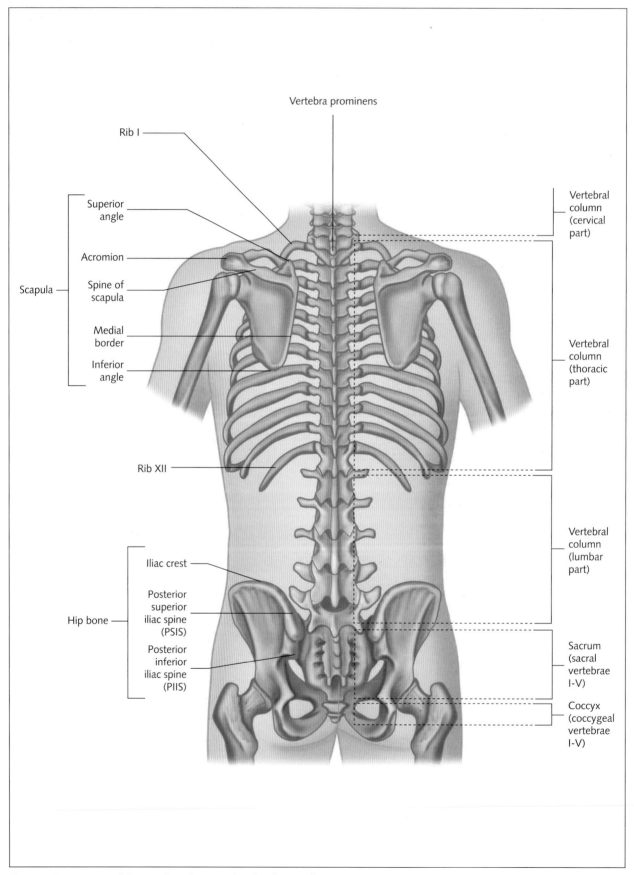

Figure 4.21 *Bones of the trunk and pectoral and pelvic girdles (posterior view)*

Appendicular Skeleton

The appendicular skeleton comprises the upper and lower extremities and their girdles—basically, the bones of the arms and legs, shoulders, and pelvis.

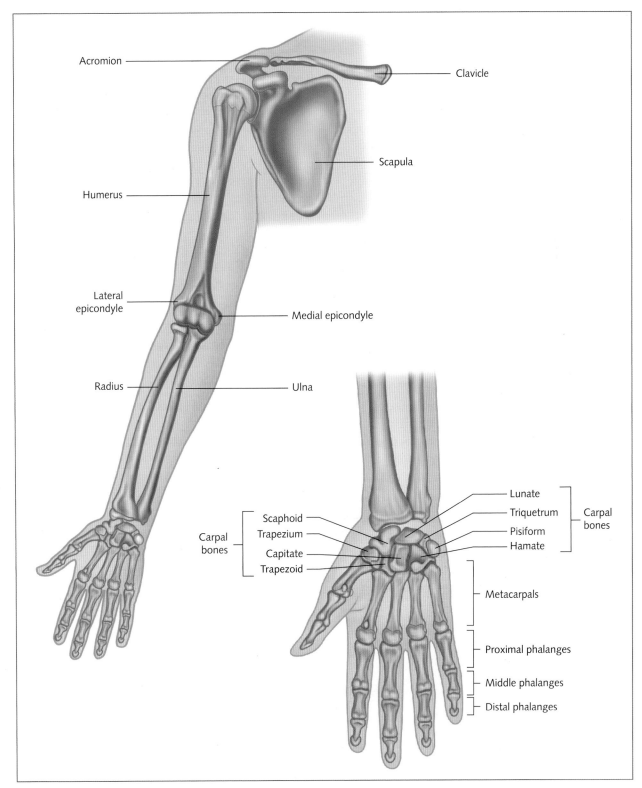

Figure 4.22 *Bones of the upper limb and shoulder girdle*

Bones of the pectoral girdle (shoulder)

The shoulder, or pectoral girdle, is made up of the **clavicle** (collar bone) and the **scapula** (shoulder blade), and these bones greatly increase the range of motion possible in the shoulder region.

The clavicle (Latin *clavis* = "key") is S-shaped, sits just below the skin at the base of the neck, and connects the upper limb to the trunk. It forms two joints: the sternoclavicular joint with the sternum, and the acromioclavicular joint with the acromion of the scapula. Both of these are diarthrotic, synovial planar joints, and the sternoclavicular joint is also classified as a pivot joint. These joints enable the shoulder joint to be highly mobile while remaining attached to the axial skeleton.

The shoulder joint (**glenohumeral joint**) is a diarthrotic, synovial ball-and-socket joint formed by the humerus and scapula. It has exceptional flexibility and more freedom of movement than any other joint in the body. It allows the following movements: flexion, extension, abduction, adduction, medial rotation, lateral rotation, and circumduction.

However, the shoulder's freedom of movement does make it prone to dislocation. It is strengthened by a group of muscles called the **rotator cuff** muscles. These surround the joint, joining the scapula to the humerus, and consist of the supraspinatus, infraspinatus, teres minor, and subscapularis muscles (see chapter 5 for more information on these muscles).

BONES OF THE PECTORAL GIRDLE	
Clavicle	This is the collarbone and it is a long, slender, double-curved bone that helps hold the arm away from the top of the thorax; it also helps prevent shoulder dislocation
Scapula	This is the shoulder blade; it is a large, flat, triangular bone

Did you know?

The clavicle is one of the most frequently broken bones in the body.

Bones of the upper limb

Bones of the arm and forearm

The upper limb is composed of four distinct anatomical regions: the shoulder, arm, forearm, and hand. It is important to differentiate between the arm and forearm. The arm only has one bone, the **humerus**, and lies between the shoulder joint (glenohumeral joint) and the elbow joint; while the forearm has two long, parallel bones, the **ulna** and **radius**, and is the region between the elbow joint and the wrist joint.

The bones of the upper limb have an important role in support and provide attachment points for the muscles. As well as furnishing strength to resist the forces and stresses acting upon the upper limbs during exercise and heavy lifting, these bones form joints that enable the wide-ranging articulation of the upper limb.

The bones of the arm and forearm meet at the elbow joint, which is classified as a hinge joint. This joint only allows for flexion and extension of the forearm.

BONES OF THE ARM AND FOREARM	
Humerus	This is the longest and largest bone of the upper limb and is the arm bone
Ulna	This bone is located on the medial aspect (little-finger side) of the forearm when the body is in the anatomical position; its proximal end is called the **olecranon**, which is commonly known as the elbow
Radius	This is located on the lateral aspect of the forearm (thumb side)

Bones of the hand

The hand contains 27 small bones and multiple joints, which can be divided into three regions: the carpals, metacarpals, and phalanges.

The **carpals** are a group of eight cube-shaped bones in the proximal region of the hand. Together these form the wrist, or *carpus*. Three of these bones (the scaphoid, lunate, and triquetrum) articulate with the distal radius to form the wrist joint. This is a diarthrotic, synovial condyloid joint that allows for flexion, extension, abduction, adduction, and circumduction.

Distally, the carpals articulate with the five **metacarpals** in the palm of the hand. These joints are referred to as carpometacarpal joints and are diarthrotic synovial joints. They form synovial planar joints at the fingers and a synovial saddle joint at the thumb. The shape of the saddle joint enables the thumb's high degree of mobility.

Fourteen **phalanges** (singular: phalanx) make up the digits. Each digit is composed of three phalanges (proximal, middle, and distal) except for the thumb which contains only a proximal phalanx and a distal phalanx. The phalanges form diarthrotic, synovial hinge joints between themselves. These are called the interphalangeal joints (IP). The joints between the phalanges and metacarpals are called the metacarpophalangeal joints (MCP) and are diarthrotic, synovial condyloid joints.

The principal role of the hand itself is grasping and manipulation.

BONES OF THE HAND	
Carpals (8)	The wrist consists of 8 small bones arranged in two irregular rows of 4 bones each, bound together by ligaments
	These bones are the: **trapezium, trapezoid, capitate, hamate, scaphoid, lunate, triquetrum,** and **pisiform**
Metacarpals (5)	The palm of the hand is formed of 5 metacarpals; they are numbered 1 to 5, starting with the thumb side of the hand
Phalanges (14)	The fingers are made up of 14 phalanges; in each finger are a proximal, middle, and distal phalange (phalanx), but in the thumb there are only a proximal and distal phalange; the thumb is sometimes called the **pollex**

Bones of the pelvic girdle (hip)

The hip, or pelvic girdle, is a strong and stable structure upon which rests the total weight of the upper body. The pelvic girdle also supports both

Infobox

Anatomy and physiology in perspective

The scaphoid is the most frequently fractured bone in the hand because we tend to put our palms down, with our hands abducted, when we fall. Unfortunately, this bone has a poor blood supply and so healing can take up to three months (Colledge et al., 2010).

the spine and the visceral organs and is a site of attachment for many muscles.

The pelvic girdle attaches the leg to the trunk of the body and is composed of two hip bones called the **innominate bones, coxal bones,** or **ossa coxae.** In a newborn baby, each of these bones is made up of three smaller bones—the **ilium, ischium,** and **pubis.** In adults these bones are fused together.

Together with the sacrum and coccyx, the pelvic girdle forms the pelvis, which is a bony, basin-like structure. The **acetabulum** is formed from fused parts of the ilium, ischium, and pubis, and is a deep socket for the head of the femur. The joint formed by the femur and the acetabulum is called the hip joint (coxal joint) and is a diarthrotic, synovial ball-and-socket joint that allows for flexion, extension, abduction, adduction, circumduction, and rotation.

The pubic bones are united anteriorly by a cartilaginous joint called the **pubic symphysis.** Posteriorly, the ilium of each hip bone connects with the sacrum at the **sacroiliac joint.**

BONES OF THE PELVIC GIRDLE	
Ilium	This large, winglike bone forms the superior portion of the hip bone; its upper border serves as a site of attachment for many muscles and is called the **iliac crest**
Ischium	This forms the inferior and posterior portion of the hip bone
Pubis	This is the most anterior part of the hip bone

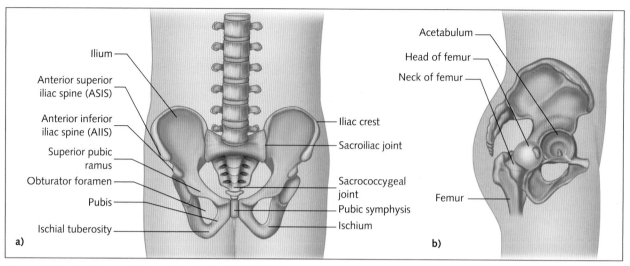

Figure 4.23 *(a) Bones of the pelvic girdle; (b) hip joint*

Bones of the lower limb

The lower limb extends from the hip to the foot and is composed of six distinct anatomical regions: the gluteal region (hip and buttocks), femoral region (thigh), knee region, leg region, talocrural region (ankle), and the foot region (foot). The bones of the lower limb are all thicker and stronger than those of the upper limb because they need to bear the weight of the entire body.

The **femur** (thigh bone) is the largest, heaviest, and strongest bone in the body and its length is approximately a quarter of a person's height. It is composed of a long body called the shaft, and two ends. The superior (proximal) end consists of a rounded head, a neck, and two trochanters. The inferior (distal) end is composed of two condyles. The shaft, or body, of the femur does not run down the thigh vertically, but is instead obliquely oriented (directed inferomedially) within the thigh—at the hip the left and right femoral heads are separated by the width of the pelvis, whereas at the knee the two lower ends are almost touching. This oblique orientation ensures a person's center of gravity runs vertically through the legs and feet when standing upright.

The head and neck of the femur project superomedially at an angle to the oblique shaft of the femur. This angle is called the angle of inclination and it allows for great mobility of the femur at the hip joint.

The knee

The knee joint is the largest joint in the body, and one of the strongest, and is actually made up of three smaller diarthrotic, synovial joints: the intermediate **patellofemoral joint** (gliding joint), and the lateral and medial **tibiofemoral joints** (modified hinge joints). Between the tibia and femur are two menisci. These are fibrocartilage discs that help to compensate for the irregular shapes of the bones and also help circulate synovial fluid.

Although the knee permits flexion and extension of the lower leg relative to the thigh as well as a small degree of medial and lateral rotation when flexed, excessive movements are restricted because of the arrangement of the anterior and posterior cruciate ligaments. The knee joint is further stabilized by the medial and lateral collateral ligaments, which prevent sideways movement and excessive rotation.

Movements at this joint are essential to many everyday activities, including walking, running, sitting, and standing; the knee joint is therefore not only strong but also flexible, and uses muscles and ligaments to withstand the stresses and strains of powerful leg movements.

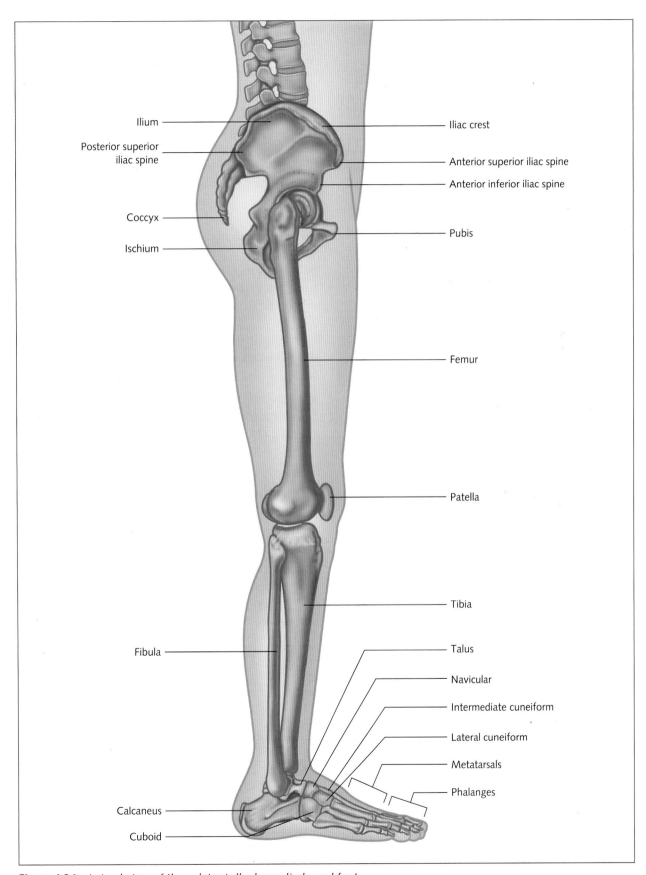

Figure 4.24 *Lateral view of the pelvic girdle, lower limb, and foot*

Bones of the leg

The **tibia** and **fibula** are the bones of the leg and their shafts are connected by a dense interosseous membrane. They articulate proximally and distally at the **tibiofibular joints**. The proximal tibiofibular joint is a diarthrotic, synovial planar joint and the distal one is an amphiarthrotic, fibrous joint. Neither of these joints has much movement and instead provides stability to the ankle. In the lower leg, the tibia bears most of the body's weight, while the fibula serves as an area for muscle attachment.

The medial malleolus of the tibia and the lateral malleolus of the fibula meet the talus of the foot at the ankle joint (**talocrural joint**). The talocrural joint is a diarthrotic, synovial hinge joint that allows for dorsiflexion and plantar flexion of the foot. A capsule sits snugly around this joint and is reinforced medially and laterally by collateral ligaments.

BONES OF THE THIGH, KNEE, AND LEG	
Femur	This is the thigh bone and it is the longest, strongest, and heaviest bone in the body
Patella	This is the kneecap and it is a sesamoid bone that is attached to the tibia by the patellar ligament; it develops in the tendon of the quadriceps femoris muscle to protect the knee joint and help maintain the position of the tendon when the knee is bent
Tibia	This is the shinbone and is the large, medial bone of the leg
Fibula	This is a thin bone that runs parallel to the tibia

Infobox

Anatomy and physiology in perspective

The knee joint is a synovial joint, and the common condition of "water on the knee" is swelling due to an excessive production of synovial fluid.

Bones of the foot

Like the bones of the hand, the bones of the foot fall into three regions: the tarsals, metatarsals, and phalanges. These are extremely strong bones that support our body weight and enable us to walk and run.

Seven tarsal bones make up the proximal region of the foot. This region can be referred to as the tarsus, posterior foot, proximal foot, or hindfoot. The talus is the only bone of the foot that articulates with the bones of the leg and it transmits about half the weight of the body to the calcaneus. The **calcaneus**, or heel bone, is the largest tarsal bone and it rests on the ground when the body assumes a standing position.

Five **metatarsal bones** make up the metatarsus, also known as the anterior, distal, or forefoot. The tarsal bones, together with the five long metatarsal bones, form the weight-bearing arches of the foot, which are reinforced by ligaments and muscles.

Extending from the distal end of the metatarsals are the **phalanges** of the toes. Their arrangement in the foot is similar to that of their counterparts in the hand.

BONES OF THE FOOT	
Tarsals (7)	The **tarsus**, or back portion, of the foot is made up of 7 tarsal bones They are the: **talus** (ankle bone), **calcaneus** (heel bone), **cuboid**, **navicular,** and three **cuneiforms** (medial, intermediate, and lateral)
Metatarsals (5)	The **metatarsus** of the foot is made up of 5 metatarsals, numbered 1 to 5, starting with the large-toe (medial) side of the foot
Phalanges (14)	The toes are made up of 14 phalanges. In each toe are a proximal, middle, and distal phalange (phalanx), but in the large toe there are only a proximal and distal phalange; the large toe is sometimes called the **hallux**

Infobox

Anatomy and physiology in perspective

A prosthesis is an artificial limb that is attached to the body as a substitute for a missing or non-functioning limb.

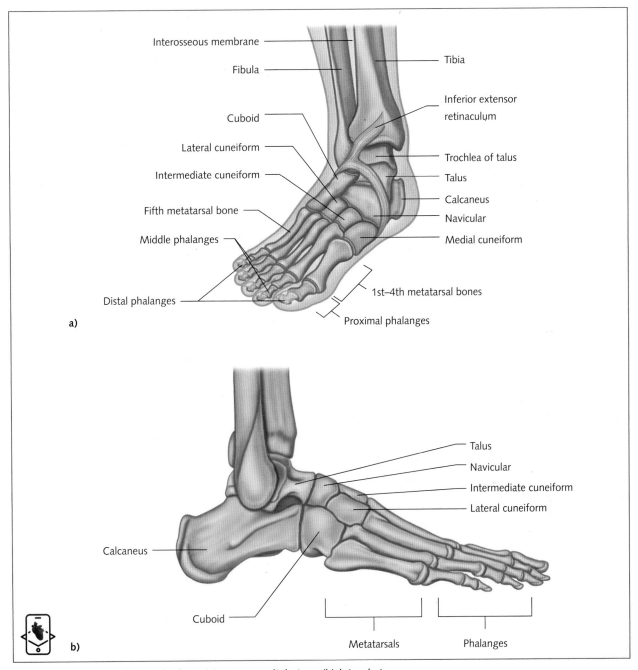

Figure 4.25 *Bones of the right foot, (a) anteromedial view; (b) lateral view*

Arches of the foot

The bones of the foot are arranged into arches that distribute the weight of the body over the entire foot. They are strong arches that give the foot its "springiness" and so enable it to support the weight of the body and provide leverage while walking. They include the:

- **Medial longitudinal arch:** This arch runs down the medial length of the foot (longitudinally) and is composed of the calcaneus, talus, navicular, all three cuneiforms, and the medial first three metatarsals.
- **Lateral longitudinal arch:** This arch runs down the lateral length of the foot (longitudinally) and is composed of the calcaneus, the cuboid, and the lateral two metatarsals.
- **Transverse arch:** This arch cuts transversely across the foot and is formed by the cuboid, the three cuneiforms, and the bases of the five metatarsals.

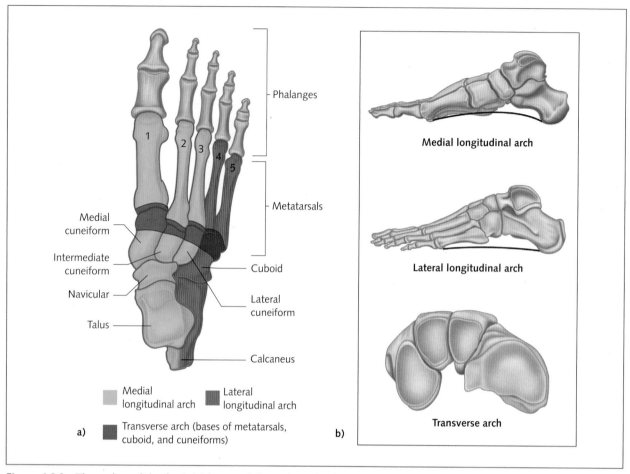

Figure 4.26 *The arches of the foot: (a) bones of the arches; (b) shapes of the arches*

Did you know?

If you are under 40 years of age, some of the bones in your body are still growing. An embryo initially has no bones, and its "skeleton" is composed entirely of fibrous connective-tissue membranes, called **mesenchyme**, and hyaline cartilage. Around the sixth or seventh week of embryonic life, ossification begins and, although bone growth in length is usually completed around 25 years of age, bones continue to thicken and be remodeled throughout life.

Take a quick look at some developmental aspects of the skeleton:

- **The head:** Babies are born with soft spots on the tops of their heads. These are called **fontanelles** and are membrane-filled spaces between the cranial bones. They enable the baby's skull to change size and shape so that it can pass through the birth canal, and also allow rapid growth of the brain during infancy. They ossify and become sutures.

- **The face:** During the first two years of life, the shape of the face changes dramatically while the brain and cranial bones expand, the teeth form, and the sinuses increase in size. The face only stops growing when you reach about 16 years of age.

- **The back:** Not only are you born with one curve in your spine that develops into four, but fusion of your sacral vertebrae only begins around the age of 16–18 years and is completed by about 30 years of age. In addition, fusion of your coccyx takes place somewhere between 20 and 30 years of age.

- **The feet:** The arches of the feet are developed by 12 or 13 years of age.

Finally, the xiphoid process of the sternum does not ossify until about the age of 40 years.

Joints

The bones of the skeleton are held together by joints. Joints are also called **articulations** and are the points of contact between bones, cartilage and bones, or teeth and bones. Without joints, our bodies would be solid structures and we would be unable to move. Thus, they function not only in holding the bones together, but also in providing movement. However, some of the joints of the body—for example, the sutures of the skull—do not allow for much movement. Instead, they form firm structures that help protect organs. Before looking at the different types of joints it helps to have an understanding of the following vocabulary:

Arthrology	The study of joints
Kinesiology	The study of the motion of the body
Cartilage	A resilient, strong connective tissue that is less hard and more flexible than bone
Ligament	A tough band of connective tissue that attaches bones to bones
Tendon	A tough band of connective tissue that attaches muscles to bones

Joints can be classified according to either their structure or their function.

Functional classification of joints

If you consider the degree of movement a joint permits, then you are looking at its functionality, and this is classified as follows:

- **Synarthroses:** These are immovable joints and are termed **synarthrotic** joints. For example, the coronal suture between the frontal and parietal bones is composed of dense fibrous connective tissue that holds the bones together and does not allow movement. These bones help form the cranium, which protects the brain.
- **Amphiarthroses:** These are slightly movable joints that permit a minimal amount of flexibility and movement. They are termed **amphiarthrotic** joints. For example, the pubic symphysis is an amphiarthrotic joint that joins the pubic bones. It allows for slight movement.
- **Diarthroses:** These are freely movable joints that permit a number of different movements.

Diarthroses enable movement because of their structure—they all have a space between the articulating bones. This space is called a **synovial cavity** (in a moment we will take an in-depth look at diarthroses). For example, the shoulder joint is a diarthrotic joint formed by the humerus and scapula. It allows for a variety of movements, including flexion, extension, abduction, adduction, medial rotation, lateral rotation, and circumduction (these movements will be described shortly).

In general, the joints of the axial skeleton are synarthrotic (immovable) or amphiarthrotic (slightly movable) and their main function is to protect the internal organs and ensure firm attachments between bones. On the other hand, the appendicular skeleton has more diarthrotic (freely movable) joints because mobility and freedom of movement are important in the limbs.

Structural classification of joints

We have looked at how joints can be classified according to their functionality (the degree of movement they permit); now let us look at how they are classified according to their structure. This takes into account the type of connective tissue that binds the joints together and whether or not there is a synovial cavity between the joints. Structurally, joints can be classified as:

- Fibrous joints
- Cartilaginous joints
- Synovial joints.

Fibrous joints

In fibrous joints bone ends are held together by fibrous (collagenous) connective tissue and there is no synovial cavity between them. Thus, they are strong joints that do not permit movement. In general, they are synarthrotic. For example, sutures are fibrous joints.

Cartilaginous joints

In cartilaginous joints, bone ends are held together by cartilage and they do not have a synovial cavity between them. Thus, these are also strong joints that permit only minimal movement. Most cartilaginous joints are amphiarthrotic, although some can be synarthrotic. For example, the pubic symphysis is a cartilaginous joint.

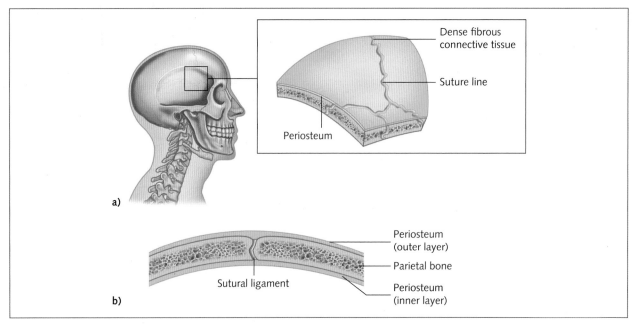

Figure 4.27 *Fibrous joint, as shown by the sutures of the skull*

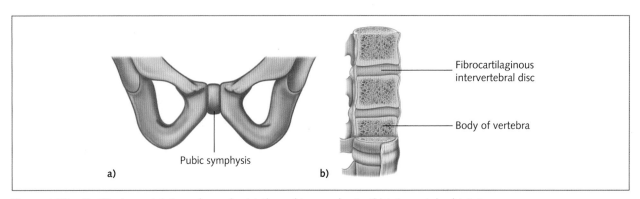

Figure 4.28 *Cartilaginous joint, as shown by (a) the pubic symphysis; (b) intervertebral joints*

Synovial joints

In synovial joints, bone ends are separated by a synovial cavity. This allows for a great deal of movement and all synovial joints are diarthrotic. For example, the knee is a synovial joint.

Synovial joints predominate in the limbs of the body and allow for a great variety of movement. There are many different types of synovial joints, but they all share some common features. Synovial joints have:

- **A synovial cavity:** This is a space that separates the articulating bones. It is the key to movement within the joints.
- **Articular cartilage:** Hyaline (articular) cartilage covers the surfaces of the articulating bones in a synovial joint. This cartilage reduces friction between the bones and helps absorb shock.

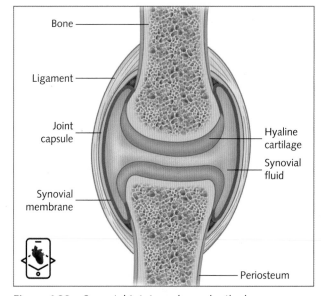

Figure 4.29 *Synovial joint, as shown by the knee*

- **Synovial capsule (articular capsule):** The entire joint is enclosed in an articular capsule made of:
  - An outer fibrous capsule of dense, irregular connective tissue that is flexible and has great tensile strength
  - An inner synovial membrane made of areolar connective tissue with elastic fibers and adipose tissue; this membrane secretes **synovial fluid**
- **Reinforcing ligaments:** The fibrous capsule is reinforced with ligaments.

Did you know?

Synovial fluid is similar in both consistency and appearance to uncooked egg white.

Synovial fluid fills the synovial cavity and:

- Lubricates the joint, thereby reducing friction
- Supplies nutrients to the articular cartilage (remember that cartilage is avascular)
- Removes waste from the articular cartilage
- Contains phagocytes that remove microbes and debris that have resulted from the general wear and tear of the joint.

In addition to the above features, some synovial joints also have:

- **Articular discs (menisci):** These are pads of fibrocartilage that lie between the articular surfaces of the bones. They help to maintain the stability of the joint and also direct the flow of synovial fluid to areas of greatest friction. Menisci are found in the knee joint.
- **Bursae:** These are sac-like structures made of connective tissue, lined with a synovial membrane and filled with synovial fluid. They cushion the movement of one structure over another and, in addition to being found inside some articular capsules, they can also be located where skin rubs over bone, between tendons and bones, between muscles and bones, and between ligaments and bones.

Synovial joints permit a range of different movements, some of which are described in the charts on the following pages.

Infobox

Anatomy and physiology in perspective

The inflammation of a synovial joint is called **synovitis** and it usually accompanies disorders such as arthritis. Signs and symptoms of synovitis include pain, tenderness, and swelling.

MOVEMENTS AT SYNOVIAL JOINTS—GENERAL

Movement	Definition
Flexion	This is the bending of a joint in which the angle between articulating bones decreases
Extension	This usually restores a body part to its anatomical position after it has been flexed, and is the straightening of a joint in which the angle between the articulating bones increases
Hyperextension	This is when a body part extends beyond its anatomical position

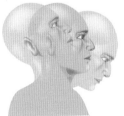

Figure 4.30 *Flexion, extension, and hyperextension*

In the classroom

Here is a simple exercise to demonstrate the movements of flexion, extension, and hyperextension. Nod your head. When your chin touches your throat, you are *flexing* your neck. When you return your head to its normal upright position, you are *extending* your neck. When you push your head backward so that your chin is facing up toward the ceiling, you are *hyperextending* your neck.

MOVEMENTS AT SYNOVIAL JOINTS—GENERAL

Movement	Definition
Abduction	This is a movement away from the midline of the body
Adduction	This is the opposite of abduction and is a movement toward the midline of the body
Circumduction	This is a circular movement of the distal end of a body part and it involves a succession of flexion–extension and abduction–adduction

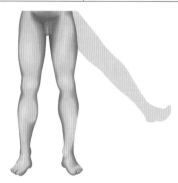

In the classroom

These common arm exercises demonstrate abduction, adduction, and circumduction. Do some star jumps. As you swing your arms up and away from your body, you are *abducting* them. Likewise, you are *abducting* your legs as you jump them outward. As you bring your arms back down toward the sides of your body, you are *adducting* them. You are also *adducting* your legs as you jump them together again. Swing your arms in a large circular movement as if you are warming up your shoulders. This circular swinging movement is *circumduction*.

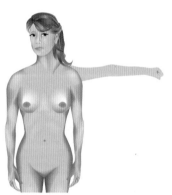

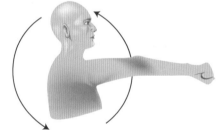

> **Study tip**
> ....
>
> **Remember:** If somebody is abducted they are kidnapped or taken away. Abduction is a movement away.
>
> When you ADDuct a body part, you are ADDing it back to your body.

Figure 4.31 *Abduction and adduction*   **Figure 4.32** *Circumduction*

MOVEMENTS AT SYNOVIAL JOINTS—GENERAL

Movement	Definition
Rotation	This is the movement of a bone in a single plane around its longitudinal axis
Medial or internal rotation	Involves the movement of the anterior surface of a bone toward the midline
Lateral or external rotation	Involves the movement of the anterior surface of a bone away from the midline

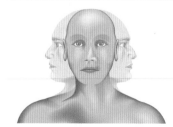

In the classroom

Turn your head from side to side as if you are saying "no." You are *rotating* your head. Now, stand in the anatomical position with your palms facing forward and turn your palms in toward your thighs so that they face backward—you have *medially rotated* your forearms. Turn your palms from facing backward to their original position in which they were facing forward—you have *laterally rotated* your forearms.

Figure 4.33 *Rotation*

MOVEMENTS AT SYNOVIAL JOINTS—FOREARM	
Movement	**Definition**
Pronation	This involves turning your palm posteriorly or inferiorly
Supination	This involves turning your palm anteriorly or superiorly

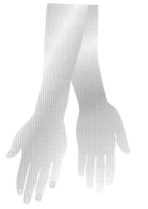

In the classroom

Stand with your arms out in front of you, with your palms facing the floor. Now turn your palms up toward the ceiling—you are *supinating* your forearm. Now turn them back down toward the floor—you are *pronating* your forearm.

Study tip

An easy way to remember the movement of supination is to imagine you are holding a bowl of soup in your hands (soup = supinate). If you pronate your forearms you will drop your soup!

Figure 4.34 *Pronation and supination*

MOVEMENTS AT SYNOVIAL JOINTS—FOOT	
Movement	**Definition**
Inversion	This is turning the sole of the foot inward
Eversion	This is the opposite of inversion, and is turning the sole of the foot outward
Dorsiflexion	This is the pulling of the foot upward toward the shin, in the direction of the dorsum
Plantar flexion	This is the opposite of dorsiflexion, and is the pointing of the foot downward, in the direction of the plantar surface

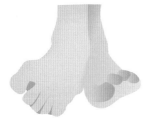

Figure 4.35 *Inversion and eversion*

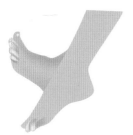

Figure 4.36 *Plantar flexion and dorsiflexion*

In the classroom

Here are a few foot exercises you can do to demonstrate inversion, eversion, dorsiflexion and plantar flexion:

Sit on the floor with your legs out straight. Roll your feet inward so that your soles are facing one another—you are *inverting* them. Now roll your feet away from one another so that your soles are facing away from each other—you are *everting* them.

Still sitting on the floor with your legs out straight, have your toes pointing up toward the ceiling. Now point your toes forward as if you are trying to touch the floor with them—you are *plantar flexing* your feet.

Then do the opposite movement, trying to pull your toes upward and back toward your shins—you are *dorsiflexing* them.

There are a number of different types of synovial joints, and they are classified according to the shapes of their articulating surfaces. They are listed in the table following.

CLASSIFICATION OF SYNOVIAL JOINTS

Name of joint	Shapes of articulating surfaces	Movements permitted		Examples
Gliding (plane)	Flat surfaces meet	Side to side Back and forth **Note:** no angular or rotary motions are permitted		Patellofemoral joint at knee Intercarpal joints Intertarsal joints Sacroiliac joint
Hinge	A convex surface fits into a concave one	Flexion Extension **Note:** movements are in a single plane only		Elbow joint Tibiofemoral joint at knee Ankle joint Interphalangeal joints
Pivot	A rounded/pointed surface fits into a ring	Rotation		Atlas and axis Ulna and radius
Condyloid (ellipsoid)	A condyle is a rounded/oval protuberance at the end of a bone and it fits into an elliptical cavity	Back and forth Flexion Extension Abduction Adduction Circumduction		Wrist joint Metacarpophalangeal joints
Saddle	A surface shaped like the legs of a rider fits into a saddle-shaped surface	Side to side Back and forth Flexion Extension	Abduction Adduction Circumduction	Thumb joint
		Opposition of thumbs (where the tip of the thumb crosses the palm and meets the tip of a finger)		
Ball and socket (spheroidal)	A ball fits into a cup-shaped socket	Flexion Extension Abduction Adduction Rotation Circumduction		Shoulder joint Hip joint

Common Pathologies of the Skeletal System

Red flags

Joint pain accompanied by:

- Swelling, warmth, discoloration
- Fever
- Cellulitis
- Skin rash or ulceration
- Loss of movement.

Disorders of the skeletal system generally involve pain, stiffness, inflammation, and weakness or loss of motion. They can be caused by a number of things, but elderly people are more prone to disorders of this system because of the process of demineralization that accompanies aging. Do not ignore severe, prolonged, or recurring joint pain as it can be symptomatic of an underlying infection, inflammatory disorder, or even tumor.

Arthritis

Arthritis is the inflammation of a joint. There are different types of arthritis:

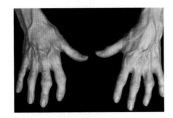

Osteoarthritis

- **Osteoarthritis (wear-and-tear arthritis):** Osteoarthritis is a degenerative joint disease caused by aging, irritation of the joints, and general wear and tear. It is a progressive disorder of movable joints, particularly weight-bearing joints such as the knees and hips, and is characterized by the deterioration of articular cartilage and the formation of spurs in the joint cavity. Signs and symptoms include pain, swelling, and a limited range of movement. Osteoarthritis is common in the elderly.
- **Psoriatic arthritis:** Psoriatic arthritis usually affects people who have psoriasis and commonly occurs as intermittent periods of joint pain with stiffness and swelling, followed by periods of remission.
- **Rheumatoid arthritis:** Rheumatoid arthritis is an autoimmune disease in which the immune system attacks its own tissues, in this case its own cartilage and joint lining. It is a chronic form of arthritis in which the synovial membrane of the joint becomes

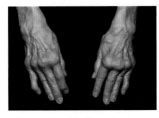

Rheumatoid arthritis

inflamed and, if left untreated, thickens and synovial fluid accumulates. The resulting pressure causes pain and tenderness. The membrane then produces an abnormal granulation tissue that adheres to the surface of the articular cartilage and sometimes erodes the cartilage completely. The exposed bone ends are then joined by fibrous tissue, which ossifies and renders the joint immovable. Rheumatoid arthritis is characterized by inflammation of the joint, swelling, pain, and loss of function. It is thought to be hereditary and can affect any age group. It normally begins in the smaller joints of the hands and feet before developing in other joints, and it is always bilateral (for example, it will attack the joints of both the left and right hands at the same time).

Bunions

Painful swelling of the joint between the great toe and the first metatarsal. A bursa, and bursitis, often develops at this joint and the great toe can become laterally displaced. This is known as **hallux valgus**. It is thought that bunions can be hereditary or caused by ill-fitting shoes.

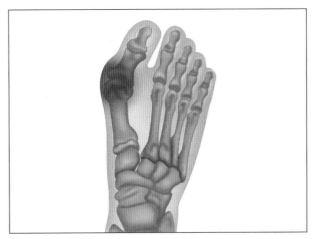

Figure 4.37 *Bunions*

Bursitis

Inflammation of a bursa and characterized by inflammation, pain, and limited movement and usually caused by overuse or irritation from unusual use. Bursitis may also be caused by injury, gout, arthritis, or some infections.

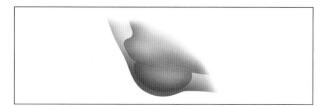

Figure 4.38 *Bursitis (shown on the elbow, olecranon bursa)*

Dislocation (luxation)

Displacement of a bone from its normal position in a joint where the bones in the joint lose contact with one another. Pain and a loss of motion usually accompany this condition.

Fractures

Break in a bone that can vary in size and severity and usually accompanied by damage to the surrounding tissue. Signs and symptoms of fractures vary but can include pain (especially when force is applied to the area), swelling, tenderness, loss of function, and bruising. There are many different types of fractures, including:

- **Simple or closed fractures:** These are clean breaks of the bone with little damage to the surrounding tissue and no break in the overlying skin.
- **Compound or open fractures:** In these fractures the bone end pierces the skin and the wound is susceptible to contamination by dirt, debris, and bacteria.
- **Comminuted fractures:** In these fractures the bone is broken into more than two pieces.
- **Impacted fractures:** These involve the bone ends being driven into each other.
- **Complicated fractures:** In these fractures the bone damages surrounding tissues and/or organs.
- **Greenstick fractures:** These fractures only occur in children and involve an incomplete break (a crack) in the bone and the bone bending.
- **Stress fractures:** These fractures are caused by the stress of a repeated activity such as walking with a heavy pack.

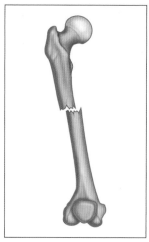

Figure 4.39 *Compound or open fracture*

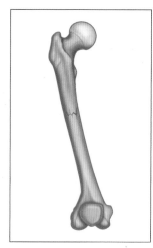

Figure 4.40 *Simple or closed fracture*

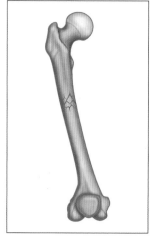

Figure 4.41 *Comminuted fracture*

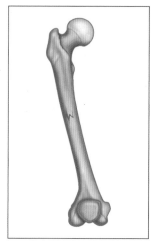

Figure 4.42 *Greenstick fracture*

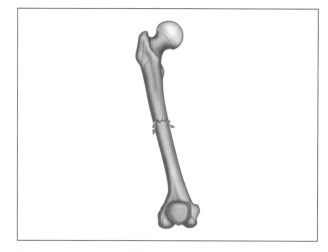

Figure 4.43 *Impacted fracture*

Gout

Gout is the build-up of uric acid and its salts in the blood and joints. Crystals accumulate in and irritate joints, and erode the cartilage. Eventually, the bones can fuse, leading to

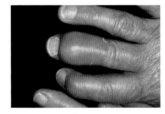

Gout

an immovable joint. Signs and symptoms include inflammation, swelling, pain, tenderness, and a loss of mobility. Gout occurs primarily in middle-aged and older males, and is suspected to be caused by diet, an abnormal gene, or environmental factors such as stress.

Osteogenesis imperfecta (brittle bone disease)

Genetic disease in which the bones are abnormally brittle. Signs can include frequent fracturing of bones, bone deformity, discoloration of the sclera of the eyes, translucent skin, possible deafness, and thin dental enamel of the teeth.

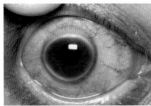

Osteogenesis imperfecta

Osteomalacia and rickets

Softening of the bones caused by their progressive demineralization due to a deficiency of vitamin D. Osteomalacia in children is known as rickets.

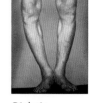

Rickets

Osteoporosis

Progressive disease in which bones lose their density and become brittle and prone to fractures. It is common in the elderly and in post-menopausal women.

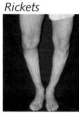

Osteoporosis

Risk factors of osteoporosis include:

- Inadequate levels of estrogen, e.g., in post-menopausal women, those who are underweight or have eating disorders, athletes, those with amenorrhea, and nursing mothers
- Prolonged use of certain drugs, e.g., alcohol, some diuretics, cortisone, and tetracycline
- Smoking
- Calcium deficiency or malabsorption
- Vitamin D deficiency
- Lack of weight-bearing exercise
- Family history of osteoporosis.

Paget's disease

Chronic bone disease where the rate at which bone is broken down and rebuilt increases to such an extent that the affected areas are abnormally enlarged and weak. Paget's disease

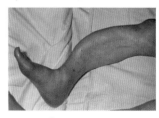

Paget's disease

has few signs or symptoms, although pain, bone enlargement, and bone deformity may occur with the cause unknown.

Sprain

Injury to a ligament in a joint characterized by considerable swelling and pain. The blood vessels, muscles, nerves, and tendons associated with the joint can also be injured.

Torn cartilage

Tearing of the menisci in the knee joint and quite common in athletes. Signs and symptoms of torn

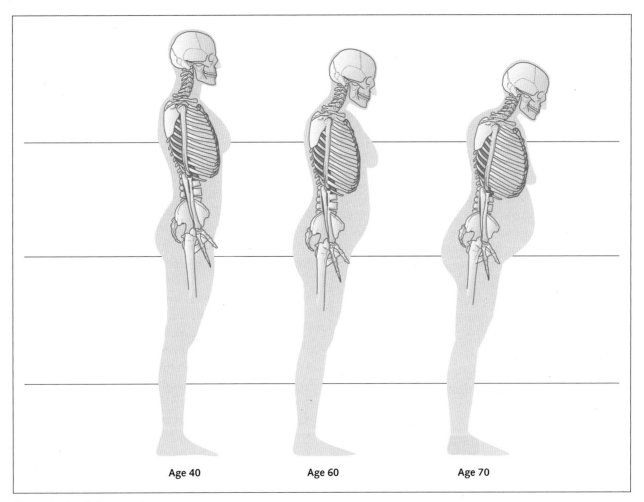

Age 40   Age 60   Age 70

Figure 4.44 *Osteoporosis*

cartilage include pain, tenderness, swelling, and limited motion.

Common pathologies of the spine

Some pathologies of the skeletal system specifically affect the vertebrae and discs of the spine. These are generally characterized by backache, spinal stiffness, and sometimes nerve disorders.

Cervical spondylosis

Involves the degeneration of the intervertebral discs and the vertebrae of the neck. It usually affects middle-aged to elderly people and it causes neck pain and possible pressure on the spinal cord. This can lead to spinal-cord compression, which can result in changes in walking such as jerky leg movements and unsteadiness, as well as weakness in the arms.

Kyphosis

An exaggerated thoracic curve that is often characterized by a hunched back, rounded shoulders, and mild, persistent back pain. Scoliosis can sometimes develop from kyphosis. Kyphosis is common in the elderly or it can be a result of rickets, osteoporosis, or poor posture.

Lordosis

An exaggerated lumbar curve that is characterized by a sway back and lower backache. It can result from excess weight around the abdomen, poor posture, or rickets, or it can be pregnancy-related.

Did you know?

In a lifetime, an average person walks approximately five times the circumference of the globe.

Prolapsed (slipped) intervertebral disc (PID)

Occurs when the disc's outer ring of fibrocartilage ruptures and its inner nucleus pulposus protrudes through this rupture and compresses a spinal nerve. A PID usually occurs if the ligaments surrounding the discs are injured or weakened and the discs are put under excess pressure. It can cause pain, numbness, and weakness along the pathway of the spinal nerve that it compresses.

Scoliosis

A lateral curvature of the spine that has few signs or symptoms, but can cause backache after sitting or standing for a long time. It can be hereditary or caused by conditions such as poor posture, having one leg shorter than the other, paralysis of the muscles on one side of the body, or chronic sciatica.

Spinal stenosis

Narrowing of the spinal canal and a cause of lower back pain and sciatica in elderly people. Spinal stenosis usually results from other diseases, such as Paget's disease or osteoarthritis.

Spondylitis

Inflammation of the joints of the spine with primary signs of pain and spinal stiffness. Different forms of spondylitis exist, the main one being **ankylosing spondylitis**. This is inflammation of the spine and large joints such as the sacroiliac joint. It develops mainly in men between the ages of 20 and 40 years and its cause is not known, although it is thought that genetics plays a role. Ankylosing spondylitis has symptom-free periods followed by flare-ups that differ in severity. Common signs and symptoms include back pain, stiffness, and muscular spasms. More severe signs and symptoms can include loss of appetite, weight loss, fatigue, anemia, and postural changes due to the fusion of sections of vertebrae.

Temporomandibular joint (TMJ) disorder

Because the temporomandibular joint is one of the most complicated joints in the body, it is prone to a number of different disorders, which are all classified as temporomandibular joint disorder or syndrome (TMJ disorder/syndrome). TMJ disorder includes symptoms such as muscle pain and tightness around the jaw, tenderness in the muscles that move the jaw, clicking of the jaw, and limitation of the movement or opening of the jaw. Associated symptoms can be

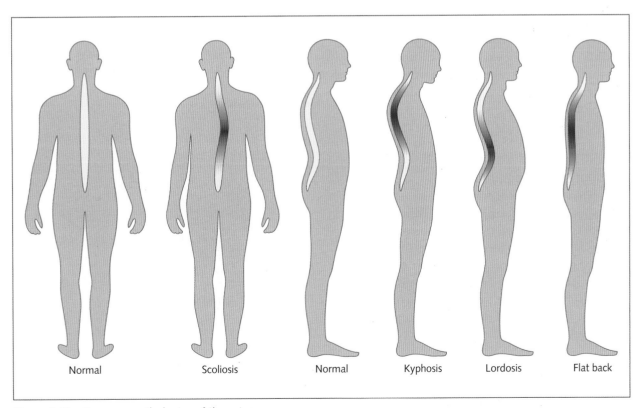

Normal   Scoliosis   Normal   Kyphosis   Lordosis   Flat back

Figure 4.45 *Common pathologies of the spine*

headaches, pain, or stiffness in the neck that radiates into the arms, dizziness, earache, and disrupted sleep. TMJ disorder can be caused by muscular tension, anatomic problems within the joints, arthritis, or psychological stress.

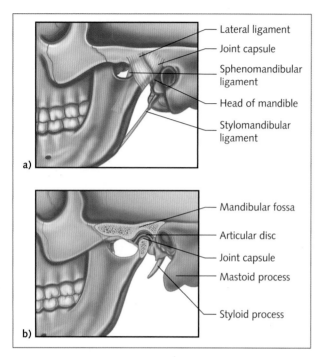

- Lateral ligament
- Joint capsule
- Sphenomandibular ligament
- Head of mandible
- Stylomandibular ligament

a)

- Mandibular fossa
- Articular disc
- Joint capsule
- Mastoid process
- Styloid process

b)

Figure 4.46 *The temporomandibular joint*

Whiplash injury

This is caused by the sudden jerking back of the head and the neck; for example, in car accidents. It is characterized by pain and stiffness resulting from damage to the ligaments, vertebrae, and sometimes spinal cord of the neck.

Common disorders of the feet

Clubfoot (talipes equinovarus)

Birth defect in which the foot is twisted out of shape. Two types exist: positional and true. **Positional clubfoot** is caused when the foot has been held in an unusual position in utero, and it can often be corrected through physical therapy after birth. **True clubfoot**, on the other hand, is usually only corrected through surgery because either the bones of the leg or foot or the muscles of the calf are structurally underdeveloped.

Hammer toes

Painful, rigid toes that are fixed in a contracted position and cannot be straightened. Usually the

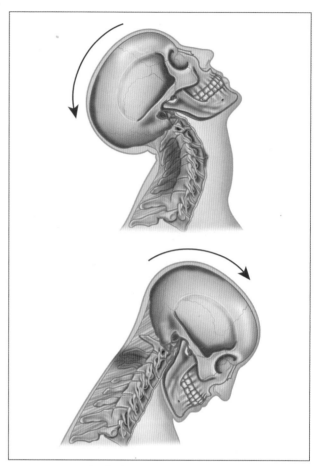

Figure 4.47 *Whiplash injury*

second, third, and fourth toes are affected. Hammer toes often accompany other foot disorders such as bunions or high arches, and can also lead to corns and nail problems. The most common cause of hammer toes is poorly fitting shoes.

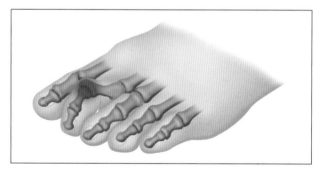

Figure 4.48 *Hammer toe*

Heel spurs

Bony growths under the heel of the foot that are usually caused by excessive pulling on the heel bone by tendons. They are not always painful, but can cause pain and difficulty in standing or walking, especially if the tissues surrounding the spur are inflamed.

Pes cavus (high arches)

The opposite of pes planus and characterized by unusually high arches in the foot. These high arches result in stiffness and limited movement of the foot, and can cause pain, calluses, and claw foot. High arches are generally inherited or can be caused by chronic illness.

Pes planus (flat foot or dropped arches)

Condition in which the arches of the foot drop and the foot spreads. Because the arches support the foot and absorb shock when the body is in motion, pes planus often results in fatigue, pain, and backache. Pes planus is sometimes hereditary but can also be the result of joint weakness, nutritional deficiencies in children, or chronic illness.

NEW WORDS	
Arthrology	The study of joints
Articulation	The point of contact between two bones; commonly called a joint
Cartilage	A resilient, strong connective tissue
Demineralization	The process through which minerals such as calcium and phosphorus are lost from the bones
Hemopoiesis	The production of blood cells and platelets
Kinesiology	The study of the motion of the body
Ligament	A tough band of connective tissue that attaches bones to bones
Osseous tissue	Bone tissue
Ossification	The process of bone formation
Osteology	The study of the structure and function of bones
Process	A bony projection or prominence
Remodeling	The process through which new bone tissue replaces old, worn out, or injured bone tissue
Tendon	A tough band of connective tissue that attaches muscles to bones

Study Outline

Functions of the skeletal system

1. Functions of the skeletal system include protection, support, shape, homeostasis of minerals, movement, energy storage, and as a site of blood cell production.

> People's Skeletal Systems Have Many Essential Bones
> Protection, Support, Shape, Homeostasis of minerals, Movement, Energy storage, Blood-cell production

2. Blood cells are produced in red bone marrow.
3. Lipids are stored in yellow bone marrow.

Anatomy of bones

Bone tissue

1. There are two types of bone tissue: compact and spongy.
2. Compact bone tissue is made up of osteons, which consist of concentric rings of lamellae through the center of which run Haversian canals, in which nerves, blood, and lymph vessels are found.
3. Compact bone functions in protection and support and is the external layer of all bones.
4. Spongy bone is a light tissue made up of lamellae arranged into trabeculae.

5. Spongy tissue contains red bone marrow, in which blood cells and platelets are produced.

Bone formation and remodeling

1. Bones are formed through the process of ossification.
2. Bones are continually replaced through the process of remodeling.

Types of bone

Bones can be classified as short, long, irregular, flat, or sesamoid.

> Skeletons Linger Inside Fluffy Shirts
> Short, Long, Irregular, Flat, Sesamoid

Structure of a long bone

1. Long bones have a long central shaft called a diaphysis, which is covered by a membrane called the periosteum.
2. The diaphysis contains the medullary/marrow cavity, which is lined by a membrane called the endosteum. This cavity contains fatty yellow bone marrow.
3. Each end of the diaphysis is called an epiphysis and is covered by articular cartilage. The epiphysis is made of spongy bone tissue, which contains red bone marrow.
4. The region where the diaphysis joins the epiphysis is the metaphysis, and in a growing bone it houses the epiphyseal plate where growth in length takes place.

Organization of the skeleton

1. The skeleton is divided into the axial and appendicular skeletons.
2. The axial skeleton consists of the bones along the center/axis of the body. These are the skull, hyoid, ribs, sternum, and the vertebrae of the spine.
3. The appendicular skeleton consists of the appendages; namely, the legs and arms and their girdles.
4. The eight bones of the cranium are: one frontal, two parietals, two temporals, one occipital, one ethmoid, one sphenoid.

> To help you remember the bones of the cranium, take a moment to picture yourself wearing a cap of fluffy pink toes. Take some time to remember this image—imagine you are looking in the mirror and seeing lots of fluffy pink toes coming out of your head. Then if you ever need to remember the bones of the cranium, simply put your fluffy pink toed cap on:
>
> Fluffy Pink **TOES**
> Frontal, Parietals, Temporals, Occipital, Ethmoid, Sphenoid

5. The 14 bones of the face are: 2 nasals, 2 maxillae, 2 zygomatics, 1 mandible, 2 lacrimals, 2 palatines, 2 inferior nasal conchae, 1 vomer.

> Virgil Can Not Make My Pet Zebra Laugh
> Vomer, inferior nasal Conchae, Nasals, Maxillae, Mandible, Palatines, Zygomatic, Lacrimals

6. The hyoid bone is found in the neck and does not articulate with any other bone.
7. The spine is composed of 33 vertebrae: 7 cervical, 12 thoracic, 5 lumbar, 5 sacral, 4 coccygeal.
8. A vertebra is composed of a thick, disc-shaped body and a vertebral arch formed by processes. The space formed by the body and arches is the vertebral foramen, through which runs the spinal cord. Transverse processes project from the sides of the arch and a spinous process projects posteriorly. These processes serve as sites of attachment for muscles. Superior and inferior articular processes form joints with the vertebrae above and below.
9. Intervertebral discs are found between the vertebrae. They are composed of the outer anulus fibrosus and the inner nucleus pulposus. These discs provide cushioning and absorb shock.
10. There are four natural curves to the spine: cervical, thoracic, lumbar, and sacral.

11. The thorax is made up of the sternum, 12 pairs of ribs, and the thoracic vertebrae. The sternum itself consists of the manubrium, body, and xiphoid process.
12. The shoulder girdle consists of the clavicle and scapula. The shoulder joint is a diarthrotic, synovial ball-and-socket joint.
13. The arm bone is the humerus. The bones in the forearm are the ulna and radius. The bones of the hand are the 8 carpals (trapezium, trapezoid, capitate, hamate, scaphoid, lunate, triquetrum, pisiform), 5 metacarpals, and 14 phalanges.

> Hands Take Crazy Things To Silly Lunch Parties
> Hamate, Trapezium, Capitate, Trapezoid, Triquetrum, Scaphoid, Lunate, Pisiform

14. The pelvic girdle consists of the ilium, ischium, and pubis. The hip joint is a diarthrotic, synovial ball-and-socket joint.
15. The thigh bone is the femur. The knee bone is the patella. The bones of the leg are the tibia and fibula. The bones of the foot are the 7 tarsals (talus, calcaneus, cuboid, navicular, 3 cuneiforms), 5 metatarsals, and 14 phalanges.
16. The foot has three arches that distribute the weight of the body over the entire foot. They are the medial and lateral longitudinal arches and the transverse arch.

Joints

Joints, or articulations, are the points of contact between bones. They hold bones together, provide movement, and protect vital organs.

Classification of joints

1. Joints can be classified according to the degree of movement they permit. This is called functional classification, and includes: synarthroses (immovable joints), amphiarthroses (slightly movable joints), and diarthroses (freely movable joints).
2. Joints can also be classified according to what type of connective tissue binds them together and whether or not there is a synovial cavity between them. This is called structural classification, and includes: fibrous joints, cartilaginous joints, and synovial joints.

Synovial joints

1. Synovial joints are joints that are lined by articular cartilage, have a synovial cavity between the articular surfaces, and are enclosed in a synovial capsule. This capsule is lined with a membrane that secretes synovial fluid, which lubricates joints and supplies nutrients to, and removes waste from, the articular cartilage. Synovial joints allow for a great deal of movement.
2. Movements at synovial joints can include flexion, extension, hyperextension, abduction, adduction, circumduction, and rotation.
3. Movements of the forearm include pronation and supination.
4. Movements of the foot include inversion, eversion, dorsiflexion, and plantar flexion.
5. Synovial joints are classified as: gliding, hinge, pivot, condyloid, saddle, or ball-and-socket.

Review

1. Name seven functions of the skeletal system.
2. Identify where in the body blood cells are produced.
3. Describe the structure and function of compact bone.
4. Describe the structure and function of spongy bone.
4. Explain what ossification is.
5. Explain what remodeling is.
6. Identify five types of bones. For each type of bone give one example.
7. Name the central shaft of a long bone.
8. Name the ends of a long bone.
9. Explain the organization of the skeleton.
10. Name the bones of the cranium.
11. Name the bones of the face.
12. Name the bone found in the neck that does not articulate with any other bones.
13. Describe the spine, giving the names of the different regions and the numbers of vertebrae found in each of these regions.
14. Name the space in a vertebra through which the spinal cord runs.
15. Describe the structure and function of an intervertebral disc.
16. Identify the bones of the thorax.
17. Describe the structure of the shoulder girdle.

18. Describe the shoulder joint and name the movements it allows.
19. Name the bones of the upper limb.
20. Name the carpals.
21. Describe the hip joint and name the movements it allows.
22. Describe the knee joint and name the movements it allows.
23. Name the bones of the lower limb.
24. Name the tarsals.
25. Explain the three arches of the foot.
26. Explain the meaning of the following words: synarthrotic, amphiarthrotic, diarthrotic.
27. Describe the following types of joints: fibrous, cartilaginous, synovial.
28. Explain the functions of synovial fluid.

Multiple-Choice Questions

1. An example of a saddle joint is:
   a. The shoulder joint
   b. The hip joint
   c. The thumb joint
   d. The elbow joint

2. Ossification is:
   a. The process by which bone is formed
   b. The process by which blood cells are formed
   c. The process in which lipids are stored
   d. The process by which cartilage is formed

3. The diaphysis is:
   a. The area at both ends of a long bone
   b. The main shaft of a long bone
   c. The lining of the ends of a long bone
   d. The lining of the main shaft of a long bone

4. How many lumbar vertebrae are there?
   a. 4
   b. 5
   c. 6
   d. 7

5. A hinge joint allows which of the following movements?
   a. Side-to-side
   b. Circumduction
   c. Supination
   d. Extension

6. What type of joint do the atlas and axis form?
   a. Pivot
   b. Saddle
   c. Ball-and-socket
   d. Hinge

7. Which of the following statements is correct?
   a. Functions of the skeletal system include protection, movement, and excretion
   b. Functions of the skeletal system include mineral homeostasis, vitamin D production, and movement
   c. Functions of the skeletal system include support, protection, and movement
   d. Functions of the skeletal system include movement and support only

8. Minerals present in bone include:
   a. Calcium and hemoglobin
   b. Calcium only
   c. Calcium and nickel
   d. Calcium and phosphorus

9. Articular cartilage is the cartilage found:
   a. Covering the ends of articulating bones
   b. Covering the bodies of articulating bones
   c. Covering synovial capsules
   d. Covering menisci

10. Which of the following movements is the opposite of inversion?
    a. Pronation
    b. Eversion
    c. Supination
    d. Opposition

5

The Muscular System

Introduction

All your body's movements are created by tiny filaments sliding to overlap one another. As they overlap, they cause a muscle to shorten, and this creates movement of the bones and joints, internal tracts, or even the heart.

The study of muscles is called **myology**, and in this chapter you will discover how your muscles work and also learn about some of the important muscles that help you move.

Student objectives

By the end of this chapter you will be able to:

- Describe the functions of the muscular system
- Describe the different muscle types, such as skeletal, cardiac, and smooth
- Identify the structure of a skeletal muscle
- Describe how a muscle contracts
- Identify the different types of muscular contraction and muscle fibers
- Identify and name the skeletal muscles
- Identify the common pathologies of the muscular system.

Did you know?

Muscles can only shorten. This means that every movement you make is a pull, not a push. Even when you are pushing something like a shopping cart, your muscles are actually still pulling on bones, not pushing.

Functions of the Muscular System

Muscles have the unique ability of shortening themselves. This is known as **contraction** and is the essential function of all muscles. Through contracting, muscles can produce movement, maintain posture, move substances within the body, regulate organ volume, and produce heat.

Movement of the skeleton (locomotion)

Skeletal muscles are a type of muscle that is mostly attached to bones by strong cords of dense connective tissue called **tendons**. When these muscles contract, they move the bones at the joints of the body and this produces movement of the skeleton. Thus, we can run, jump, and even somersault. Some skeletal muscles are not attached to bones. Instead, they are attached to skin. These are the muscles of the face and they enable us to smile, frown, and reveal our inner emotions.

Maintenance of posture

When we are awake, certain skeletal muscles are always partially contracted to keep our bodies in an upright position. For example, the muscles of the neck maintain a sustained partial contraction to keep our heads upright. Muscle tendons also surround, protect, and stabilize joints, thus stabilizing body positions.

Movement of substances and the regulation of organ volume

In addition to skeletal muscle, there are two other types of muscle: **smooth** and **cardiac** (more on these in a minute). All three types of muscle function in moving substances within the body and in regulating organ control and volume. For example:

- **Skeletal muscle:** Skeletal muscle contracts to help return venous blood to the heart and to move lymph through the lymphatic vessels.
- **Cardiac muscle:** The heart is made up of cardiac muscle tissue, which contracts to pump blood around the body. Cardiac muscle also helps regulate blood pressure.

- **Smooth (visceral) muscle:** Smooth muscle lining hollow tracts of the body contracts to move food through the gastrointestinal tract, moves urine through the urinary tract, and moves a baby through the birthing canal.

Heat production

Skeletal muscles release a lot of energy as they contract. This energy takes the form of heat, which is considered a by-product of muscle contraction. The heat generated by muscular contraction is used to maintain our normal body temperature. If the body needs to increase its temperature, skeletal muscles contract involuntarily (shiver) to increase heat production. The generation of heat in the body is called **thermogenesis**.

In the classroom

Take a moment to think back to the functions of the skin and remember how smooth muscles also play a role in helping to maintain normal body temperatures by vasodilation and vasoconstriction.

Muscle Tissue

Types of muscle tissue

There are three different types of muscle tissue, which differ in their anatomy, location, and function and in what they are controlled by (figure 5.1).

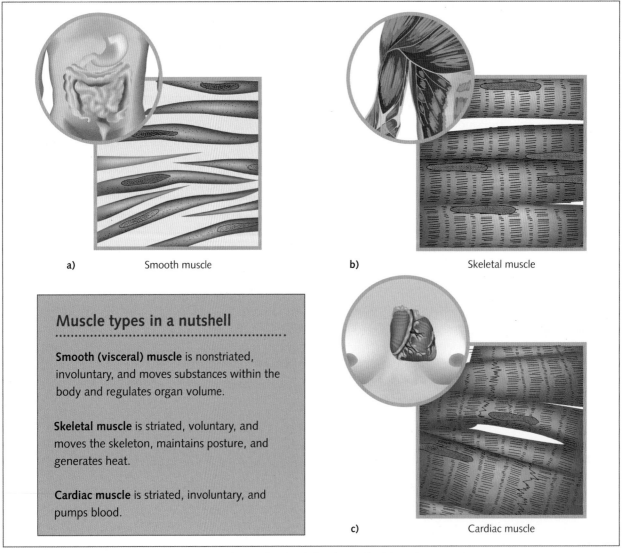

a) Smooth muscle

b) Skeletal muscle

Muscle types in a nutshell

Smooth (visceral) muscle is nonstriated, involuntary, and moves substances within the body and regulates organ volume.

Skeletal muscle is striated, voluntary, and moves the skeleton, maintains posture, and generates heat.

Cardiac muscle is striated, involuntary, and pumps blood.

c) Cardiac muscle

Figure 5.1 *Types of muscle tissue, (a) smooth muscle; (b) skeletal muscle; (c) cardiac muscle*

- **Anatomy (striated/non-striated):** Muscle tissue is either **striated** or **non-striated**. When looked at under a microscope, striated tissue is made up of light and dark bands.
- **Location:** The type of muscle tissue often depends on where it is in the body, or what it is attached to.
- **Function:** Different muscle tissues have very specific functions. For example, cardiac muscle tissue functions only in contracting the heart.

- **Control (voluntary/involuntary):** Muscle tissue is under either **voluntary** or **involuntary** control. Voluntary muscle is under conscious control, while involuntary muscle is not under conscious control. Most involuntary muscles are controlled by neurotransmitters and hormones. Some also contain **autorhythmic cells**, which are self-excitable cells.

CHARACTERISTICS OF THE THREE TYPES OF MUSCLE TISSUE

Type	Anatomy	Location	Function	Control
Skeletal muscle	Muscle fibers: • Are striated • Are generally long and cylindrical-shaped (although some are circular) • Have multiple nuclei and many mitochondria • Are strengthened and reinforced by connective tissue • Connect to tendons	Attached by tendons to bones, skin, or other muscles	• Enables movement of the skeleton • Enables movement of lymph and venous blood • Maintains posture • Produces heat	Voluntary
Cardiac muscle	Muscle fibers: • Are striated • Are arranged in spiral-shaped bundles of branching cells	Forms most of the heart	• Pumps blood around the body • Helps regulate blood pressure	• Involuntary • Contracts at a steady rate set by a "pacemaker" that is adjusted by neurotransmitters and hormones
Smooth muscle (visceral muscle)	Muscle fibers: • Are non-striated, which is why they are called smooth • Are spindle-shaped • Have a single nucleus • Are arranged in sheets or layers that alternately contract and relax to change the size or shape of structures	Forms the walls of hollow internal structures such as blood vessels, the gastrointestinal tract, and the bladder	• Moves substances through tracts • Regulates organ volume	• Involuntary • Contracts auto-rhythmically and is controlled by neurotransmitters and hormones

Skeletal Muscle

Now that you have a basic understanding of the functions and types of muscle tissue, we will take a look at skeletal muscles and see how they work together with the skeleton to produce movement. But before we go any further, here is some important vocabulary that describes the characteristics of muscle tissue:

Excitability (irritability)	The ability of muscle cells (and also nerve cells) to respond to stimuli
Conductivity	The ability of muscle cells to move action potentials along their plasma membranes
Action potentials	An electrical change that occurs on the membrane of a muscle fiber in response to a nerve impulse
Contractility	The ability of muscles to contract and shorten
Extensibility	The ability of muscles to extend and lengthen
Elasticity	The ability of muscles to return to their original shape after contracting or extending

Structure of a skeletal muscle

It is often easier to understand how something works if you know what it is made of. So, before we look at exactly how a muscle contracts, let us slowly break a muscle down into its smallest components.

Study tip

When learning about muscles, remember that:

myo- = muscle
sarco- = flesh

Connective tissue: The outer protection of a muscle

Lining the walls of the body, and holding the muscles and limbs together, is a dense, irregular connective tissue called **fascia** (fascia also surrounds and protects organs of the body).

Fascia:

- Separates muscles into different functional groups and fills spaces between muscles, thus allowing free movement of the muscles
- Supports the nerves, blood, and lymphatic vessels that serve the muscles.

Beneath the fascia lie muscles. Looking at a muscle under a microscope, you will see hundreds of muscle fibers surrounded and held together by connective tissue. This connective tissue surrounds, protects

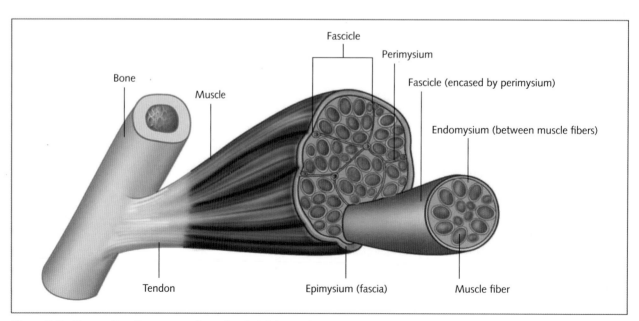

Figure 5.2 *Connective tissue wrappings of a skeletal muscle*

and reinforces the fibers because, although they are capable of producing great power, they are still quite fragile cells that can be damaged. Three types of dense, irregular connective tissue protect and strengthen a muscle:

- The **epimysium:** This is the outermost layer that encircles the whole muscle.
- The **perimysium:** This surrounds bundles of 10–100 muscle fibers. These bundles are called **fascicles.**
- The **endomysium:** This surrounds each individual muscle fiber within the fascicle. It contains many blood capillaries so that each muscle fiber has a good supply of blood, which brings oxygen and nutrients to the muscles and removes their waste products.

Together, the epimysium, perimysium, and endomysium extend beyond the muscle fibers and become tendons or **aponeuroses.** Tendons are cylindrical cords of connective tissue that attach muscles to the periosteum of bones. Aponeuroses are flat, sheet-like tendons that attach muscles to the periosteum of bones or to the skin.

> ### In the classroom
> ....
>
> Take a few minutes to review the structure and functions of a cell discussed in chapter 2. This will help you to understand the structure of a skeletal fiber, which is essentially a type of cell. Take note that because muscle fibers require energy to contract, they contain many mitochondria.

Muscle fibers: The inner cells of a skeletal muscle

Each muscle fiber within the fascicle is a single cell that has similar properties to the generalized animal cell you learnt about in chapter 2. However, there are slight variations (mainly in the vocabulary):

- A muscle cell is called a **muscle fiber** or **myofiber.**
- The fiber is a long, cylindrical shape.
- The plasma membrane is called the **sarcolemma.**

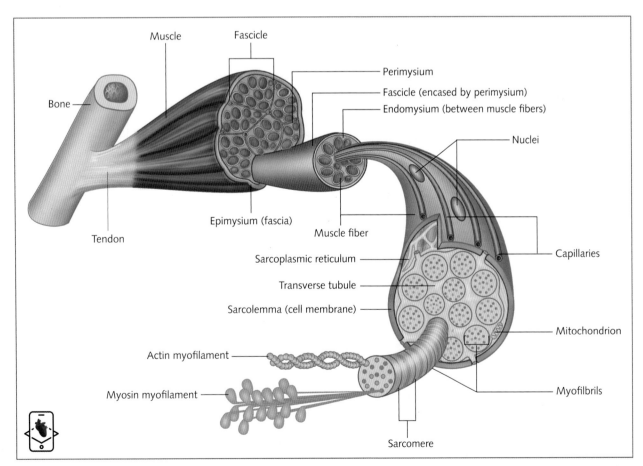

Figure 5.3 *Structure of a skeletal muscle*

- The cytoplasm is called the **sarcoplasm**.
- There are many nuclei in a muscle fiber and they are located at its periphery, out of the way of the contractile elements (described shortly).
- There are many mitochondria, which lie in rows throughout the fiber and are close to the muscle proteins that use adenosine triphosphate (ATP) during contraction.
- Long, threadlike organelles nearly fill the sarcoplasm. These are called **myofibrils** and are the contractile elements of skeletal muscles. They are made of filaments called **myofilaments** that are arranged into compartments called **sarcomeres**. Sarcomeres are the basic functional units of skeletal muscles and we will study them in detail shortly.
- The endoplasmic reticulum of muscle fibers is called the **sarcoplasmic reticulum** and it stores calcium, which is necessary for muscular contraction.

> **Did you know?**
> ....
>
> Some muscle fibers are as long as 12 in (30 cm).

> **Did you know?**
> ....
>
> A woman's muscles are naturally smaller than a man's. This is because a woman has fewer muscle fibers and less ability to store glycogen and convert it into energy.

Sarcomeres: The basic functional units of a skeletal muscle

We have now broken down a muscle by removing its outer covering of protective connective tissue

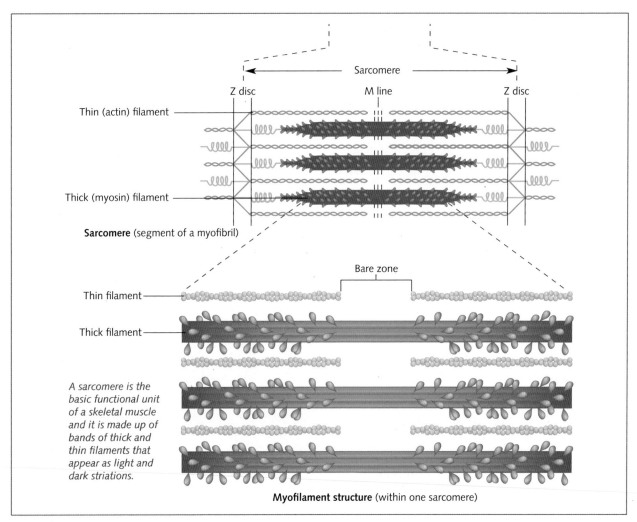

Thin (actin) filament

Thick (myosin) filament

Sarcomere (segment of a myofibril)

Z disc　　M line　　Z disc

Sarcomere

Bare zone

Thin filament

Thick filament

A sarcomere is the basic functional unit of a skeletal muscle and it is made up of bands of thick and thin filaments that appear as light and dark striations.

Myofilament structure (within one sarcomere)

Figure 5.4 *Structure of a sarcomere*

and breaking down its cell, or fiber, into its different components. As mentioned above, one of the components of a muscle fiber is a myofibril, which is the contractile element of a skeletal muscle. Myofibrils are made up of myofilaments, which are arranged in compartments called sarcomeres. We will now look at a sarcomere.

A sarcomere is the basic functional unit of a striated muscle fiber. In other words, it contains the filaments that move to overlap one another and cause a muscle to shorten.

Sarcomeres contain three types of filaments:

- **Thick filaments:** Thick filaments contain molecules of the protein **myosin**, which are shaped like two golf clubs twisted together:
  - The handles of the clubs form the tails of the molecules and point toward the center of the sarcomere
  - The heads of the clubs form the heads of the molecules and are called **myosin heads** or **cross-bridges**. These extend toward the thin filaments
  - The molecules lie parallel to one another
- **Thin filaments:** Thin filaments contain the proteins **actin**, **tropomyosin**, and **troponin**. These molecules have irregular shapes but appear together as a chain of twisted molecules. On each molecule is a **myosin-binding site** where myosin heads can attach to bring about contraction. When a muscle is relaxed, these sites are blocked by a tropomyosin-troponin complex so that myosin cannot bind to them.
- **Elastic filaments:** Elastic filaments contain the protein **titin** (**connectin**), which helps stabilize the position of the thick filaments.

Sarcomeres are made up of two different regions, or bands, which give skeletal muscles their striated appearance:

- **A-band:** The A-band is a darker area composed mainly of thick filaments with only a few thin filaments that have overlapped into the area. In the center of the A-band is a narrow **H-zone** that contains thick filaments only. It is divided by an **M-line** of protein molecules that hold the thick filaments together.

- **I-band:** The I-band is a lighter area composed of thin filaments only.

Sarcomeres are separated from one another by **Z-discs** (**Z-lines**), which are narrow regions of dense material.

Muscle Contraction

How do muscles contract?

Muscles shorten when the thick and thin filaments in the sarcomere slide past one another. This is known as the **sliding-filament mechanism**. Let's take a look at what starts this sliding and how exactly it works:

- **Relaxed muscle:** When a muscle is relaxed the myosin-binding sites on each actin molecule are covered by a tropomyosin-troponin complex. Thus, the myosin heads cannot bind with the actin molecules. ATP is attached to ATP-binding sites on the myosin heads and it is split into ADP and P (a phosphate group). This means that energy has been transferred from the ATP to the myosin heads. They are in an energized or activated state ready to bind to the myosin-binding sites on the actin molecules as soon as the spaces become available.
- **A nerve impulse starts the process:** A nerve impulse from the central nervous system triggers the release of a neurotransmitter called **acetylcholine** (refer to chapter 6 for further details). This neurotransmitter in turn triggers a **muscle action potential**, which is an electrical change that occurs on the membrane of the muscle fiber. This muscle action potential travels along the sarcolemma and causes the release of calcium, which is stored in the sarcoplasmic reticulum of the fiber.

Study tip

Just a reminder: ATP stands for adenosine triphosphate, and this is the main energy-transferring molecule in the body.

- **Calcium frees up the myosin-binding sites:** Calcium binds with the troponin on the myosin-binding sites and causes the tropomyosin-troponin complex to move away from the sites. This frees up the sites so that the myosin can bind with the actin.

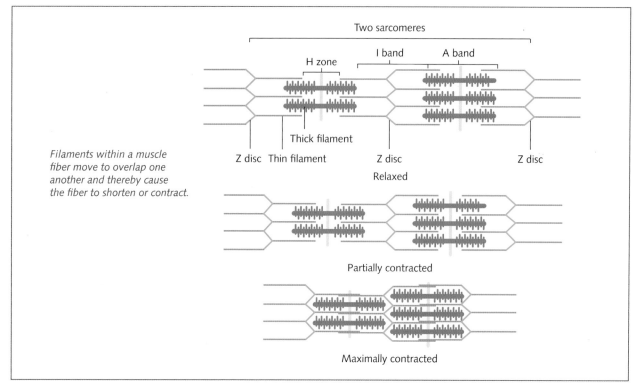

Filaments within a muscle fiber move to overlap one another and thereby cause the fiber to shorten or contract.

Figure 5.5 *The sliding-filament mechanism*

- **Myosin binds to actin in a power stroke:** A "power-stroke" occurs when the myosin heads bind to the myosin-binding sites on the actin and change their shape by swivelling their heads toward the center of the sarcomere. It is this change in shape that draws the thin filaments past the thick filaments. The thin filaments slide inward toward the H-zone. The thick filaments remain in the same place. This inward sliding causes the Z-discs to come toward each other, and the entire sarcomere shortens even though the actual lengths of the thin and thick filaments do not change. The sarcomere shortens, the muscle fibers shorten, the whole muscle shortens and pulls on a bone—thus, movement is generated.
- **Myosin heads detach from actin:** After the power stroke, ATP binds to the myosin heads at ATP-binding sites. This causes the heads to detach themselves from the actin. The ATP on the myosin heads is then split by an enzyme and it transfers its energy to the myosin heads so they are once again in an activated state and ready to combine with another site further along the thin filament.
- **The cycle begins again:** The above cycle begins again and continues as long as ATP and calcium are present.

Muscle contraction in a nutshell

Contraction is all about the myosin heads of thick filaments binding to sites on thin actin filaments and pulling these filaments inward. A nerve impulse, ATP, and calcium are needed.

How do muscles relax?

Two processes take place to stop muscle contraction:

- **Acetylcholine is broken down:** An enzyme breaks down acetylcholine and this stops any further muscle action potentials. Therefore, calcium is no longer released.
- **Calcium levels drop:** Calcium levels drop and there is no longer enough calcium available to bind with the troponin. Thus, the tropomyosin-troponin complex moves back over the myosin-binding sites on the actin and so prevents the myosin heads from binding with the actin.

The thin filaments, therefore, slip back into their relaxed position and no further contraction takes place.

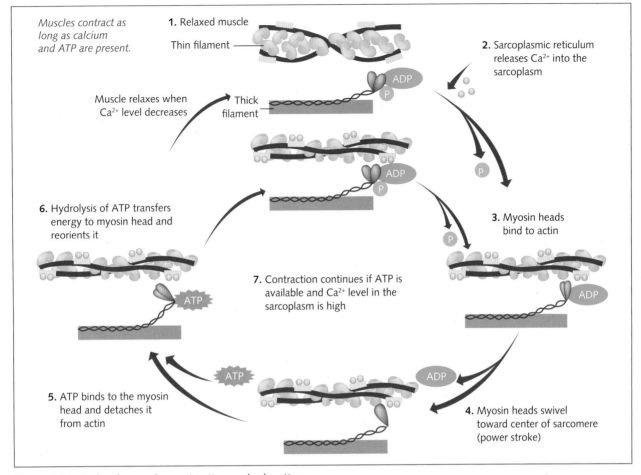

Muscles contract as long as calcium and ATP are present.

1. Relaxed muscle

Thin filament

2. Sarcoplasmic reticulum releases Ca^{2+} into the sarcoplasm

Muscle relaxes when Ca^{2+} level decreases

Thick filament

6. Hydrolysis of ATP transfers energy to myosin head and reorients it

3. Myosin heads bind to actin

7. Contraction continues if ATP is available and Ca^{2+} level in the sarcoplasm is high

5. ATP binds to the myosin head and detaches it from actin

4. Myosin heads swivel toward center of sarcomere (power stroke)

Figure 5.6   *Cycle of muscular contraction and relaxation*

Did you know?

During maximum muscle contraction, the distance between the Z-discs can be halved.

Infobox

Anatomy and physiology in perspective

Have you ever tried to lift or push a really heavy object and noticed that no matter how much tension is in your muscles, you are not generating any movement? This is because muscular contraction is taking place, but no shortening of the muscles is occurring. Why not? This is because the myosin heads are swivelling and generating force, but the thin filaments are not sliding inward. This is called an isometric contraction (more on this later).

Infobox

Anatomy and physiology in perspective

To understand the workings of the sliding-filament mechanism, picture yourself jogging on a treadmill. As one foot hits the belt it pushes it backward, then the other foot hits the belt and pushes it backward. These strokes are repeated again and again until the belt is moving smoothly. All the time, however, you are staying in the same place. Now, imagine you are the thick filament, your feet are the myosin heads and the belt of the treadmill is the thin filament. As each myosin head (foot) connects with the thin filament (belt), it moves it backward toward the H-zone. Each repeated movement moves the thin filament more smoothly. Meanwhile, the thick filament (you) is staying in the same place. Don't forget … your legs, the myosin heads, need a constant supply of energy to keep going.

Did you know?

When a person dies, calcium leaks out of the sarcoplasmic reticulum and binds with troponin, causing the tropomyosin-troponin complex to move off the myosin-binding sites. The myosin heads are, therefore, able to bind with the actin and contraction occurs. However, because the person is dead, there is no ATP available to activate the release of the myosin heads from the actin and so the muscles are in a permanent state of contraction. This is called **rigor mortis**. It lasts about 24 hours, until the tissues begin to degenerate.

Types of muscular contraction

Muscle tone

Even when we think our muscles are completely relaxed, a few of the muscles fibers are still involuntarily contracted. This constant contraction gives muscles their firmness, or tension. This is called **muscle tone**, or **tonus**. Tone is essential for maintaining posture and keeping our bodies in an upright position. Here are some more terms associated with muscle tone:

Atony	A lack of muscle tone
Atrophy	The wasting away of muscles; muscles decrease in size
Hypotonia	A loss of muscle tone; muscles appear loose and flattened, and are described as **hypotonic**
Hypertonia	An increase in muscle tone; muscles appear stiff or rigid, and are described as **hypertonic**.

Isotonic and isometric contractions

Most physical activities include two types of contraction: isotonic and isometric.

- **Isotonic contractions:** Isotonic contractions are regular contractions in which muscles shorten and create movement, while the tension in the muscle

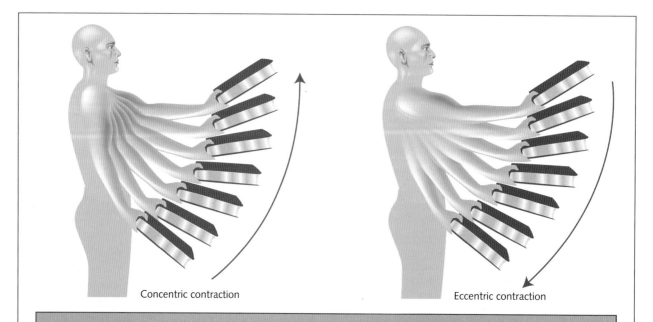

Concentric contraction

Eccentric contraction

In the classroom

Pick a book up off your desk and bring it up toward your face. The muscle in your arm is shortening and reducing the angle at your elbow joint. It is performing a concentric contraction. Now replace the book on the table. The muscle in your arm is still contracting even though it is lengthening. It is performing an eccentric contraction.

Figure 5.7 *Isotonic contraction*

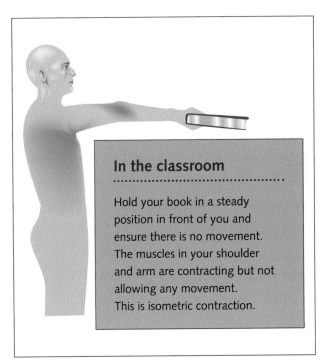

In the classroom

Hold your book in a steady position in front of you and ensure there is no movement. The muscles in your shoulder and arm are contracting but not allowing any movement. This is isometric contraction.

Figure 5.8 *Isometric contraction*

remains constant. They improve muscle strength and joint mobility and come in two forms:

- **Concentric contractions:** These are always toward the center and are contractions in which the muscle shortens and generates a movement that decreases the angle at a joint
- **Eccentric contractions:** These are always away from the center and are contractions in which muscles lengthen

- **Isometric contractions:** In isometric contractions, the muscle contracts but it does not shorten and no movement is generated. This type of contraction stabilizes some joints while others are moved. It also improves muscle tone.

Infobox

Anatomy and physiology in perspective

When people lift weights they are performing both isotonic and isometric contractions. As they are lifting the weights their muscles are contracting isotonically, and as they are holding the weights in place their muscles are contracting isometrically.

Muscle metabolism

Muscles need energy in the form of ATP to contract. They obtain this energy in a number of different ways, including:

- **The phosphagen system:** Muscles store a small amount of ATP in their fibers and are able to convert it into energy through what is called the phosphagen system. However, this is only enough energy to last for around 15 seconds of maximal muscular activity.
- **Glycolysis:** Once the ATP inside the fibers has been used up, muscles break down glucose through a process called glycolysis. This process does not need oxygen and is called an **anaerobic** process. Through glycolysis, glucose is broken down into **pyruvic acid** (**pyruvate**) and ATP. The ATP is used by the muscles, while the pyruvic acid enters the mitochondria of the muscle fiber, where it needs oxygen to be broken down completely. If there is not enough oxygen present to completely break down the pyruvic acid, then it is converted into **lactic acid**. Lactic acid can diffuse out of the skeletal muscles into the blood and be used by heart muscle fibers and kidney and liver cells to produce ATP. However, some lactic acid does accumulate in the muscle tissues and blood and can cause muscle fatigue and soreness.
- **Aerobic respiration:** If there is enough oxygen present, then the pyruvic acid is completely oxidized into carbon dioxide, water, ATP, and heat.

This process is called **cellular respiration** or **biological oxidation**. Aerobic respiration provides energy for activities of longer than 10 minutes, as long as there is an adequate supply of oxygen and nutrients.

Where do the muscles get their glucose and oxygen from?

Glucose: Carbohydrates are broken down into glucose and stored in the body as **glycogen**. Glycogen can be stored in both the liver and the muscles.

Oxygen: Oxygen is supplied to muscle fibers in two forms. Firstly, it is stored in the muscle cells themselves in the form of **myoglobin**, and, secondly, it is stored in the blood in the form of **hemoglobin**.

Infobox

Anatomy and physiology in perspective

Athletes performing short sprints, such as the 100 m, produce ATP anaerobically, while those running longer distances, such as the 5000 m, produce most of it aerobically. Those running marathons basically produce all the ATP they need aerobically.

Did you know?

After your first year of life, the growth of your muscles is due to the enlargement of the existing cells and not an increase in the number of cells.

Why do muscles sometimes stop working?

If a muscle, or group of muscles, is overstimulated it can become progressively weaker until it no longer responds to any stimulus and cannot maintain its contractions. This is called **muscle fatigue**. Muscle fatigue can occur for a number of reasons, including:

- An insufficient supply of oxygen or glycogen
- A build-up of lactic acid
- A failure of action potentials to release adequate acetylcholine.

Muscle fiber types

Not all muscle fibers are identical, and they differ not only in their appearance (color and size), but also in the way in which they produce ATP, how quickly they contract, and how quickly they fatigue.

There are three different types of muscle fiber: **slow oxidative, fast oxidative,** and **fast glycolytic.** Most muscles are composed of a combination of all three types. The proportions of the types of fiber are dependent on the usual activity of the muscle. For example, postural muscles that do not need to contract quickly but that do need to maintain a constant, fatigue-resistant contraction contain a large proportion of slow oxidative fibers, which are very resistant to fatigue. The following table explains the different types of fibers.

Infobox

Anatomy and physiology in perspective

Marathon runners can sometimes collapse when their muscles suddenly stop working. This is an example of true muscle fatigue. Their muscles have literally stopped contracting owing to a lack of oxygen and glucose and a build-up of lactic acid.

Runners (or people who do other forms of strenuous exercise) are also usually seen to breathe heavily for a long time after they have stopped exercising. This is because they need to recover oxygen to restore the body to its resting condition by making ATP reserves, eliminating accumulated lactic acid, repairing tissues, and cooling the body down. This heavy breathing is called **recovery oxygen consumption**, or recovering the **oxygen debt**.

Did you know?

The color of muscle fibers varies according to the amount of **myoglobin** found in them. Like hemoglobin, myoglobin is a red-colored, iron-containing protein that binds to oxygen and so provides oxygen to muscle fibers.

- **Red muscle fibers:** These have a high myoglobin content and also have more mitochondria and more blood capillaries than white muscle fibers.
- **White muscle fibers:** These have a low myoglobin content and also have fewer mitochondria and blood capillaries than red muscle fibers.

Study tip

Before learning your muscles, review the charts "Movements at Synovial Joints" in chapter 4. This will help you to understand and visualize the different actions of the muscles.

MUSCLE FIBER TYPES			
Features	**Type I: Slow-twitch**	**Type II: Fast-twitch**	
	Type I: Slow oxidative	*Type IIA: Fast oxidative*	*Type IIB: Fast glycolytic*
Color	Red	Red to pink	White
Diameter of fiber	Smallest	Medium	Largest
Oxygen supply	Contains large amounts of myoglobin (therefore red), many mitochondria, and many blood capillaries	Contains large amounts of myoglobin (therefore red to pink), many mitochondria, and many blood capillaries	Has a low myoglobin content (therefore white), few mitochondria, and few blood capillaries
ATP production	Generates ATP by aerobic processes (therefore called oxidative fibers)	Generates ATP by aerobic processes (therefore called oxidative fibers)	Generates ATP by anaerobic processes (glycolysis); therefore, cannot supply the muscle continuously with ATP
Contraction velocity	Splits ATP slowly and therefore has a slow contraction velocity	Splits ATP quickly and therefore has a fast contraction velocity	Due to its large diameter, it splits ATP very fast and therefore has a strong, rapid contraction velocity
Fatigue resistance	Very resistant to fatigue	Resistant to fatigue, but not as much as type 1	Fatigues easily
Activities	Maintaining posture and endurance activities	Walking and running	Fast movements, such as throwing a ball

Muscles of the Body

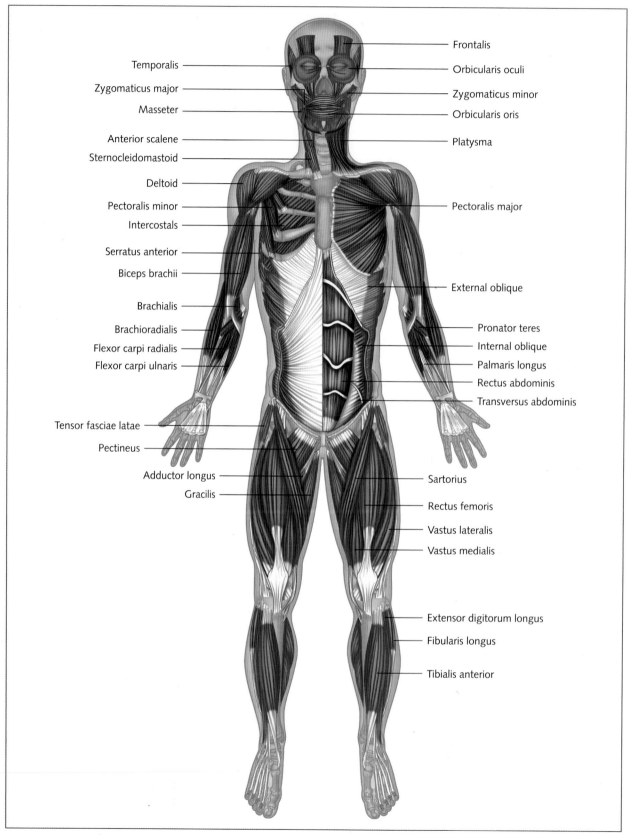

Figure 5.9 *Overview of the skeletal muscles (anterior view)*

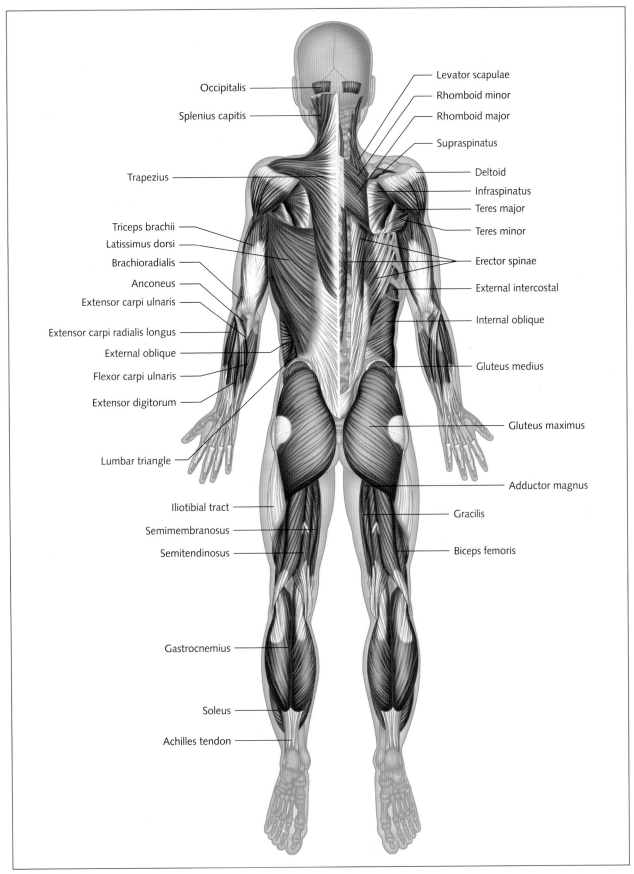

Figure 5.10 *Overview of the skeletal muscles (posterior view)*

Skeletal Muscles and Movement

How skeletal muscles produce movement

Before looking at the different skeletal muscles that make up the muscular system, it is necessary to understand how they produce movement. A muscle is usually attached to two bones that form a joint, and when the muscle contracts, it pulls the movable bone toward the stationary bone. All muscles have at least two attachments:

- **Origin:** The point where the muscle attaches to the stationary bone is called the origin.
- **Insertion:** The point where the muscle attaches to the moving bone is called the insertion. During contraction, the insertion usually moves toward the origin.

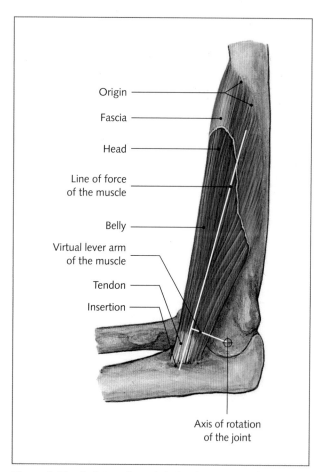

Origin
Fascia
Head
Line of force
of the muscle
Belly
Virtual lever arm
of the muscle
Tendon
Insertion

Axis of rotation
of the joint

Figure 5.11   *Relationship of skeletal muscles to bones*

Muscles only shorten when they contract and thus can only pull, never push. Therefore, most body movements are the result of two or more muscles acting together or against each other so that whatever one muscle does, another muscle can undo. For example, one muscle contracts to bend your elbow and another muscle contracts to pull it straight again.

This means that muscles at joints are usually arranged in opposing pairs of flexors–extensors, abductors–adductors, and so on. These pairs are also accompanied by other muscles to ensure that movements are smooth and efficient.

- The muscle responsible for causing a particular movement is called the **prime mover**, or **agonist**.
- The muscle that opposes this movement is called the **antagonist**. It relaxes and lengthens in a controlled way to ensure the movement is performed smoothly by the prime mover.
- Additional muscles at the joint ensure a steady movement and help the prime mover function effectively. These muscles are called **synergists** and they are usually found alongside the prime mover.
- Specialized synergists stabilize the bone of the prime mover's origin so that it can act efficiently. These muscles are called **fixators**, or **stabilizers**.

In the classroom

Flex your forearm at your elbow joint. Two specific muscles are at work here: your biceps brachii is contracting. It is the prime mover. In opposition to this, your triceps brachii muscle is lengthening. It is the antagonist.

Now extend your forearm at your elbow joint. Once again, two muscles are working here but this time it is your triceps brachii that is contracting and that is now the prime mover. The biceps brachii is lengthening and is the antagonist.

Study tip

Muscle names often reflect a muscle's characteristics. So, when you are trying to learn them be aware of how their names describe their:

- **Shape:** The trapezius is shaped like a trapezium.
- **Direction:** The obliques run diagonal to the midline.
- **Position:** The tibialis is found next to the tibia bone.
- **Movement:** The flexor digitorum longus flexes the toes.
- **Number of origins:** The biceps brachii has two heads (bi = 2, ceps = heads).
- **Attachments:** The carpi radialis is attached to the carpum (carpum = wrist).
- **Size:** The gluteus maximus is the largest of the gluteal muscles.
- **Origin and insertion:** The sternocleidomastoid originates on the sternum and clavicle and inserts on the mastoid process.

Muscles of the face and scalp

Muscles of facial expression

The muscles of facial expression are a group of very superficial muscles that usually originate in the fascia or bones of the skull and insert into the skin. They move the skin and enable us to express emotions such as surprise, fear, happiness, and sadness.

Occipitofrontalis, sometimes called **epicranius**, plays an important role in facial expression, such as raising the eyebrows and wrinkling the forehead. It comprises two muscle bellies (or **gasters**), right and left, positioned opposite each other, from the front to the back of the skull, with a flat tendinous tissue called the **galea aponeurotica** linking the two. The anterior portion is the **frontal belly**, while the posterior portion is the **occipital belly**.

The **orbicularis oculi** and **levator palpebrae** function in moving the eyelids and protecting the eye. For example, the orbicularis oculi can cause the eyelids to close involuntarily or blink if an object is brought too close to the eye.

Frowning, wrinkling your nose, or flaring your nostrils involves the muscles found in the center of your face and around your nose. These include the **procerus** and **nasalis**.

The **orbicularis oris** is a sphincter muscle that encircles the mouth and enables you to close or purse your lips and move them when speaking. It is also important because it serves as the insertion for some of the other facial muscles that are responsible for moving the lips. Muscles that move the lips include the **levator labii superioris, zygomaticus (major and minor), risorius, depressor anguli oris, depressor labii inferioris,** and **mentalis. Buccinator** is an important muscle in smiling as well as in mastication. It keeps the cheek taut, preventing it from folding and being injured when chewing.

The **platysma** is included in the facial muscles of expression because it moves the lower lip. It does, however, also move the lower jaw and draw the skin of the chest upward, so is often also included with the neck muscles. It is a large, flat muscle that often stands out after a runner has finished a hard race.

Muscles of mastication

The muscles of mastication include **masseter, temporalis,** and **pterygoids;** these muscles work together to move the mandible (lower jaw) and are involved in biting and chewing.

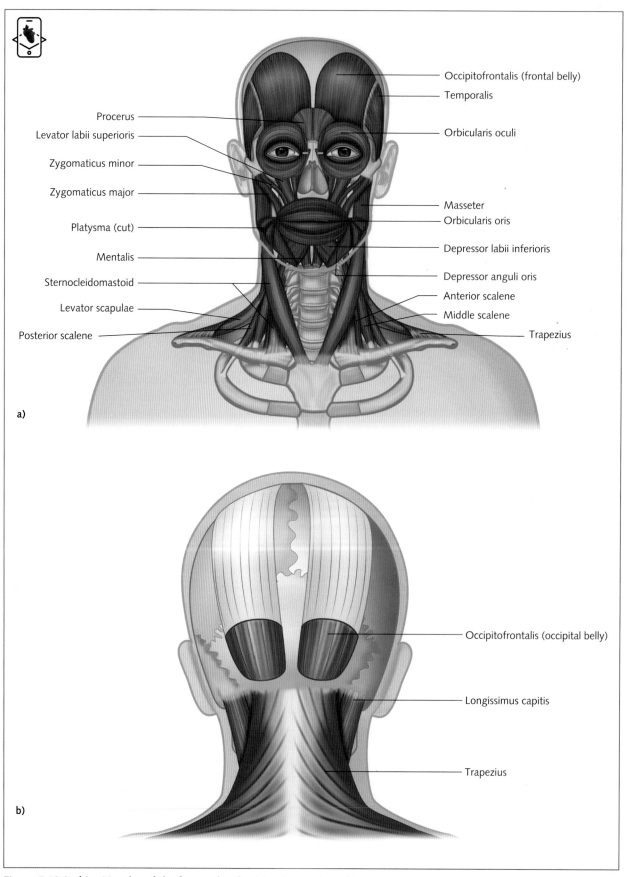

Figure 5.12 (a–b) *Muscles of the face and scalp, (a) anterior view; (b) posterior view*

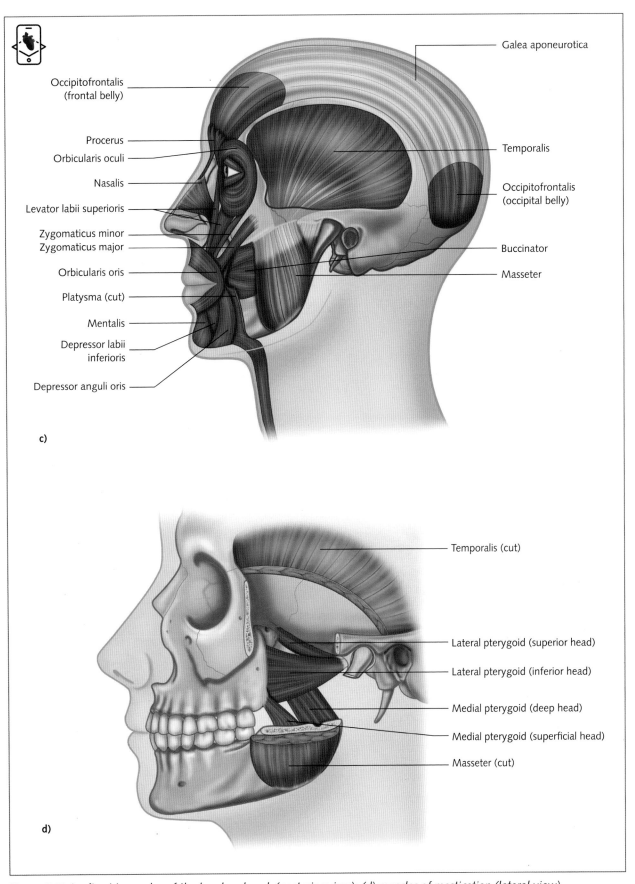

Figure 5.12 (c–d) *(c) muscles of the head and neck (posterior view); (d) muscles of mastication (lateral view)*

FACE AND SCALP MUSCLES

Muscle	Origin	Insertion	Nerve	Action
Scalp				
Occipitofrontalis	*Frontal belly:* skin of eyebrows *Occipital belly:* lateral two-thirds of superior nuchal line of occipital bone. Mastoid process of temporal bone	Galea aponeurotica	Facial nerve (VII)	*Frontal belly:* raises eyebrows and wrinkles skin of forehead horizontally *Occipital belly:* pulls scalp backward
Temporoparietalis	Fascia above ear	Lateral border of galea aponeurotica	Facial nerve (VII)	Tightens scalp. Raises ears
Ear				
Superior auricular	Fascia in temporal region above ear	Superior part of ear	Facial nerve (VII)	Elevates ear
Anterior auricular	Anterior part of temporal fascia	Into helix of ear	Facial nerve (VII)	Draws ear forward and upward
Posterior auricular	Mastoid process of temporal bone	Posterior part of ear	Facial nerve (VII)	Pulls ear backward and upward
Eyelids				
Orbicularis oculi	*Orbital part:* frontal bone. Frontal process of maxilla. Medial palpebral ligament *Palpebral part:* medial palpebral ligament	*Orbital part:* circular path around orbit, returning to origin *Palpebral part:* lateral palpebral raphe	Facial nerve (VII)	*Orbital part:* strongly closes eyelids *Palpebral part:* gently closes eyelids
Levator palpebrae superioris	Root of orbit (lesser wing of sphenoid bone)	Skin of upper eyelid	Oculomotor nerve (III)	Raises upper eyelid
Corrugator supercilii	Medial end of superciliary arch of frontal bone	Deep surface of skin under medial half of eyebrows	Facial nerve (VII)	Draws eyebrows medially and downward
Nose				
Procerus	Fascia over nasal bone. Upper part of lateral nasal cartilage	Skin between eyebrows	Facial nerve (VII)	Produces wrinkles over bridge of nose
Nasalis	*Transverse part:* maxilla just lateral to nose *Alar part:* maxilla over lateral incisor	*Transverse part:* joins muscle of opposite side across bridge of nose *Alar part:* alar cartilage of nose	Facial nerve (VII)	*Transverse part:* compresses nasal aperture *Alar part:* draws cartilage downward and laterally

FACE AND SCALP MUSCLES

Muscle	Origin	Insertion	Nerve	Action
Nose (continued)				
Depressor septi nasi	Maxilla above medial incisor	Nasal septum and ala	Facial nerve (VII)	Pulls the nose inferiorly
Mouth				
Depressor anguli oris	Oblique line of mandible	Skin at corner of mouth	Facial nerve (VII)	Pulls corner of mouth downward and laterally
Depressor labii inferioris	Anterior part of oblique line of mandible	Skin of lower lip	Facial nerve (VII)	Pulls lower lip downward and laterally
Mentalis	Mandible inferior to incisor teeth	Skin of chin	Facial nerve (VII)	Protrudes lower lip and pulls up skin of chin
Risorius	Fascia over masseter muscle	Skin at corner of mouth	Facial nerve (VII)	Retracts corner of mouth
Zygomaticus major	Posterior part of lateral surface of zygomatic bone	Skin at corner of mouth	Facial nerve (VII)	Pulls corner of mouth upward and laterally
Zygomaticus minor	Anterior part of lateral surface of zygomatic bone	Upper lip just medial to corner of mouth	Facial nerve (VII)	Elevates upper lip
Levator labii superioris	*Angular head:* zygomatic bone and frontal process of maxilla *Infraorbital head:* lower border of orbit	*Angular head:* greater alar cartilage, upper lip, and skin of nose *Infraorbital head:* muscles of upper lip	Facial nerve (VII)	Raises upper lip. Dilates nostril
Levator anguli oris	Canine fossa of maxilla	Skin at corner of mouth	Facial nerve (VII)	Elevates corner of mouth
Orbicularis oris	Muscle fibers surrounding opening of mouth	Skin and fascia at corner of mouth	Facial nerve (VII)	Closes lips. Protrudes lips
Buccinator	Posterior parts of maxilla and mandible; pterygomandibular raphe	Blends with orbicularis oris and into lips	Facial nerve (VII)	Presses cheek against teeth. Compresses distended cheeks
Mastication				
Masseter	Zygomatic arch and maxillary process of zygomatic bone	Lateral surface of ramus of mandible	Trigeminal nerve (V)	Elevation of mandible

FACE AND SCALP MUSCLES

Muscle	Origin	Insertion	Nerve	Action
Mastication (continued)				
Temporalis	Bone of temporal fossa. Temporal fascia	Coronoid process of mandible. Anterior margin of ramus of mandible	Trigeminal nerve (V)	Elevation and retraction of mandible
Lateral pterygoid	*Superior head:* roof of infratemporal fossa *Inferior head:* lateral surface of lateral plate of pterygoid process	*Superior head:* capsule and articular disc of temporomandibular joint *Inferior head:* neck of mandible	Trigeminal nerve (V)	Protrusion and side-to-side movements of mandible
Medial pterygoid	*Deep head:* medial surface of lateral pterygoid plate of pterygoid process. Pyramidal process of palatine bone *Superficial head:* tuberosity of maxilla and pyramidal process of palatine bone	Medial surface of ramus and angle of mandible	Trigeminal nerve (V)	Elevation and side-to-side movement of mandible

Muscles of the neck

There are a number of muscles found in the neck. **Sternocleidomastoid (SCM)** is one of the largest and most superficial neck muscles. SCM is shaped like a strap and plays an important role in moving the head. It is often affected in whiplash injury and can also cause headaches and neck pain. SCM is also a useful landmark, as it divides each side of the neck into two regions: the anterior triangle and posterior triangle (also called the anterior and lateral cervical regions).

The **anterior triangle** is situated at the front of the neck. The muscles in the anterior triangle are divided according to where they lie in relation to the hyoid bone, i.e., above (supra-) or below (infra-). The **suprahyoid muscles** each have different actions, but in general they all assist elevation of the hyoid bone, an action involved in swallowing. The four **infrahyoid muscles** can be divided into two groups: superficial and deep, and their function is to steady the hyoid bone, fixing it so that the suprahyoid muscles can act.

The **posterior triangle** is an anatomical area located in the lateral aspect of the neck. There are many muscles that make up the borders and floor of this region. One significant muscle is the **omohyoid**, which is split into two bellies by a tendon. The inferior belly crosses the posterior triangle, traveling in a superomedial direction and splitting the triangle into two. The muscle then crosses underneath SCM, to enter the anterior triangle. A number of vertebral muscles form the floor of the posterior triangle, including **splenius capitis**, **levator scapulae**, and the **scalene** muscles.

The **scalene** muscles comprise three paired muscles (anterior, middle, and posterior), and as well as forming part of the floor of the posterior triangle, they act as accessory muscles of respiration and perform flexion at the neck.

The **anterior scalene** muscle lies on the lateral aspect of the neck, deep to the prominent SCM muscle.

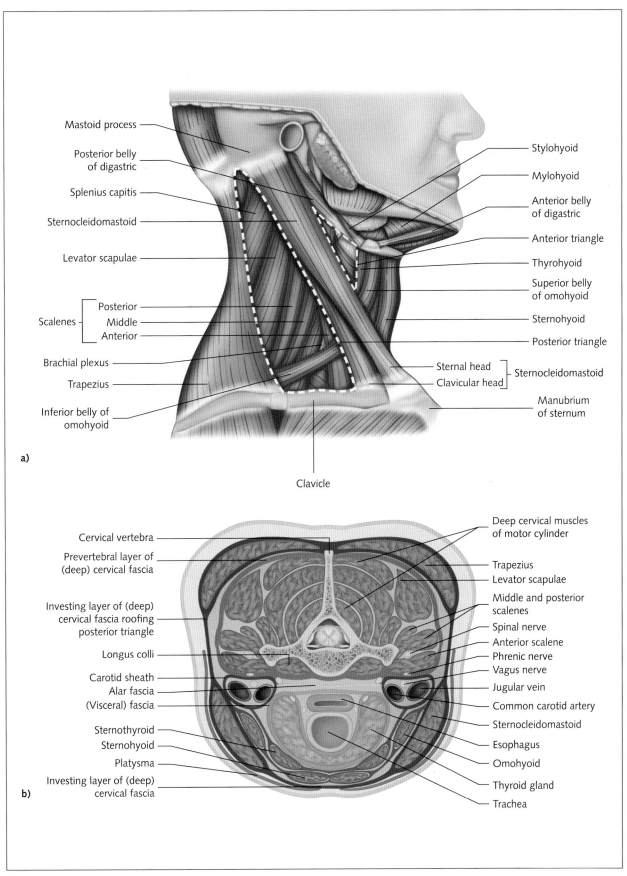

Figure 5.13 *Muscles of the neck, (a) lateral view; (b) cross-section*

It inserts into the first rib. The **middle scalene**, the largest and longest of the three scalenes, has several long, thin muscle bellies arising from the cervical spine; these bellies converge into one large belly, which inserts into the first rib. And, finally, the **posterior scalene** is the smallest and deepest of the scalene muscles; unlike the anterior and middle scalene muscles, it inserts into the second rib.

NECK MUSCLES				
Muscle	**Origin**	**Insertion**	**Nerve**	**Action**
Platysma	Subcutaneous fascia of upper quarter of chest	Subcutaneous fascia and muscles of chin and jaw. Inferior border of mandible	Facial nerve (VII)	Pulls lower lip from corner of mouth downward and laterally. Draws skin of chest upward
Anterior Triangle—Suprahyoid Muscles				
Mylohyoid	Mylohyoid line on inner surface of mandible	Median fibrous raphe and adjacent part of hyoid bone	Mylohyoid nerve from inferior alveolar branch of mandibular nerve (V_3)	Depresses mandible when hyoid is fixed. Elevates and pulls hyoid forward when mandible is fixed. Supports and elevates floor of oral cavity
Geniohyoid	Inferior mental spine on inner surface of mandible	Hyoid bone	Branch from ventral ramus of C1 carried along hypoglossal nerve (XII)	Protrudes and elevates hyoid bone. Depresses mandible if hyoid bone is fixed
Stylohyoid	Base of styloid process of temporal bone	Hyoid bone	Facial nerve (VII)	Pulls hyoid bone upward and backward, thereby elevating tongue
Digastric	*Anterior belly:* digastric fossa on inner side of lower border of mandible *Posterior belly:* mastoid notch on medial side of mastoid process of temporal bone	Body of hyoid bone via a fascial sling over an intermediate tendon	*Anterior belly:* mylohyoid nerve, from mandibular nerve (V_3) *Posterior belly:* facial nerve (VII)	*Anterior belly:* raises hyoid bone. Opens mouth by lowering mandible *Posterior belly:* pulls hyoid upward and back
Anterior Triangle—Infrahyoid Muscles				
Sternohyoid	Posterior aspect of sternoclavicular joint, and adjacent manubrium of sternum	Lower border of hyoid bone (medial to insertion of omohyoid)	Ventral rami of C1 to 3 through the ansa cervicalis	Depresses hyoid bone after swallowing

NECK MUSCLES

Muscle	Origin	Insertion	Nerve	Action
Anterior Triangle—Infrahyoid Muscles (*continued*)				
Sternothyroid	Posterior surface of manubrium of sternum	Oblique line on outer surface of thyroid cartilage	Ventral rami of C1 to 3 through the ansa cervicalis	Draws larynx downward
Thyrohyoid	Oblique line of outer surface of thyroid cartilage	Lower border of body and greater horn of hyoid bone	Fibers from ventral ramus of C1 carried along hypoglossal nerve (XII)	Raises thyroid and depresses hyoid bone
Omohyoid	*Inferior belly:* upper border of scapula medial to the scapular notch *Superior belly:* intermediate tendon	*Inferior belly:* intermediate tendon *Superior belly:* lower border of hyoid bone, lateral to insertion of sternohyoid	Ventral rami of C1 to 3 through ansa cervicalis	Depresses and fixes hyoid bone
Prevertebral and Lateral Vertebral Muscles				
Longus colli	*Superior oblique:* transverse processes of C3–5 *Inferior oblique:* anterior surface of bodies of T1, 2, maybe T3 *Vertical:* anterior surface of bodies of T1–3 and C5–7	*Superior oblique:* anterior arch of atlas *Inferior oblique:* transverse processes of C5–6 *Vertical:* transverse processes of C2–4	Ventral rami of cervical nerves C2–6	Flexes neck anteriorly and laterally and slight rotation to opposite side
Longus capitis	Transverse processes of C3–6	Inferior surface of basilar part of occipital bone	Ventral rami of cervical nerves C1–3, (C4)	Flexes head
Rectus capitis anterior	Anterior surface of lateral mass of atlas and its transverse process	Inferior surface of basilar part of occipital bone	Branches from ventral rami of cervical nerves C1, 2	Flexes head at atlanto-occipital joint
Rectus capitis lateralis	Transverse process of atlas	Jugular process of occipital bone	Branches from ventral rami of cervical nerves C1, 2	Flexes head laterally to same side. Stabilizes atlanto-occipital joint

NECK MUSCLES				
Muscle	**Origin**	**Insertion**	**Nerve**	**Action**
Posterior Triangle				
Scalenes	*Anterior:* anterior tubercles of transverse processes of C3–6 *Middle:* transverse processes of C2–7 *Posterior:* posterior tubercles of transverse processes of C4–6	*Anterior:* scalene tubercle and upper surface of 1st rib *Middle:* upper surface of 1st rib, behind groove for subclavian artery *Posterior:* upper surface of 2nd rib	*Anterior:* ventral rami of cervical nerves C4–7 *Middle:* ventral rami of cervical nerves C3–7 *Posterior:* ventral rami of lower cervical nerves C5–7	*Acting on both sides:* flex neck; raise 1st or 2nd rib during active respiratory inhalation *Acting on one side:* side flex and rotate neck
Sternocleidomastoid	*Sternal head:* upper part of anterior surface of manubrium of sternum *Clavicular head:* upper surface of medial third of clavicle	*Sternal head:* lateral one-half of superior nuchal line of occipital bone *Clavicular head:* outer surface of mastoid process of temporal bone	Accessory nerve (XI) and branches from ventral rami of cervical nerves C2, 3 (C4)	*Bilateral contraction:* draws head forward (protracts); raises sternum, and consequently ribs, during deep inhalation *Unilateral contraction:* flexes head to same side; rotates head to opposite side

Muscles of the trunk

Muscles of the anterior thorax

The muscles of the anterior thorax can be divided into muscles that move the shoulder and arm and muscles used in breathing. We will firstly look at the muscles of breathing and then the muscles of the abdominal wall, before going into detail of the muscles that move the shoulder.

Muscles of breathing

The **diaphragm** is the most important muscle of breathing (respiration), as well as serving as an important anatomical landmark that separates the thorax from the abdomen. Structurally, it consists of two parts—a peripheral muscle and a central tendon. The **peripheral muscle** arises from the sternum, ribs, and vertebrae, to converge and form a **central tendon**. During quiet inspiration, the diaphragm accounts for the major part of inspiratory effort.

The **external intercostal** and **internal intercostal** muscles are attached to the ribs and contract and relax to alter the size of the thoracic cavity.

When people are struggling to breathe—for example, during an asthma attack—they also use the sternocleidomastoid and scalenes (see muscles of the neck). These muscles are referred to as the *accessory muscles of respiration*.

Muscles of the abdominal wall

Four pairs of flat, sheet-like muscles make up the abdominal wall. These muscles are the **rectus abdominis, external oblique, internal oblique,** and **transversus abdominis**. Together with the iliopsoas (discussed later), these muscles are crucial to supporting and stabilizing the lower back. A weakness in these core muscles can often lead to injury of the lumbar spine.

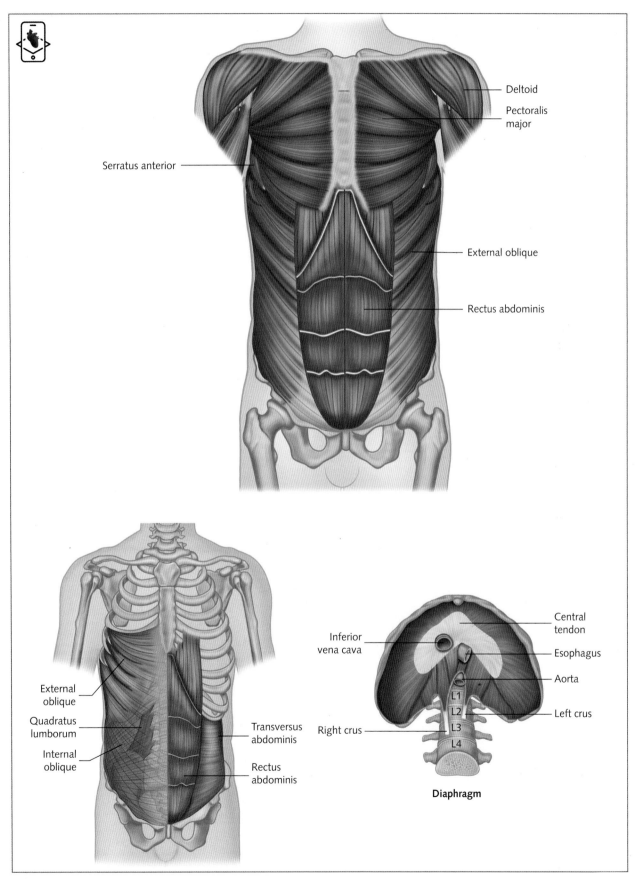

Figure 5.14 *Muscles of the anterior abdominal wall*

Muscles of the anterior thorax that move the shoulder and arm

The muscles that move the shoulder (pectoral girdle) are divided into anterior and posterior groups. They function mainly in stabilizing the scapula, which acts as the point of origin for many of the muscles that move the humerus. Anterior muscles that move the shoulder girdle include the **subclavius, pectoralis minor**, and **serratus anterior**.

Note: Certain terms are used when describing movements of the shoulder (and also the mandible). These terms are:

- **Protraction:** Forward movement of the shoulder on a plane parallel to the ground
- **Retraction:** The opposite of protraction: a backward movement on a plane parallel to the ground
- **Elevation:** Lifting the shoulders upward
- **Depression:** Dropping the shoulders downward.

The **pectoralis major** is the large muscle of the chest and, together with the pectoralis minor, it forms the front wall of the armpit. This muscle helps move the arm, and when it is very tight it can restrict expansion of the chest.

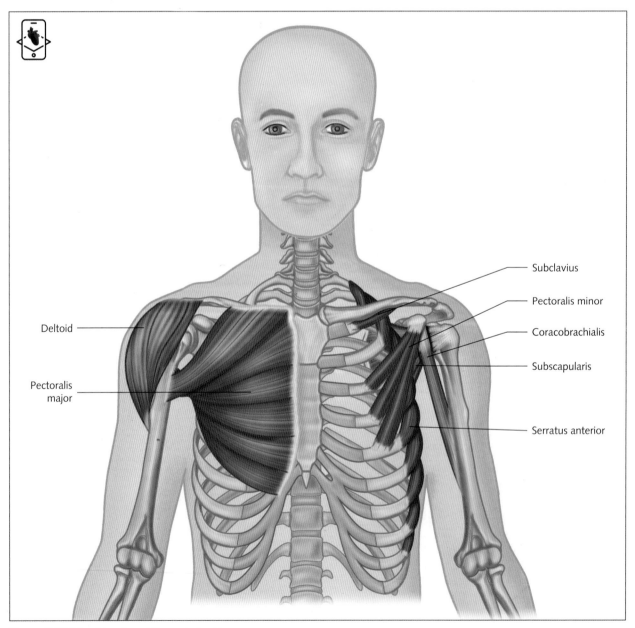

Deltoid

Pectoralis major

Subclavius

Pectoralis minor

Coracobrachialis

Subscapularis

Serratus anterior

Figure 5.15 (a) *Muscles of the anterior thorax*

Muscles of the shoulder

Muscles of the shoulder originate in both the back and the anterior thorax and are as follows:

- Muscles of the back that move the shoulder—**trapezius, levator scapulae, rhomboid major, rhomboid minor, latissimus dorsi**, and the **rotator cuff** muscles (discussed below)
- Muscles of the anterior thorax that move the shoulder—**subclavius, pectoralis minor**, and **serratus anterior** (refer to figure 5.15 (a)).

Rotator cuff

Four muscles work together to hold the head of the humerus in the glenoid cavity of the scapula. These muscles are **subscapularis, supraspinatus, infraspinatus**, and **teres minor**.

Together, their tendons form the rotator cuff, which encircles the ball-and-socket joint of the shoulder and strengthens and reinforces it.

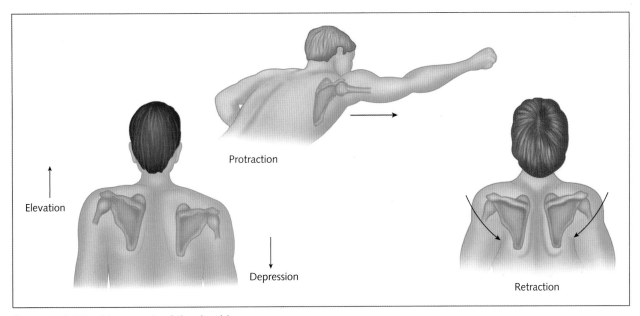

Figure 5.15 (b) *Movements of the shoulder*

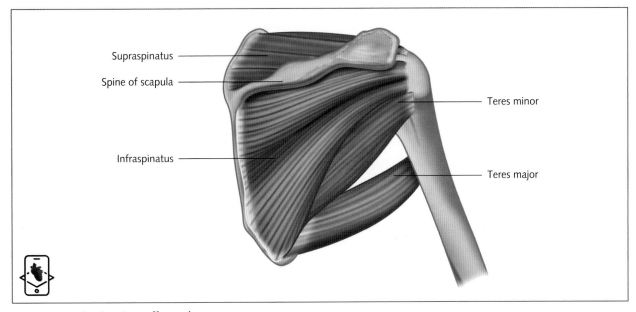

Figure 5.16 (a) *Rotator cuff muscles*

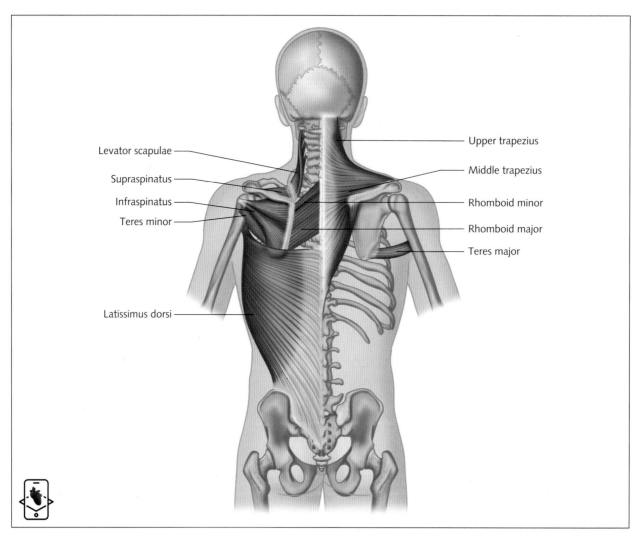

Figure 5.16 (b) *Muscles of the shoulder (posterior view)*

THORAX, ANTERIOR ABDOMINAL, AND SHOULDER MUSCLES				
Muscle	**Origin**	**Insertion**	**Nerve**	**Action**
Muscles of the Thorax				
Intercostals	*External:* lower border of a rib *Internal:* upper border of a rib and costal cartilage *Innermost:* superior border of each rib	*External:* upper border of rib below *Internal:* lower border of rib above *Innermost:* inferior border of the preceding rib	The corresponding intercostal nerves	Contract to stabilize ribcage during movements of trunk. Prevent intercostal space from bulging out or sucking in during respiration. Act to fix the position of the ribs during respiration (innermost only)

THORAX, ANTERIOR ABDOMINAL, AND SHOULDER MUSCLES

Muscle	Origin	Insertion	Nerve	Action
Muscles of the Thorax (*continued*)				
Diaphragm	*Sternal portion:* back of xiphoid process *Costal portion:* inner surfaces of lower 6 ribs and their costal cartilages *Lumbar portion:* L1–3. Medial and lateral lumbocostal arches	All fibers converge and attach onto a central tendon	Phrenic nerve (ventral rami) C3–5	Forms floor of thoracic cavity. Pulls central tendon downward during inhalation
Muscles of the Anterior Abdominal Wall				
Obliques	*External:* muscular slips from the outer surfaces of the lower 8 ribs *Internal:* iliac crest. Lateral two-thirds of inguinal ligament. Thoracolumbar fascia	*External:* lateral lip of iliac crest. Aponeurosis ending in linea alba *Internal:* inferior borders of bottom three or four ribs. Linea alba via an abdominal aponeurosis. Pubic crest and pectineal line	*External:* ventral rami of T5–12 *Internal:* ventral rami of T7–12 and L1	*Both together:* compress abdomen, helping to support abdominal viscera against pull of gravity. Contraction of one side alone side flexes trunk to that side and rotates it to the opposite side *Internal:* contraction of one side alone side flexes and rotates trunk
Transversus abdominis	Anterior two-thirds of iliac crest. Lateral third of inguinal ligament. Thoracolumbar fascia. Costal cartilages of lower 6 ribs	Aponeurosis ending in linea alba. Pubic crest and pectineal line	Ventral rami of T7–12 and L1	Compresses abdomen
Rectus abdominis	Pubic crest, pubic tubercle, and symphysis pubis	Anterior surface of xiphoid process. 5th to 7th costal cartilages	Ventral rami of T5–12	Flexes lumbar spine and pulls ribcage down. Stabilizes pelvis during walking
Muscles of the Posterior Abdominal Wall				
Quadratus Lumborum	Transverse process of L5 vertebra. Posterior part of iliac crest. Iliolumbar ligament	Medial part of lower border of 12th rib. Transverse processes of L1–4	Ventral rami of T12, L1–4	Side flexes vertebral column. Fixes 12th rib during deep respiration. Helps extend lumbar part of vertebral column and gives it lateral stability

THORAX, ANTERIOR ABDOMINAL, AND SHOULDER MUSCLES

Muscle	Origin	Insertion	Nerve	Action
Muscles of the Posterior Abdominal Wall (*continued*)				
Iliopsoas	*Psoas major:* transverse processes of L1–5. Bodies of T12–L5 and intervertebral discs between each vertebra *Iliacus:* Superior two-thirds of iliac fossa. Anterior sacroiliac and iliolumbar ligaments. Upper lateral part of sacrum	Lesser trochanter of femur	*Psoas major:* ventral rami of L1–3 *Iliacus:* femoral nerve L2–4	Main flexors of hip joint. Flex and laterally rotate thigh. Bring leg forward in walking or running
Muscles Attaching the Upper Limb to the Trunk				
Trapezius	Medial third of superior nuchal line of occipital bone. External occipital protuberance. Ligamentum nuchae. Spinous processes and supraspinous ligaments of C7 and T1–12	Superior edge of crest of spine of scapula. Medial border of acromion. Posterior border of lateral one-third of clavicle	*Motor supply:* accessory nerve (XI) *Sensory supply (proprioception):* ventral rami of cervical nerves C3 and 4	Powerful elevator of the scapula; rotates the scapula during abduction of humerus above horizontal. Middle fibers retract scapula. Lower fibers depress scapula
Levator scapulae	Transverse processes of C1, 2, and posterior tubercles of transverse processes of C3, 4	Posterior surface of medial border of scapula from superior angle to root of spine of scapula	Ventral rami of C3 and C4 spinal nerves and dorsal scapular nerve (C5)	Elevates scapula. Helps retract scapula. Helps side flex neck
Rhomboids	*Minor:* spinous processes of C7, T1. Lower part of ligamentum nuchae *Major:* spinous processes of T2–5 and intervening supraspinous ligaments	*Minor:* posterior surface of medial border of scapula at the root of spine of scapula *Major:* posterior surface of medial border of scapula from the root of spine of scapula to the inferior angle	Dorsal scapular nerve C4, 5	Elevate and retract scapula
Serratus anterior	Lateral surfaces of upper 8 or 9 ribs and deep fascia covering the related intercostal spaces	Anterior surface of medial border of scapula	Long thoracic nerve C5–7	Rotates scapula for abduction and flexion of arm. Protracts scapula

THORAX, ANTERIOR ABDOMINAL, AND SHOULDER MUSCLES

Muscle	Origin	Insertion	Nerve	Action
Muscles Attaching the Upper Limb to the Trunk (*continued*)				
Pectoralis minor	Outer surfaces of 3rd to 5th ribs, and fascia of the corresponding intercostal spaces	Coracoid process of scapula	Medial pectoral nerve C5, (6), 7, 8, T1	Draws tip of shoulder downward. Protracts scapula. Raises ribs during forced inspiration
Subclavius	1st rib at junction between rib and costal cartilage	Groove on inferior surface of middle one-third of clavicle	Nerve to subclavius C5, 6	Draws tip of shoulder downward. Pulls clavicle medially to stabilize sternoclavicular joint
Pectoralis major	*Clavicular head:* anterior surface of medial half of clavicle *Sternocostal head:* anterior surface of sternum. First 7 costal cartilages. Sternal end of 6th rib. Aponeurosis of external oblique	Lateral lip of intertubercular sulcus of humerus	Medial and lateral pectoral nerves: *clavicular head:* C5, 6; *sternocostal head:* C6–8, T1	Flexion, adduction, and medial rotation of arm at glenohumeral joint. *Clavicular head:* flexion of extended arm. *Sternocostal head:* extension of flexed arm
Latissimus dorsi	Spinous processes of lower 6 thoracic vertebrae and related interspinous ligaments; via thoracolumbar fascia to the spinous processes of lumbar vertebrae, related interspinous ligaments, and iliac crest. Lower 3 or 4 ribs	Twists to insert into the floor of intertubercular sulcus of humerus, just below the shoulder joint	Thoracodorsal nerve C6–8	Adduction, medial rotation, and extension of the arm at the glenohumeral joint. Assists in forced inspiration by raising lower ribs
Muscles of the Shoulder Joint				
Deltoid	*Anterior fibers:* anterior border of lateral one-third of clavicle. *Middle fibers:* lateral margin of acromion process. *Posterior fibers:* inferior edge of crest of spine of scapula	Deltoid tuberosity of humerus	Axillary nerve C5, 6	Major abductor of the arm; anterior fibers assist in flexing the arm; posterior fibers assist in extending the arm
Supraspinatus	Medial two-thirds of supraspinous fossa of scapula and deep fascia that covers the muscle	Most superior facet on the greater tubercle of humerus	Suprascapular nerve C5, 6	Initiates abduction of arm to 15 degrees at glenohumeral joint

THORAX, ANTERIOR ABDOMINAL, AND SHOULDER MUSCLES				
Muscle	**Origin**	**Insertion**	**Nerve**	**Action**
Muscles of the Shoulder Joint (*continued*)				
Infraspinatus	Medial two-thirds of infraspinous fossa of scapula and deep fascia that covers the muscle	Middle facet on posterior surface of greater tubercle of humerus	Suprascapular nerve C5, 6	Lateral rotation of arm at glenohumeral joint
Teres minor	Upper two-thirds of a strip of bone on posterior surface of scapula immediately adjacent to lateral border of scapula	Inferior facet on greater tubercle of humerus	Axillary nerve C5, 6	Lateral rotation of arm at glenohumeral joint
Subscapularis	Medial two-thirds of subscapular fossa	Lesser tubercle of humerus	Upper and lower subscapular nerves C5, 6, (7)	Medial rotation of arm at glenohumeral joint
Teres major	Oval area on lower third of posterior surface of inferior angle of scapula	Medial lip of intertubercular sulcus on anterior surface of humerus	Lower subscapular nerve C5–7	Medial rotation and extension of arm at glenohumeral joint

Muscles of the back

The muscles of the back can be divided into:

- **Superficial:** Associated with movements of the shoulder
- **Intermediate:** Associated with movements of the thoracic cage and respiration
- **Deep:** Associated with movements of the vertebral column.

The superficial and intermediate muscles are classified as **extrinsic muscles,** and are involved in moving the upper limbs and thoracic wall. The deep muscles are classified as **intrinsic muscles** and they act on the vertebral column, maintaining posture and producing movement.

Superficial layer

The superficial extrinsic back muscles form the V-shaped musculature associated with the middle and upper back, and include the **trapezius, latissimus dorsi, levator scapulae,** and **rhomboids** (pp. 160–161).

The superficial intrinsic back muscles are located on the posterolateral portions of the neck covering deeper muscles. There are two muscles in this group—**splenius capitis** and **splenius cervicis**—which laterally flex, rotate, and extend the head and neck.

Intermediate layer

The **erector spinae,** also called **sacrospinalis,** forms the intermediate layer of the deep intrinsic muscles. The erector spinae is actually made up of three sets of muscles organized in parallel columns and is important in maintaining posture. It is often the muscle you injure when you lift a heavy object without bending your knees first.

Deep layer

Underneath the erector spinae muscles is another layer of muscles that help to support posture and assist the intermediate muscles in moving the spine.

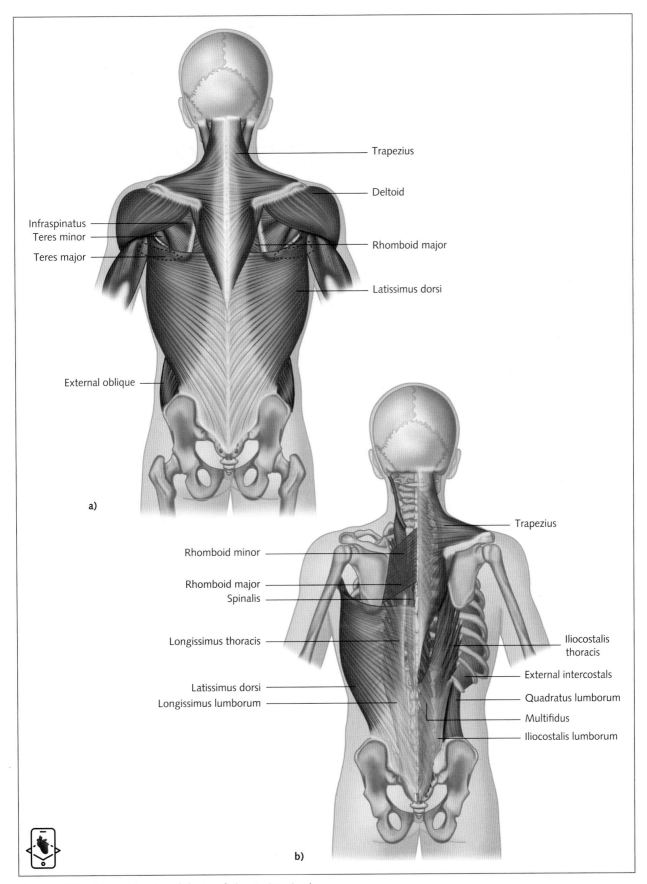

Figure 5.17 (a & b) *Muscles of the trunk (posterior view)*

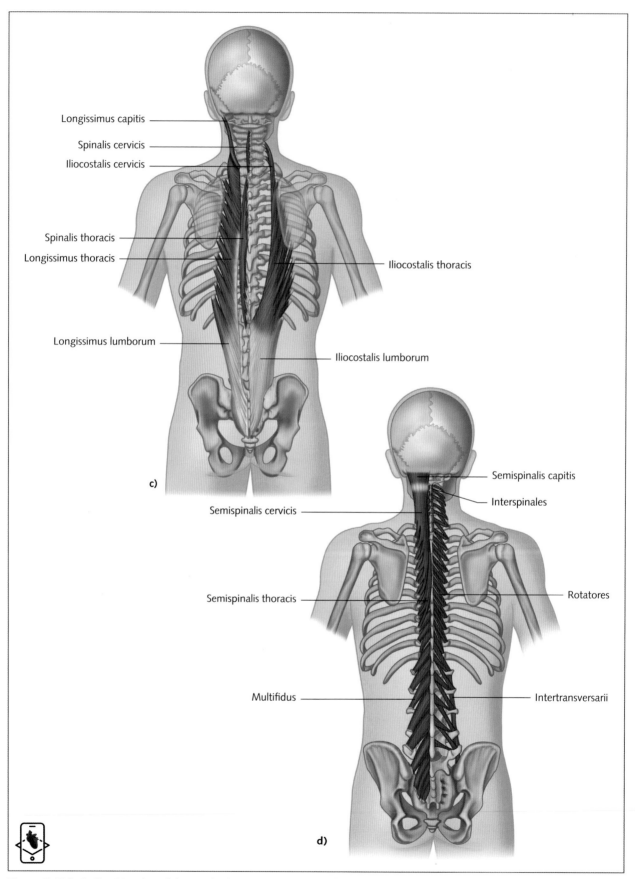

Figure 5.17 (c & d) *Muscles of the trunk, c) erector spinae muscles; d) transversospinalis muscles*

Muscles of the back that move the shoulder and arm

The **trapezius**, **levator scapulae**, and **rhomboid** muscles help to stabilize the scapula, which functions as a point of origin for many muscles. These muscles are easily affected by stress and can become hypertonic, causing neck pain, shoulder stiffness, and headaches.

Muscles located on the back that move the arm can be divided into those that originate on the scapula and those that originate on the axial skeleton.

The muscles originating on the scapula include the muscles of the rotator cuff (discussed earlier), which strengthen and reinforce the shoulder joint. More muscles originate on the scapula but are located on the arm itself. These are discussed in the section "Muscles of the arm and forearm."

The pectoralis major (discussed as a muscle of the anterior thorax) and latissimus dorsi originate on the axial skeleton. Together with the **subscapularis** and **teres major**, the **latissimus dorsi** forms the posterior wall of the armpit and moves the humerus.

MUSCLES THAT MOVE THE VERTEBRAL COLUMN				
Muscle	**Origin**	**Insertion**	**Nerve**	**Action**
Erector Spinae—Iliocostalis Portion				
Iliocostalis portion	*Lumborum:* sacrum, spinous processes of L1–5 and T11–12 and their supraspinous ligaments. Iliac crest *Thoracis:* angles of lower 6 ribs *Cervicis:* angles of ribs 3 to 6	*Lumborum:* angles of lower 6 or 7 ribs *Thoracis:* angles of upper 6 ribs and transverse process of C7 *Cervicis:* transverse processes of C4–6	Dorsal rami of cervical, thoracic, and lumbar spinal nerves	Extends and side flexes vertebral column. Draws ribs down for forceful inhalation (thoracis only)
Erector Spinae—Longissimus Portion				
Longissimus portion	*Thoracis:* blends with iliocostalis in lumbar region and is attached to transverse processes of lumbar vertebrae *Cervicis:* transverse processes of T1–5 *Capitis:* transverse processes of T1–5. Articular processes of C4–7	*Thoracis:* transverse processes of T1–12. Area between tubercles and angles of lower 9 or 10 ribs *Cervicis:* transverse processes of C2–6 *Capitis:* posterior margin of mastoid process of temporal bone	Dorsal rami of C1–S1	Extends and side flexes vertebral column. Draws ribs down for forceful inhalation (thoracis only). Extends and rotates head (capitis only)
Erector Spinae—Spinalis Portion				
Spinalis portion	*Thoracis:* spinous processes of T11–12 and L1–2 *Cervicis:* ligamentum nuchae. Spinous process of C7 *Capitis:* usually blends with semispinalis capitis	*Thoracis:* spinous processes of T1–8 *Cervicis:* spinous process of C2 *Capitis:* with semispinalis capitis	Dorsal rami of spinal nerves C2–L3	Extends vertebral column. Helps maintain correct curvature of spine in standing and sitting positions. Extends head (capitis only)

MUSCLES THAT MOVE THE VERTEBRAL COLUMN				
Muscle	Origin	Insertion	Nerve	Action
Spinotransversales Group				
Splenius capitis and splenius cervicis	*Capitis:* lower part of ligamentum nuchae. Spinous processes of C7 and T1–4 *Cervicis:* spinous processes of T3–6	*Capitis:* posterior aspect of mastoid process of temporal bone. Lateral part of superior nuchal line, deep to attachment of sternocleidomastoid *Cervicis:* posterior tubercles of transverse processes of C1–3	*Capitis:* dorsal rami of middle cervical nerves *Cervicis:* dorsal rami of lower cervical nerves	*Acting on both sides:* extend head and neck *Acting on one side:* side flex neck; rotate head to same side as contracting muscle
Transversospinales Group				
Semispinalis	*Thoracis:* transverse processes of T6–10 *Cervicis:* transverse processes of T1–6 *Capitis:* transverse processes of C4–T7	*Thoracis:* spinous processes of C6–T4 *Cervicis:* spinous processes of C2–5 *Capitis:* between superior and inferior nuchal lines of occipital bone	Dorsal rami of thoracic and cervical spinal nerves	Extends thoracic and cervical parts of vertebral column. Assists in rotation of thoracic and cervical vertebrae. Semispinalis capitis extends and assists in rotation of the head
Multifidus	Sacrum, origin of erector spinae, PSIS, mammillary processes of all lumbar vertebrae. Transverse processes of all thoracic vertebrae. Articular processes of lower 4 cervical vertebrae	Base of spinous processes of all vertebrae from L5 to C2	Dorsal rami of spinal nerves	Extension, side flexion, and rotation of vertebral column
Rotatores	Transverse process of each vertebra	Base of spinous process of adjoining vertebra above	Dorsal rami of spinal nerves	Rotate and assist in extension of vertebral column

Muscles of the arm and forearm

The humerus bone is moved by a number of muscles that all originate on the trunk of the body. Only two of them, the pectoralis major and latissimus dorsi discussed previously, originate on the axial skeleton. All the other muscles that move the humerus originate on the scapula, including the rotator cuff muscles, also previously discussed.

The shoulder joint is capable of a large variety of movements including flexion, extension, abduction, adduction, medial rotation, lateral rotation, and circumduction. It has more freedom of movement than any other joint in the body.

Muscles located on the arm that move the forearm

Some of the muscles located on the arm move the forearm. They originate on the scapula or humerus, pass over the elbow joint and insert into the radius and ulna. The elbow joint is a hinge joint and therefore capable of only flexion and extension. Thus, the

MUSCLES OF THE ARM

Muscle	Origin	Insertion	Nerve	Action
Muscles of the Arm—Anterior Compartment				
Biceps brachii	*Long head:* supraglenoid tubercle of scapula *Short head:* tip of coracoid process	Radial tuberosity	Musculocutaneous nerve C5, 6	Powerful flexor of forearm at elbow joint. Supinates forearm
Brachialis	Anterior aspect of humerus (medial and lateral surfaces) and adjacent intermuscular septae	Tuberosity of ulna	Musculocutaneous nerve C5, 6	Flexor of forearm at elbow joint
Coracobrachialis	Tip of coracoid process	Medial aspect of humerus at mid-shaft	Musculocutaneous nerve C5–7	Flexor of arm at glenohumeral joint
Muscles of the Arm—Posterior Compartment				
Triceps brachii	*Long head:* infraglenoid tubercle of scapula *Medial and lateral heads:* Posterior surface of humerus	Posterior part of olecranon process of ulna	Radial nerve C6–8	Extends forearm at elbow joint

muscles that move the forearm can be categorized into flexors and extensors. Some of these muscles also allow pronation and supination of the forearm at the wrist.

The arm is divided by a fascial layer known as the medial and lateral intermuscular septa; this layer divides the arm into anterior and posterior compartments. These compartments contain muscles that are innervated by the same nerve and perform the same action.

Brachialis and **biceps brachii** lie anteriorly and are the major flexors at the elbow. The three-headed **triceps brachii** muscle lies posteriorly and is the major extensor of the elbow, together with **anconeus**. Both biceps brachii and **supinator** act as the **supinators** of the forearm, whereas **pronator teres** and **pronator quadratus** are the major **pronators**.

Muscles that move the wrist

The muscles of the forearm move the wrist and can be divided into anterior and posterior compartments. The tendons of these muscles are held close to the bones by strong fibrous bands called retinacula. The **flexor retinaculum** (transverse carpal ligament)

is found on the palmar surface of the carpal bones, while the **extensor retinaculum** (dorsal carpal ligament) is found over the dorsal surface of the carpal bones.

The anterior compartment contains the **forearm flexors**, arranged in superficial, intermediate, and deep layers:

- **Superficial:** Four superficial muscles are attached proximally to the medial epicondyle of the humerus by a common flexor tendon. These muscles are the **pronator teres, flexor carpi radialis, palmaris longus,** and **flexor carpi ulnaris** and they pronate the forearm and flex the wrist, fingers, and thumb.
- **Intermediate:** This consists of one muscle, the **flexor digitorum superficialis**. It flexes the fingers.
- **Deep:** This comprises three muscles, the **flexor digitorum profundus, flexor pollicis longus,** and **pronator quadratus**.

Following a similar pattern of superficial and deep layers, but this time arising from the lateral

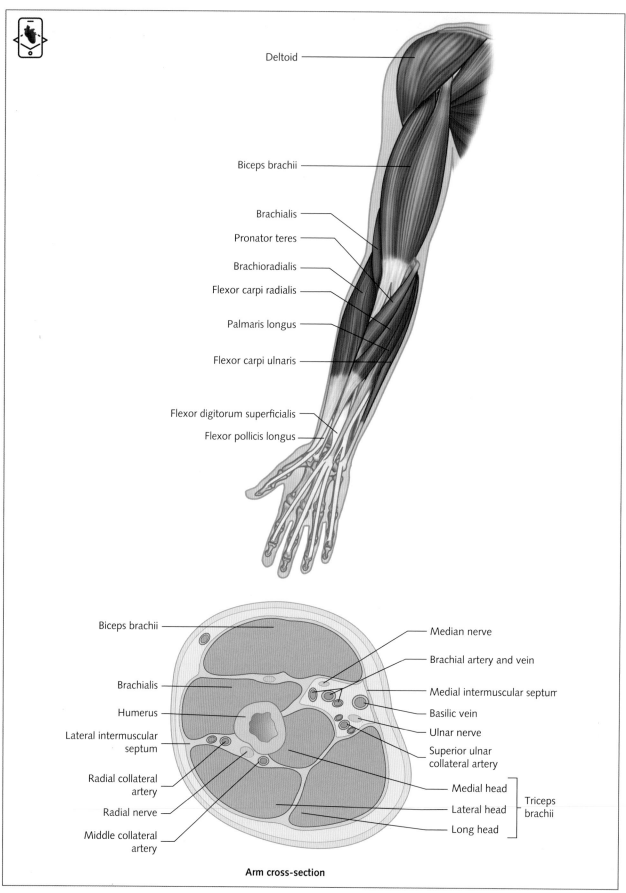

Deltoid

Biceps brachii

Brachialis

Pronator teres

Brachioradialis

Flexor carpi radialis

Palmaris longus

Flexor carpi ulnaris

Flexor digitorum superficialis

Flexor pollicis longus

Biceps brachii

Brachialis

Humerus

Lateral intermuscular septum

Radial collateral artery

Radial nerve

Middle collateral artery

Median nerve

Brachial artery and vein

Medial intermuscular septum

Basilic vein

Ulnar nerve

Superior ulnar collateral artery

Medial head

Lateral head — Triceps brachii

Long head

Arm cross-section

Figure 5.18 (a) *Muscles of the upper limb (anterior view)*

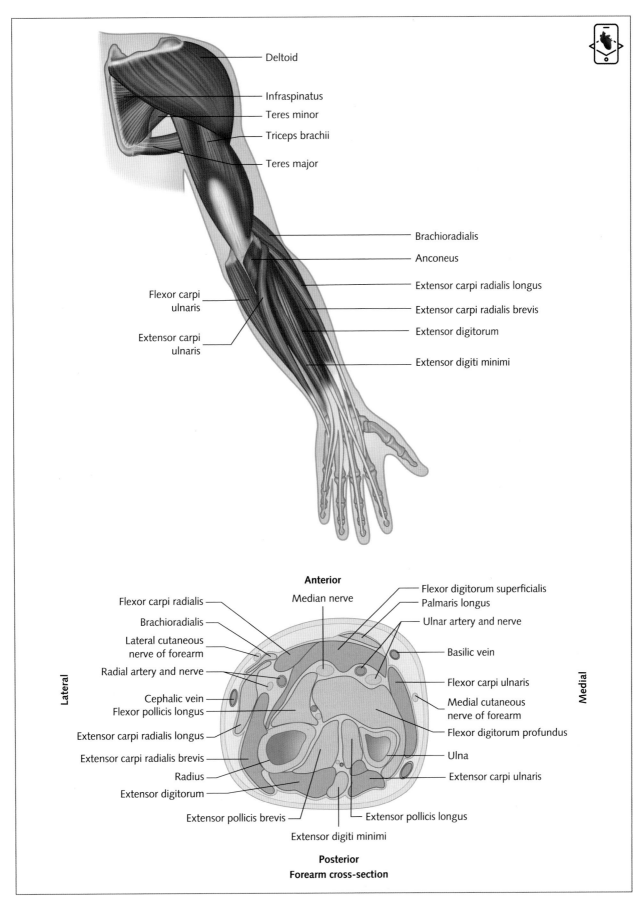

Deltoid

Infraspinatus

Teres minor

Triceps brachii

Teres major

Brachioradialis

Anconeus

Extensor carpi radialis longus

Extensor carpi radialis brevis

Extensor digitorum

Extensor digiti minimi

Flexor carpi ulnaris

Extensor carpi ulnaris

Anterior

Median nerve

Flexor digitorum superficialis

Palmaris longus

Ulnar artery and nerve

Flexor carpi radialis

Brachioradialis

Lateral cutaneous nerve of forearm

Radial artery and nerve

Basilic vein

Flexor carpi ulnaris

Medial cutaneous nerve of forearm

Cephalic vein

Flexor pollicis longus

Flexor digitorum profundus

Extensor carpi radialis longus

Extensor carpi radialis brevis

Radius

Ulna

Extensor carpi ulnaris

Extensor digitorum

Extensor pollicis brevis

Extensor pollicis longus

Extensor digiti minimi

Lateral

Medial

Posterior

Forearm cross-section

Figure 5.18 (b) *Muscles of the upper limb (posterior view)*

epicondyle, the posterior compartment contains the **extensors** of the wrist and fingers, which act as antagonists to the flexor muscles. In general, the extensors are somewhat weaker than the flexor muscles that they work against.

MUSCLES OF THE FOREARM

Muscle	Origin	Insertion	Nerve	Action
Muscles of the Anterior Compartment of the Forearm—Superficial Layer				
Flexor carpi unaris	*Humeral head:* medial epicondyle *Ulnar head:* olecranon and posterior border of ulna	Pisiform. Hook of hamate. Base of 5th metacarpal	Ulnar nerve C7, 8, T1	Flexes and adducts wrist
Palmaris longus	Medial epicondyle of humerus	Palmar aponeurosis of hand	Median nerve C(6), 7, 8	Flexes wrist joint. Tenses palmar fascia
Flexor carpi radialis	Medial epicondyle of humerus	Bases of 2nd and 3rd metacarpals	Median nerve C6, 7	Flexes and abducts wrist joint
Pronator teres	*Humeral head:* medial epicondyle and adjacent supra-epicondylar ridge *Ulnar head:* medial border of coronoid process	Mid-lateral surface of radius	Median nerve C6, 7	Pronates forearm
Muscles of the Anterior Compartment of the Forearm—Intermediate Layer				
Flexor digitorum superficialis	*Humero-ulnar head:* medial epicondyle. Adjacent border of coronoid process *Radial head:* oblique line of radius	Four tendons that insert into the sides of the middle phalanges of the four fingers	Median nerve C8, T1	Flexes proximal interphalangeal joints of the index, middle, ring, and little fingers
Muscles of the Anterior Compartment of the Forearm—Deep Layer				
Flexor digitorum profundus	Medial and anterior surfaces of ulna. Medial half of interosseous membrane	Four tendons that attach to the palmar surfaces of the distal phalanges of the index, middle, ring, and little fingers	*Medial half:* ulnar nerve C8, T1 *Lateral half:* anterior interosseous branch of median nerve C8, T1	Flexes distal interphalangeal joints of the index, middle, ring, and little fingers
Flexor pollicis longus	Anterior surface of shaft of radius. Radial half of interosseous membrane	Palmar surface of base of distal phalanx of thumb	Anterior interosseous branch of median nerve C(6), 7, 8	Flexes interphalangeal joint of thumb

MUSCLES OF THE FOREARM

Muscle	Origin	Insertion	Nerve	Action
Muscles of the Anterior Compartment of the Forearm—Deep Layer (*continued*)				
Pronator quadratus	Linear ridge on distal anterior surface of ulna	Distal anterior surface of radius	Anterior interosseous branch of median nerve C7, 8	Pronation
Muscles of the Posterior Compartment of the Forearm—Superficial Layer				
Brachioradialis	Proximal part of lateral supraepicondylar ridge and adjacent intermuscular septum	Lower surface of distal end of radius	Radial nerve C5, 6	Accessory flexor of elbow joint when forearm is midpronated
Extensor carpi radialis longus	Distal part of lateral supraepicondylar ridge and adjacent intermuscular septum	Dorsal surface of base of 2nd metacarpal	Radial nerve C6, 7	Extends and abducts wrist
Extensor carpi radialis brevis	Lateral epicondyle and adjacent intermuscular septum	Dorsal surface of base of 2nd and 3rd metacarpals	Radial nerve C7, 8	Extends and abducts wrist
Extensor digitorum	Lateral epicondyle and adjacent intermuscular septum and deep fascia	Four tendons that insert via extensor hoods into the dorsal aspects of the bases of the middle and distal phalanges of the index, middle, ring, and little fingers	Posterior interosseous nerve C7, 8	Extends the index, middle, ring, and little fingers
Extensor digiti minimi	Lateral epicondyle and adjacent intermuscular septum together with extensor digitorum	Extensor hood of little finger	Posterior interosseous nerve C6, 7, 8	Extends little finger
Extensor carpi unaris	Lateral epicondyle and posterior border of ulna	Tubercle on base of medial side of 5th metacarpal	Posterior interosseous nerve C6, 7, 8	Extends and adducts wrist
Anconeus	Lateral epicondyle	Olecranon process and proximal posterior surface of ulna	Radial nerve C6, 7, 8	Abduction of ulna in pronation. Accessory extensor of elbow joint

MUSCLES OF THE FOREARM				
Muscle	Origin	Insertion	Nerve	Action
Muscles of the Posterior Compartment of the Forearm—Deep Layer				
Supinator	*Superficial part:* lateral epicondyle. Radial collateral and anular ligaments *Deep part:* supinator crest of ulna	Lateral surface of radius superior to the anterior oblique line	Deep branch of the radial nerve C7, 8	Supination
Abductor pollicis longus	Posterior surfaces of ulna and radius. Intervening interosseous membrane	Lateral side of base of 1st metacarpal	Posterior interosseous nerve C7, 8	Abducts carpometacarpal joint of thumb; accessory extensor of thumb
Extensor pollicis brevis	Posterior surface of radius. Adjacent interosseous membrane	Base of dorsal surface of proximal phalanx of thumb	Posterior interosseous nerve C7, 8	Extends metacarpophalangeal joint of thumb
Extensor pollicis longus	Posterior surface of ulna. Adjacent interosseous membrane	Dorsal surface of base of distal phalanx of thumb	Posterior interosseous nerve C7, 8	Extends interphalangeal joint of thumb
Extensor indicis	Posterior surface of ulna. Adjacent interosseous membrane	Extensor hood of index finger	Posterior interosseous nerve C7, 8	Extends index finger

Muscles of the hand

The principal role of the hand itself is grasping and manipulation, with the muscle groups involved termed extrinsic and intrinsic. The **extrinsic muscles** originate more proximally in the forearm and insert into the hand as long tendons to provide crude movements. The **intrinsic muscles**, located within the hand itself, are responsible for fine control of the complicated movements of the fingers, and are compartmentalized as follows:

- The **thenar eminence** is a raised area of firm tissue found on the radial side/lateral surface of the palm of the hand, beneath the thumb. It is responsible for opposition of the thumb and is composed of the three thenar muscles, which make up the thenar compartment (namely, the **abductor pollicis brevis**, **flexor pollicis brevis**, and the **opponens pollicis**), as well as the **adductor pollicis**, which forms the **adductor compartment**.
- The **hypothenar eminence** (or **hypothenar compartment**) is an area of soft tissue found on the ulnar side of the palm, beneath the little finger. It is composed of three muscles that move the little finger. Namely, the **abductor digiti minimi**, **flexor digiti minimi brevis**, and **opponens digiti minimi**.
- The **central compartment** is composed of the **lumbricals** and the **long flexor tendons**.
- The **interosseous compartments** are located between the metacarpals and contain the **interossei**.

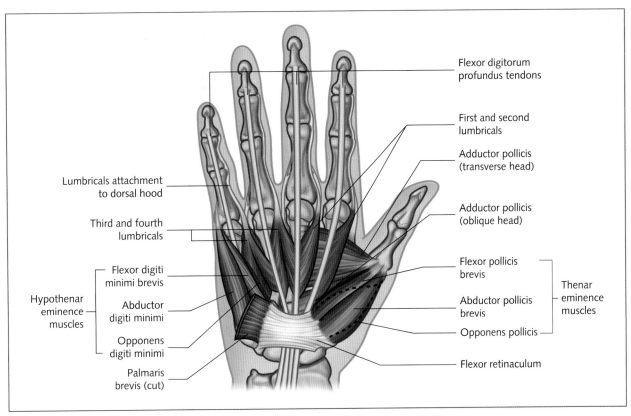

Figure 5.19 *Muscles of the hand (palmar view)*

MUSCLES OF THE HAND

Muscle	Origin	Insertion	Nerve	Action
Palmaris brevis	Palmar aponeurosis. Flexor retinaculum	Skin on ulnar border of hand	Superficial branch of ulnar nerve C(7), 8, T1	Improves grip
Dorsal interossei	Adjacent sides of metacarpals	Extensor hood and base of proximal phalanges of index, middle, and ring fingers	Deep branch of ulnar nerve C8, T1	Abduction of index, middle, and ring fingers at metacarpophalangeal joints
Palmar interossei	Sides of metacarpals	Extensor hoods of the thumb, index, ring, and little fingers and proximal phalanx of thumb	Deep branch of ulnar nerve C8, T1	Adduction of the thumb, index, ring, and little fingers at metacarpophalangeal joints
Adductor pollicis	*Transverse head:* palmar surface of 3rd metacarpal *Oblique head:* capitate and bases of 2nd and 3rd metacarpals	Base of proximal phalanx of thumb and extensor hood of thumb	Deep branch of ulnar nerve C8, T1	Adducts thumb

MUSCLES OF THE HAND

Muscle	Origin	Insertion	Nerve	Action
Lumbricals	Tendons of flexor digitorum profundus	Extensor hoods of index, ring, middle, and little fingers	*Lateral lumbricals:* digital branches of median nerve *Medial lumbricals:* deep branch of ulnar nerve	Extend interphalangeal joints and simultaneously flex metacarpophalangeal joints
Muscles of the Hand—Hypothenar Eminence				
Abductor digiti minimi	Pisiform, pisohamate ligament, and tendon of flexor carpi ulnaris	Proximal phalanx of little finger	Deep branch of ulnar nerve C(7), 8, T1	Abducts little finger at metacarpophalangeal joint
Opponens digiti minimi	Hook of hamate. Flexor retinaculum	Entire length of medial border of 5th metacarpal	Deep branch of ulnar nerve C(7), 8, T1	Laterally rotates 5th metacarpal
Flexor digiti minimi brevis	Hook of hamate. Flexor retinaculum	Proximal phalanx of little finger	Deep branch of ulnar nerve C(7), 8, T1	Flexes little finger at metacarpophalangeal joint
Muscles of the Hand—Thenar Eminence				
Abductor pollicis brevis	Tubercles of trapezium and scaphoid and adjacent flexor retinaculum	Proximal phalanx and extensor hood of thumb	Recurrent branch of median nerve C8, T1	Abducts thumb at metacarpophalangeal joint
Opponens pollicis	Flexor retinaculum. Tubercle of trapezium	Entire length of radial border of 1st metacarpal	Recurrent branch of median nerve C8, T1	Medially rotates thumb
Flexor pollicis brevis	Flexor retinaculum. Tubercle of trapezium	Proximal phalanx of thumb	Recurrent branch of median nerve C8, T1	Flexes thumb at metacarpophalangeal joint

Muscles of the hip

The muscles of the hip joint move the femur. They generally originate on the hip bones and insert on the femur. Some of them cross both the hip and knee joints to insert on the tibia and fibula. The hip joint is a ball-and-socket joint that allows for flexion, extension, abduction, adduction, circumduction, and rotation. In addition to functioning in movement, the muscles of the lower limb are important in maintaining posture and stability. These muscles are generally large and powerful.

Psoas major and **iliacus** are the only anterior muscles that move the femur and, because they are located in the hip and lower-back region, they are often considered muscles of the trunk. Together they form the **iliopsoas**, which is the main hip flexor and lower-back stabilizer. Lower-back and hip problems often develop if this muscle is hypertonic.

The posterior muscles that move the femur include the **gluteals, piriformis, obturators, gemelli**, and **quadratus femoris**. Not all of these muscles are discussed here. The **gluteus maximus** muscle is the heaviest muscle in the body and, together with the **gluteus medius** and **minimus**, it forms the buttock. Imbalances in these muscles can lead to lower-back, hip, and knee problems.

Tensor fasciae latae is a deep lateral muscle that has a long tendon called the fascia lata tendon. This joins the tendon of the gluteus maximus muscle to form a structure known as the iliotibial tract (ITT) or iliotibial band (ITB).

Muscles of the thigh

The muscles located in the thigh generally originate in the hip bones, cross the knee joint, and insert into the leg (tibia and fibula). They permit flexion, extension, and slight rotation of the leg and are categorized into medial, anterior, and posterior compartments. These compartments are separated by deep fascia.

The medial compartment of the thigh is called the adductor compartment because the muscles within it all adduct the femur. These muscles include the adductors, pectineus, and gracilis, and they are the muscles affected when you pull or strain your groin.

The anterior compartment of the thigh is called the extensor compartment because all the muscles within it extend the leg. Some of the muscles also flex the thigh (namely, the rectus femoris and sartorius). The anterior compartment includes the quadriceps femoris and sartorius muscles. The quadriceps femoris (often referred to as the quads) is made up of four distinct parts: the rectus femoris and the three vasti muscles. Their tendon, the quadriceps tendon, attaches to the patella.

The posterior compartment of the thigh is called the flexor compartment because its muscles flex the leg. Most of them also extend the thigh. The flexor compartment is composed of three muscles with long, stringlike tendons that are collectively called the hamstrings. These muscles are the biceps femoris, semitendinosus, and semimembranosus.

MUSCLES OF THE HIP AND THIGH				
Muscle	Origin	Insertion	Nerve	Action
Muscles of the Gluteal Region				
Gluteus maximus	Outer surface of ilium and posterior surface of sacrum and coccyx (over sacroiliac joint)	Posterior aspect of iliotibial tract. Gluteal tuberosity of proximal femur	Inferior gluteal nerve L5, S1, 2	Powerful extensor of flexed femur at hip joint. Lateral stabilizer of hip and knee joints. Laterally rotates and abducts thigh
Tensor fasciae latae	Lateral aspect of crest of ilium between ASIS and tubercle of the crest	Iliotibial tract	Superior gluteal nerve L4, 5, S1	Stabilizes the knee in extension
Gluteus medius	External surface of ilium between anterior and posterior gluteal lines	Oblique ridge on lateral surface of greater trochanter	Superior gluteal nerve L4, 5, S1	Abducts femur at hip joint. Medially rotates thigh
Gluteus minimus	External surface of ilium between anterior and inferior gluteal lines	Anterolateral border of greater trochanter	Superior gluteal nerve L4, 5, S1	Abducts, medially rotates, and may assist in flexion of hip joint
Piriformis	Anterior surface of sacrum between anterior sacral foramina	Medial side of superior border of greater trochanter	Branches from sacral nerves S1, 2	Laterally rotates extended femur at hip joint. Abducts flexed femur at hip joint

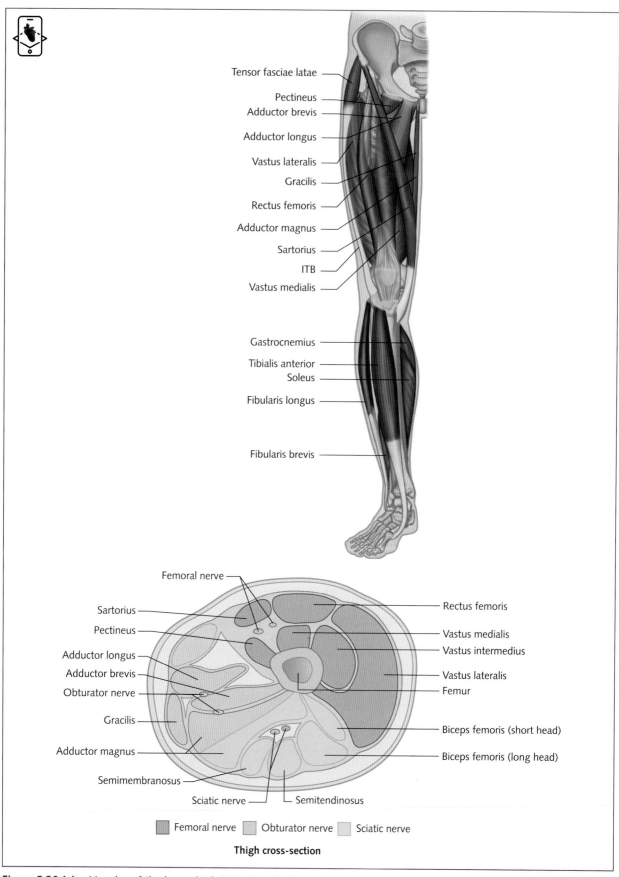

Figure 5.20 (a) *Muscles of the lower limb (anterior view)*

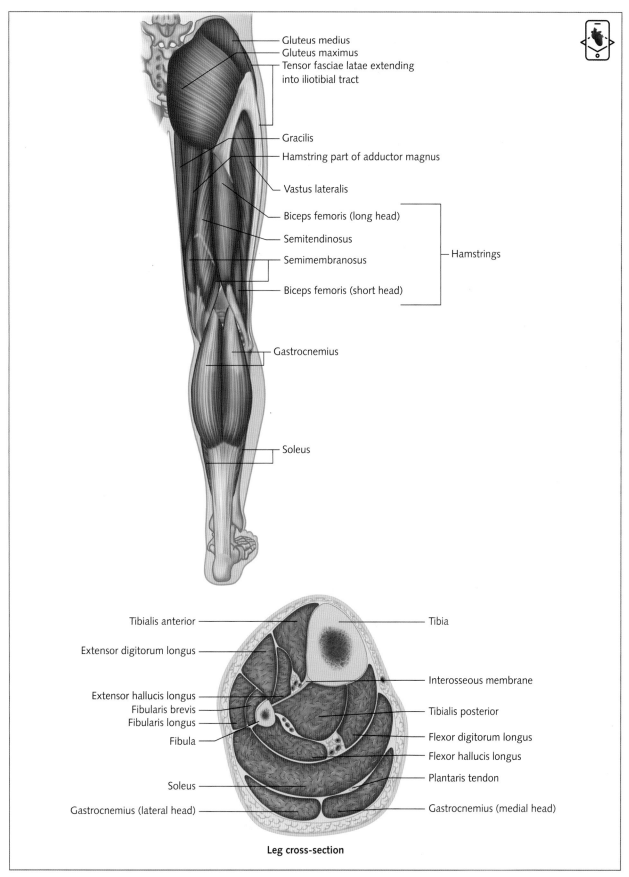

Gluteus medius
Gluteus maximus
Tensor fasciae latae extending into iliotibial tract
Gracilis
Hamstring part of adductor magnus
Vastus lateralis
Biceps femoris (long head)
Semitendinosus
Semimembranosus
Biceps femoris (short head)
Hamstrings
Gastrocnemius
Soleus

Tibialis anterior
Extensor digitorum longus
Extensor hallucis longus
Fibularis brevis
Fibularis longus
Fibula
Soleus
Gastrocnemius (lateral head)

Tibia
Interosseous membrane
Tibialis posterior
Flexor digitorum longus
Flexor hallucis longus
Plantaris tendon
Gastrocnemius (medial head)

Leg cross-section

Figure 5.20 (b) *Muscles of the lower limb (posterior view)*

MUSCLES OF THE HIP AND THIGH

Muscle	Origin	Insertion	Nerve	Action
Muscles of the Gluteal Region (*continued*)				
Deep lateral hip rotators	*Obturator internus:* inner surface of ischium, pubis, and ilium *Gemellus superior:* external surface of ischial spine *Gemellus inferior:* upper aspect of ischial tuberosity *Quadratus femoris:* lateral edge of ischium just anterior to ischial tuberosity	Greater trochanter of femur (except quadratus femoris, which inserts just behind and below the others)	*Obturator internus and gemellus superior:* nerve to obturator internus, L5, S1 *Gemellus inferior and quadratus femoris:* nerve to quadratus femoris, L5, S1, (2)	Laterally rotate hip joint. Abduct flexed femur at hip joint. Help hold head of femur in acetabulum
Muscles of the Anterior Compartment of the Thigh				
Sartorius	Anterior superior iliac spine	Medial surface of tibia just inferomedial to tibial tuberosity	Femoral nerve L2, 3, (4)	Flexes the thigh at the hip joint. Flexes the leg at the knee joint
Quadriceps femoris	*Rectus femoris:* straight head: AIIS; reflected head: groove above acetabulum (on ilium) *Vasti group:* upper half of shaft of femur	Patella, then via patellar ligament, into the tibial tuberosity	Femoral nerve L2, 3, 4	*Rectus femoris:* flexes the thigh at the hip joint and extends leg at the knee joint *Vasti group:* extend leg at the knee joint
Muscles of the Medial Compartment of the Thigh				
Gracilis	A line on the external surfaces of the pubis, the inferior pubic ramus, and ramus of the ischium	Medial surface of proximal shaft of tibia	Obturator nerve L2, 3	Adducts thigh at hip joint. Flexes leg at knee joint
Pectineus	Pecten pubis and adjacent bone of pelvis	Oblique line, from base of lesser trochanter to linea aspera of femur	Femoral nerve L2, 3	Adducts and flexes thigh at hip joint
Obturator externus	External surface of obturator membrane and adjacent bone	Trochanteric fossa	Posterior division of obturator nerve L3, 4	Laterally rotates thigh at hip joint

MUSCLES OF THE HIP AND THIGH

Muscle	Origin	Insertion	Nerve	Action
Muscles of the Medial Compartment of the Thigh (*continued*)				
Adductors	Anterior part of the pubic bone (ramus). Adductor magnus also takes its origin from the ischial tuberosity	Entire length of femur, along linea aspera and medial supracondylar line to adductor tubercle on medial epicondyle of femur	*Magnus:* obturator nerve L2, 3, 4. Sciatic nerve L2, 3, 4 *Brevis:* obturator nerve L2, 3 *Longus:* obturator nerve L2, 3, 4	Adduct and medially rotate thigh at hip joint
Muscles of the Posterior Compartment of the Thigh				
Hamstrings	Ischial tuberosity. Biceps femoris (short head only): lateral lip of linea aspera	*Semimembranosus:* groove and adjacent bone on medial and posterior surface of medial tibial condyle *Semitendinosus:* medial surface of proximal tibia *Biceps femoris:* head of fibula	Sciatic nerve L5, S1, 2	Flex leg at knee joint Semimembranosus and semitendinosus extend thigh at hip joint, medially rotate thigh at hip joint, and leg at knee joint Biceps femoris extends and laterally rotates thigh at hip joint and laterally rotates leg at knee joint

Muscles of the leg

The muscles located in the leg generally originate in the tibia and fibula (sometimes in the femur or knee capsule), cross the ankle joint, and insert on the foot. Like the muscles of the thigh, the muscles of the leg are divided into three compartments that are separated by deep fascia: the anterior, posterior, and lateral compartments. In addition, the posterior compartment may be further subdivided into superficial, intermediate, and deep layers.

The **anterior** or **extensor compartment** of the leg contains muscles that extend (dorsiflex) the foot at the ankle joint and extend the toes. Its tendons are held firmly to the ankle by the **transverse ligament** of the ankle (**superior extensor retinaculum**) and the **cruciate ligament** of the ankle (**inferior extensor retinaculum**). There are four muscles within this group. **Tibialis anterior** dorsiflexes and inverts the foot at the ankle joint. **Extensor hallucis longus** and **extensor digitorum longus** extend the toes and help dorsiflex the ankle. **Fibularis tertius** works with extensor digitorum longus to dorsiflex the foot at the ankle joint and, together with muscles in the lateral compartment, helps evert the foot.

The **posterior** or **flexor compartment** of the leg contains the muscles that plantar flex the foot and flex the toes. These are commonly known as the **calf muscles** and are arranged in three layers, like an onion skin.

The most superficial layer contains the **gastrocnemius, soleus,** and **plantaris** muscles, which join to form the **Achilles tendon** (**calcaneal tendon**), the strongest tendon in the body. The gastrocnemius has two heads, and together with the one head of the

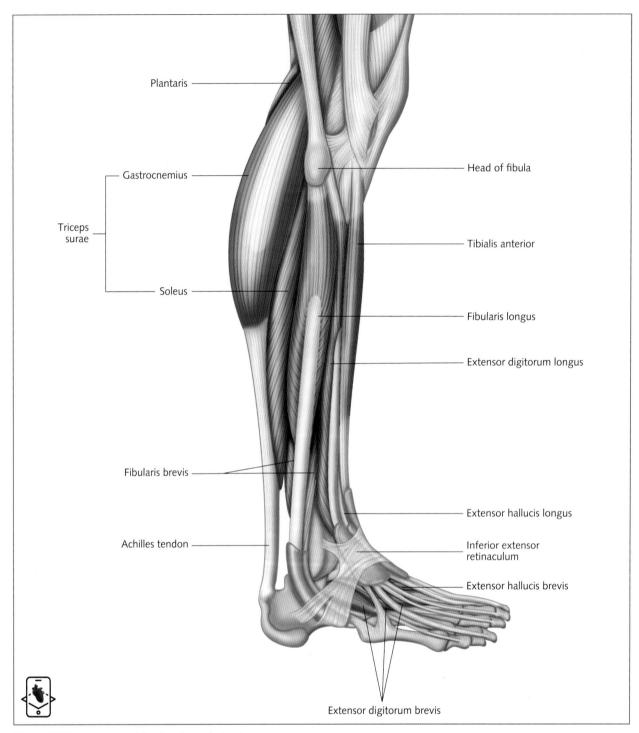

Figure 5.21 *Muscles of the leg (lateral view)*

soleus, is also referred to as the **triceps surae**. The word *triceps* means "three-headed" and the word *surae* means "of the calf."

The soleus is the deepest of these muscles and arises from the soleal line on the tibia and from the back of the fibula. It is so named as it is fish shaped. The gastrocnemius forms the bulk of the muscle mass of

the calf and forms the posterior muscular wall of the knee. It arises from two heads, one from each of the medial and lateral femoral condyles. On the inner aspect of the lateral head of this muscle the small muscular belly of the plantaris arises from the femur but soon narrows to form a delicate tendon (the longest tendon in the body). All three muscles are plantar flexors of the foot at the ankle joint, with gastrocnemius and plantaris also aiding flexion of the knee.

The intermediate layer comprises **flexor hallucis longus** (FHL) and **flexor digitorum longus** (FDL). Both of these muscles plantar flex the foot at the ankle joint; FHL flexes the distal phalanx of the big toe and supports the medial longitudinal arch of the foot and FDL flexes the distal phalanges of the lateral four toes and supports the lateral longitudinal arch of the foot.

The **tibialis posterior** and **popliteus** muscles form the deepest of these layers. Popliteus arises above the much larger tibialis posterior, which itself arises from the tibia, fibula, and the interosseous membrane. Tibialis posterior plantar flexes the foot at the ankle joint, helping to maintain the medial longitudinal arch of the foot, and with the aid of its anterior component, tibialis anterior, it is also an invertor of the foot.

Situated in the **lateral group** are the **fibulares** muscles: **fibularis longus** arises from the upper part of the fibula, and **fibularis brevis** from lower down the fibula. Both muscles plantar flex the foot at the ankle joint but are principally evertors of the ankle.

MUSCLES OF THE LEG				
Muscle	**Origin**	**Insertion**	**Nerve**	**Action**
Muscles of the Anterior Compartment of the Leg				
Tibialis anterior	Lateral surface of tibia and adjacent interosseous membrane	Medial and inferior surfaces of medial cuneiform and adjacent surfaces on base of 1st metatarsal	Deep fibular nerve L4, 5	Dorsiflexes foot at ankle joint. Inverts foot
Extensor digitorum longus	Proximal one-half of medial surface of fibula and related surface of lateral tibial condyle	Along dorsal surface of the 4 lateral toes. Each tendon divides to attach to bases of middle and distal phalanges	Deep fibular nerve L5, S1	Extends lateral four toes and dorsiflexes foot
Extensor hallucis longus	Middle one-half of medial surface of fibula and adjacent interosseous membrane	Base of distal phalanx of great toe	Deep fibular nerve L5, S1	Extends great toe. Dorsiflexes foot
Fibularis tertius	Distal part of medial surface of fibula	Dorsomedial surface of base of 5th metatarsal	Deep fibular nerve L5, S1	Dorsiflexes and everts foot
Muscles of the Posterior Compartment of the Leg—Superficial Layer				
Gastrocnemius	*Medial head:* posterior surface of distal femur just superior to medial condyle *Lateral head:* upper posterolateral surface of lateral femoral condyle	Posterior surface of calcaneus via the Achilles tendon	Tibial nerve S1, 2	Plantar flexes foot. Flexes knee

MUSCLES OF THE LEG

Muscle	Origin	Insertion	Nerve	Action
Muscles of the Posterior Compartment of the Leg—Superficial Layer (*continued*)				
Soleus	Posterior aspect of fibular head and adjacent surfaces of neck and proximal shaft. Soleal line and medial border of tibia. Tendinous arch between tibial and fibular attachments	Posterior surface of calcaneus via the Achilles tendon	Tibial nerve S1, 2	Plantar flexes foot
Plantaris	Lower part of lateral supracondylar line of femur and oblique popliteal ligament of knee joint	Posterior surface of calcaneus via the Achilles tendon	Tibial nerve S1, 2	Plantar flexes foot. Flexes knee
Muscles of the Posterior Compartment of the Leg—Intermediate Layer				
Flexor digitorum longus	Medial side of posterior surface of tibia, below soleal line	Plantar surfaces of bases of distal phalanges of lateral 4 toes	Tibial nerve S2, 3	Flexes lateral four toes
Flexor hallucis longus	Lower two-thirds of posterior surface of fibula and adjacent interosseous membrane	Plantar surface of base of distal phalanx of great toe	Tibial nerve S2, 3	Flexes great toe, and is important in the final propulsive thrust of foot during walking
Muscles of the Posterior Compartment of the Leg—Deep Layer				
Tibialis posterior	Posterior surfaces of interosseous membrane and adjacent regions of tibia and fibula	Mainly to tuberosity of navicular and adjacent region of medial cuneiform	Tibial nerve L4, 5	Inverts and plantar flexes foot
Popliteus	Lateral femoral condyle	Posterior surface of proximal tibia	Tibial nerve L4, 5, S1	Stabilizes and unlocks the knee joint
Muscles of the Lateral Compartment of the Leg				
Fibularis longus	Upper two-thirds of lateral surface of fibular head, fibula, and occasionally lateral tibial condyle	Lateral side of distal end of medial cuneiform. Base of 1st metatarsal	Superficial fibular nerve L5, S1, 2	Everts and plantar flexes foot
Fibularis brevis	Lower two-thirds of lateral surface of shaft of fibula	Lateral tubercle at base of 5th metatarsal	Superficial fibular nerve L5, S1, 2	Everts foot

Muscles of the foot

The muscles acting on the foot can be divided into the extrinsic and intrinsic muscles. The **extrinsic muscles** arise from the anterior, lateral, and posterior compartments of the leg. They are mainly responsible for eversion, inversion, and plantar flexion of the foot.

The **intrinsic muscles** are located within the foot and are responsible for the fine motor actions of the foot.

There are two intrinsic muscles located on the **dorsum** (top) of the foot. They primarily extend the toes, but also assist some of the extrinsic muscles in their actions.

There are 10 intrinsic muscles on the **plantar aspect/ sole** of the foot. They act collectively to stabilize the arches of the foot, and individually to control movement of the digits. The sole can be described as consisting of an aponeurosis and then four muscle layers.

The **plantar aponeurosis**, also called the **plantar fascia**, is a fibrous flat sheet that lies deep to the superficial fascia of the sole and covers the first layer of muscles. The muscular layers of the sole are:

- First layer: **abductor hallucis**, **flexor digitorum brevis**, and **abductor digiti minimi**
- Second layer: **quadratus plantae** and **lumbricals**
- Third layer: **flexor hallucis brevis**, **adductor hallucis**, and **flexor digiti minimi brevis**
- Fourth layer: **dorsal** and **plantar interossei**.

Like the hand, the foot has lumbrical and interosseous muscles, but their functions are far less important.

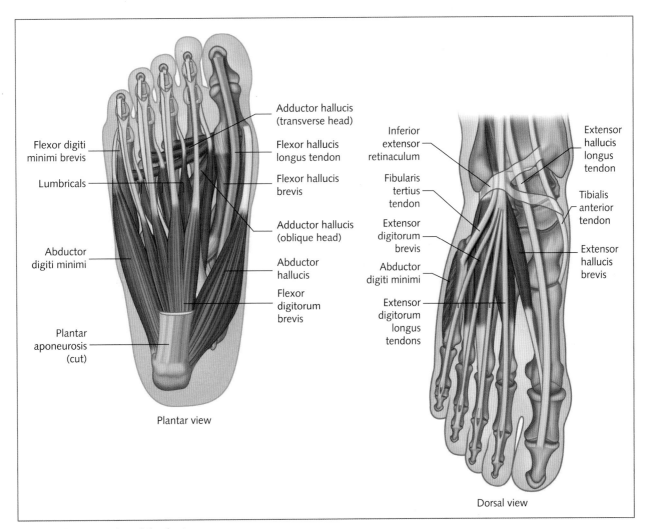

Flexor digiti minimi brevis

Lumbricals

Abductor digiti minimi

Plantar aponeurosis (cut)

Adductor hallucis (transverse head)

Flexor hallucis longus tendon

Flexor hallucis brevis

Adductor hallucis (oblique head)

Abductor hallucis

Flexor digitorum brevis

Plantar view

Inferior extensor retinaculum

Fibularis tertius tendon

Extensor digitorum brevis

Abductor digiti minimi

Extensor digitorum longus tendons

Extensor hallucis longus tendon

Tibialis anterior tendon

Extensor hallucis brevis

Dorsal view

Figure 5.22 *Muscles of the foot*

MUSCLES OF THE FOOT

Muscle	Origin	Insertion	Nerve	Action
Muscles of the Sole of the Foot—First Layer				
Abductor hallucis	Medial process of calcaneal tuberosity	Medial side of base of proximal phalanx of great toe	Medial plantar nerve from tibial nerve S1–3	Abducts and flexes great toe at metatarsophalangeal joint
Flexor digitorum brevis	Medial process of calcaneal tuberosity and plantar aponeurosis	Sides of plantar surfaces of middle phalanges of lateral 4 toes	Medial plantar nerve from tibial nerve S1–3	Flexes lateral four toes at proximal interphalangeal joint
Abductor digiti minimi	Lateral and medial processes of calcaneal tuberosity, and band of connective tissue connecting calcaneus with base of 5th metatarsal	Lateral side of base of proximal phalanx of little toe	Lateral plantar nerve from tibial nerve S1–3	Abducts 5th toe at metatarsophalangeal joint
Muscles of the Sole of the Foot—Second Layer				
Quadratus plantae	Medial surface of calcaneus and lateral process of calcaneal tuberosity	Lateral border of tendon of flexor digitorum longus in proximal sole of foot	Lateral plantar nerve from tibial nerve S1–3	Flexes distal phalanges of 2nd to 5th toes
Lumbricals	*1st lumbrical:* medial side of tendon of flexor digitorum longus associated with 2nd toe *2nd to 4th lumbricals:* adjacent tendons of flexor digitorum longus	Medial free margins of extensor hoods of 2nd to 5th toes	*1st lumbrical:* medial plantar nerve from tibial nerve *Lateral three lumbricals:* lateral plantar nerve from tibial nerve S2, 3	Flex metatarsophalangeal joint and extend interphalangeal joints
Muscles of the Sole of the Foot—Third Layer				
Flexor hallucis brevis	Medial part of plantar surface of cuboid, and adjacent part of lateral cuneiform. Tendon of tibialis posterior	Lateral and medial sides of base of proximal phalanx of great toe	Medial plantar nerve from tibial nerve S1, 2	Flexes metatarsophalangeal joint of great toe
Adductor hallucis	*Transverse head:* ligaments associated with metatarsophalangeal joints of lateral 3 toes *Oblique head:* bases of 2nd to 4th metatarsals; sheath covering fibularis longus tendon	Lateral side of base of proximal phalanx of great toe	Lateral plantar nerve from tibial nerve S2, 3	Adducts great toe at metatarsophalangeal joint

MUSCLES OF THE FOOT				
Muscle	Origin	Insertion	Nerve	Action
Muscles of the Sole of the Foot—Third Layer (*continued*)				
Flexor digiti minimi brevis	Base of 5th metatarsal and sheath of fibularis longus tendon	Lateral side of base of proximal phalanx of little toe	Lateral plantar nerve from tibial nerve S2, 3	Flexes little toe at metatarsophalangeal joint
Muscles of the Sole of the Foot—Fourth Layer				
Dorsal interossei	Sides of adjacent metatarsals	Extensor hoods and bases of proximal phalanges of 2nd to 4th toes	Lateral plantar nerve from tibial nerve; 1st and 2nd dorsal interossei also innervated by deep fibular nerve S2, 3	Abduct 2nd to 4th toes at metatarsophalangeal joints. Resist extension of metatarsophalangeal joints and flexion of interphalangeal joints
Plantar interossei	Bases and medial sides of 3rd–5th metatarsals	Extensor hoods and bases of proximal phalanges of 3rd–5th toes	Lateral plantar nerve from tibial nerve S2, 3	Adduct third to fifth toes at metatarsophalangeal joints. Resist extension of metatarsophalangeal joints and flexion of interphalangeal joints
Muscles of the Dorsal Aspect of the Foot				
Extensor digitorum brevis	Superolateral surface of calcaneus	Lateral sides of tendons of extensor digitorum longus of 2nd to 4th toes	Deep fibular nerve S1, 2	Extends 2nd to 4th toes
Extensor hallucis brevis	Superolateral surface of calcaneus	Base of proximal phalanx of great toe	Deep fibular nerve S1, 2	Extends metatarsophalangeal joint of great toe

Common Pathologies of the Muscular System

The health of the muscular system is essential to the functioning of the body. Muscle pain (myalgia) can be caused by infections, inflammation, injury, neuropathy, medication, or alcoholism. Certain disorders, such as muscular dystrophy, are inherited. In general, muscular disorders are accompanied by pain, tenderness, inflammation, and limited movement.

Red flags

Please also refer to the "Red flags" section of the skeletal system in chapter 4:

- Progressive muscular weakness
- Loss of function.

Study tip

Key words to remember:

- **Lumbago:** Pain in the muscles and joints of the lower back
- **Myalgia:** Muscular pain
- **Myositis:** Muscle-tissue inflammation
- **Myopathy:** Muscle-tissue disease
- **Rheumatism:** Pain, stiffness, and inflammation in the joints and/or muscles.

Infobox

Anatomy and physiology in perspective: How do skeletal muscles heal?

Skeletal-muscle cells do not have much potential to divide but, if injured, they can be replaced by new cells derived from dormant stem cells called **satellite cells**. However, if there is more damage to the muscle than the satellite cells can cope with, fibrosis occurs. This is the replacement of muscle fibers by scar tissue, which is a fibrous connective tissue that does not allow much movement and which can restrict movement at joints.

Infobox

Anatomy and physiology in perspective

Medications known to have adverse musculoskeletal effects include steroids, statins, ACE-inhibitors, antiepileptics, and immunosuppressants.

Disorders of muscles, bursae, and tendons

Fibromyalgia

Term used to describe a group of disorders that are all characterized by aching, stiffness, and pain in the soft tissue (muscles, tendons, and ligaments) coupled with pain resulting from gentle finger pressure applied at specific "tender spots." Different types of fibromyalgia exist and their causes are not always known, although it tends to affect women more than men. The different types are all usually aggravated by physical or mental stress, fatigue, strain, or overuse. **Lumbago** is fibromyalgia of the lumbar region. It can be caused by general tension, a slipped disc, or a strained muscle or ligament.

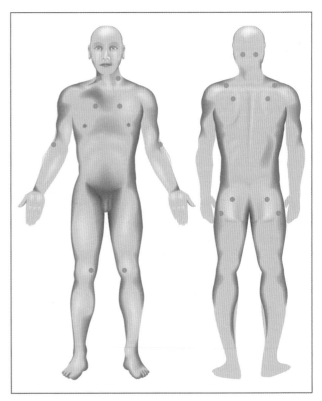

Figure 5.23 *Fibromyalgia—finding the tender points*

Fibrositis (muscular rheumatism)

Inflammation of the fibrous connective tissue and characterized by inflammation, pain, and stiffness.

Ganglion cyst

Fluid-filled growth that usually develops near joints or tendon sheaths on the hand or foot. The cause of ganglion cysts is unknown and although they can be removed by surgery, they can also disappear over time.

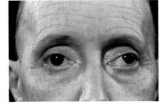

Ganglion cyst

Muscular dystrophies

Group of inherited muscle-destroying diseases that lead to muscle weakness. They are generally characterized by a progressive atrophy of the skeletal muscle due to the degeneration of individual muscle fibers.

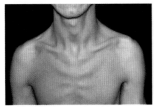
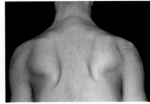

Muscular dystrophy (anterior)   *Muscular dystrophy (posterior)*

Myasthenia gravis

Autoimmune disease characterized by a weakness of skeletal muscles that is a result of impaired communication between nerves and muscles. More common

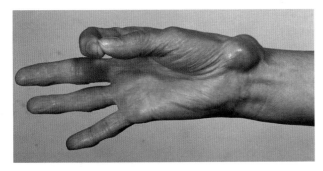

Myasthenia gravis

among women, symptoms may include drooping eyelids, weak eye muscles, double vision, extreme fatigue, difficulty in speaking and swallowing, and weakness of the arms and legs. Myasthenia gravis often occurs in exacerbations (periods in which signs and symptoms worsen) and sign/symptom-free periods.

Poliomyelitis (polio)

Contagious viral infection of the nervous system that results in muscle weakness and sometimes paralysis. Its initial signs and symptoms include a general feeling of malaise, fever, headaches, muscle pain, and a stiff neck and back. These may progress into weakness or paralysis of the muscles.

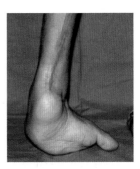

Poliomyelitis (polio)

Rupture

Tearing of muscle fascia that is generally accompanied by pain and swelling.

Spasm

Abnormal, involuntary muscular contraction that may occur as part of another disorder or as a localized condition.

A cramp is a type of spasm, as is a tic (twitching of the eyelid or facial muscles). **Cramp** is a common muscular disorder that can affect healthy, active people as much as it affects other groups of people. It is characterized by a sudden, painful contraction of a muscle or group of muscles, and it can happen during sleep and during or after exercise. There are a number of theories as to what causes cramps, including insufficient stretching before exercise, an inadequate blood flow to the muscles, low blood levels of electrolytes, and excess intake of caffeine or nicotine.

Strain

Overstretching of a muscle that is characterized by pain, swelling, and sometimes restricted movement.

Tetanus (lockjaw)

Infectious bacterial disease characterized by muscle stiffness, spasms, and rigidity in the jaw and neck. If not treated, these spasms can move into the back and chest and eventually affect the entire body.

Sports injuries and repetitive strain injury (RSI)

Most often caused by overuse of specific muscles during sport or exercise, or when repeating movements while performing a regular activity, e.g., typing. Muscles can also be overused when structural abnormalities, such as an unequal length of legs, place extra stress on other parts of the body.

Infobox

Anatomy and physiology in perspective

Most sports injuries are best treated as soon as possible with the RICE method. This involves:

Rest, **I**ce, **C**ompression, **E**levation

The injured area is rested immediately and ice is applied to the area to reduce swelling and pain. A compress such as a bandage is applied, and the area is then elevated to help limit further swelling. In addition to this, it is important to give the injured area enough time to heal itself properly before returning to the sporting activity.

Carpal tunnel syndrome

Compression of the median nerve as it passes through the wrist and is often caused by repetitive, forceful

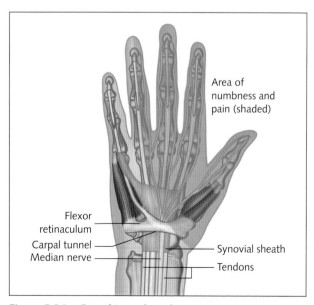

Figure 5.24 *Carpal tunnel syndrome*

use of the wrist when it is in the wrong position. Also common in pregnancy, diabetes, rheumatoid arthritis, and people who have an underactive thyroid gland. Carpal tunnel syndrome is characterized by numbness and tingling of the thumb and first three fingers, and the thumb also tends to be weak. The little finger is often symptom-free.

Frozen shoulder (adhesive capsulitis)

Inflammation of the shoulder joint and is characterized by chronic, painful stiffness. It has many causes, such as injury to the shoulder or a stroke. It can also develop slowly for no apparent reason.

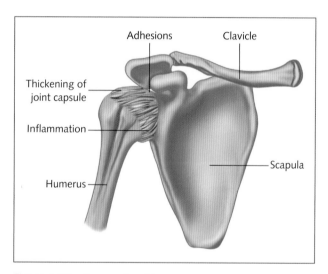

Figure 5.25 *Frozen shoulder*

Did you know?

Adhesions are bands of scar tissue that join two surfaces of the body that are usually separate.

Golfer's elbow (medial epicondylitis)

Damage to the tendons on the inside of the elbow that bend the wrist toward the palm. Symptoms include pain on the palmar side of the forearm from the elbow toward the wrist, and it can be caused by movements that bend the wrist toward the palm with excessive force. These include certain golf swings, tennis serves, throwing javelins, or even carrying a heavy suitcase.

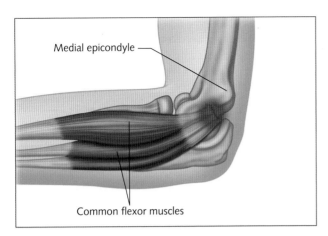

Figure 5.26 *Golfer's elbow*

Housemaid's knee (prepatellar bursitis)

Inflammation of the bursa in front of the kneecap characterized by inflammation and pain and is usually a result of frequent kneeling.

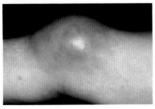

Housemaid's knee

Shin splints

Term used to describe pain along the tibia. It may occur in the anterior and lateral muscles of the shin (anterolateral shin splints) or the posterior and medial muscles (posteromedial shin splints). Where the pain is felt will depend on the muscles affected. Generally, shin splints is initially characterized by

pain on movement. If left untreated, the pain will occur when the shins are touched. Shin splints can result from running on hard surfaces with poorly supportive shoes, or from having an imbalance in the size of opposing muscles.

Tendinitis

Inflammation of a tendon and is usually a result of overuse or repetitive use. However, it can sometimes be caused by a bacterial infection or result from another disorder of the musculoskeletal system. It is characterized by inflammation, pain, and tenderness when moved or touched.

Achilles tendinitis is inflammation of the Achilles tendon, and it is common in runners as it can be caused by excessive uphill or downhill running. It can also be caused by a number of different functional abnormalities, including tight hamstrings and high arches. It is essential that the injury is rested and allowed to heal fully before exercise is resumed.

Tenosynovitis is tendinitis accompanied by inflammation of the tendon sheath.

Tennis elbow (lateral epicondylitis)

Damage to the tendons of the lateral, or outer, border of the elbow. Symptoms include pain in the elbow and on the outer, back side of the forearm, and it is often caused by improper backhand tennis techniques (hence the name), having weak shoulder and wrist muscles, or repetitive extension of the wrist.

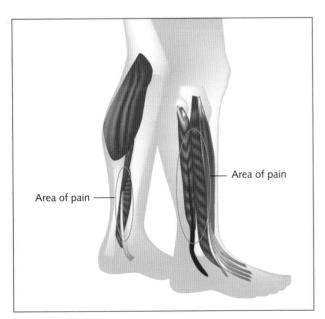

Figure 5.27 *Shin splints*

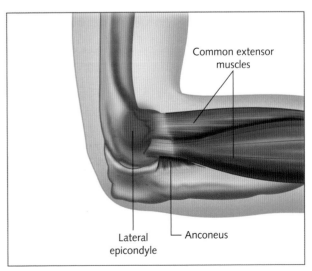

Figure 5.28 *Tennis elbow*

NEW WORDS	
Action potential	An electrical charge that occurs on the membrane of a muscle cell in response to a nerve impulse
Aerobic	Requiring oxygen
Agonist	The muscle responsible for causing a movement (prime mover)
Anaerobic	Not requiring oxygen
Antagonist	The muscle that opposes the movement caused by the prime mover; it relaxes and lengthens in a controlled way to ensure the movement is performed smoothly by the prime mover
Aponeurosis	A flat, sheet-like tendon that attaches muscles to bone, to skin, or to another muscle
Atony	The lack of muscle tone
Atrophy	The wasting away of muscles
Autorhythmic cells	Muscle or nerve cells that generate an impulse without an external stimulus, i.e., they are self-excitable
Conductivity	The ability of muscle cells to move action potentials along their plasma membranes
Contractility	The ability of muscles to contract and shorten
Depression (of the shoulders)	Dropping the shoulders downward
Elasticity	The ability of muscles to return to their original shape after contracting or extending
Elevation (of the shoulders)	Lifting the shoulders upward
Excitability	The ability of muscle or nerve cells to respond to stimuli
Extensibility	The ability of muscles to extend and lengthen
Fascia	Connective tissue that surrounds and protects organs, lines walls of the body, holds muscles together, and separates muscles
Fatigue (of muscles)	A muscle's inability to respond to stimulus or maintain contractions
Fibrosis	The replacement of connective tissue by scar tissue
Fixators	Muscles that stabilize the bone of the prime mover's origin so that it can act efficiently (stabilizers)
Glycolysis	The cellular process through which glucose is split into pyruvic acid and ATP
Hypertonia	An increase in muscle tone; muscles are described as hypertonic
Hypotonia	The loss of muscle tone; muscles are described as hypotonic
Insertion	The point where a muscle attaches to the moving bone of a joint
Irritability	The ability of muscle or nerve cells to respond to stimuli

NEW WORDS	
Myoglobin	A protein that binds with oxygen and carries it to muscle cells
Myology	The study of muscles
Origin	The point where a muscle attaches to the stationary bone of a joint
Prime mover	The muscle responsible for causing a movement (agonist)
Protraction	A forward movement of the shoulder or mandible on a plane parallel to the ground
Retraction	The opposite of protraction; a backward movement on a plane parallel to the ground
Stabilizers	Muscles that stabilize the bone of the prime mover's origin so that it can act efficiently (fixators)
Striated	Having the appearance of light and dark bands, or striations
Synergists	Muscles that help the prime mover
Tendon	A strong cord of dense connective tissue that attaches muscles to bones, to the skin, or to other muscles
Thermogenesis	The generation of heat in the body
Tone (tonus)	The partial contraction of a resting muscle

Study Outline

Functions of the muscular system

Functions of the muscular system include locomotion, maintenance of posture, movement of substances, regulation of organ volumes, and heat production.

> **SHLOP**
> Substances moved, Heat produced, Locomotion, Organ volume controlled, Posture

Muscle tissue

Types of muscle tissue

1. There are three different types of muscle tissue: skeletal, cardiac, and smooth (visceral).
2. Skeletal muscle is striated and voluntary, and functions in moving the skeleton, maintaining posture, and generating heat.
3. Cardiac muscle is striated and involuntary, and functions in pumping blood around the body.

4. Smooth (visceral) muscle is non-striated and involuntary, and functions in moving substances within the body and regulating organ volume.

> Suzie Violently Strips, Clair Innocently Strips, Sarah Innocently does Nothing
> Skeletal, Voluntary, Striated—Cardiac, Involuntary, Striated—Smooth, Involuntary, Non-striated

Structure of a skeletal muscle

Connective tissue: The outer protection of a muscle

1. Fascia separates muscles into different functional groups and supports the nerves and blood and lymphatic vessels that serve the muscles.
2. Muscles are surrounded, protected, and reinforced by three types of connective tissue: epimysium, perimysium, and endomysium.
3. The epimysium is the outermost layer of connective tissue that encircles the whole muscle.

4. The perimysium surrounds bundles of muscle fibers called fascicles.
5. The endomysium surrounds each individual muscle fiber within a fascicle.
6. All three types of connective tissue extend beyond the muscle to become tendons or aponeuroses. These join the muscles to the periosteum of bones or to the skin or other muscles.

Muscle fibers: The inner cells of a skeletal muscle

1. The cell of a muscle is called a fiber. Its membrane is the sarcolemma, its cytoplasm is the sarcoplasm, and its endoplasmic reticulum is the sarcoplasmic reticulum.
2. Muscle fibers are multi-nucleated and also have many mitochondria.
3. Muscle fibers contain myofibrils, which are the contractile elements of the muscle. They are made up of myofilaments and are arranged into sarcomeres.

Sarcomeres: The basic functional units of a skeletal muscle

1. A sarcomere contains the filaments that move to overlap one another and cause a muscle to shorten.
2. They contain three types of filaments: thick, thin, and elastic filaments.
3. Thick filaments contain myosin.
4. Thin filaments contain actin, tropomyosin, and troponin. They also contain the myosin-binding sites for myosin.
5. Elastic filaments contain titin (connectin) and help stabilize the position of the thick filaments.
6. Sarcomeres are made up of two bands, which give muscles their striated appearance: the A-band and the I-band.
7. The A-band is dark and contains mainly thick filaments. In the center of the A-band is the H-zone, which contains thick filaments only. The H-zone is divided by an M-line of protein molecules that holds the thick filaments together.
8. The I-band is a light area containing thin filaments only.
9. Sarcomeres are separated from one another by Z-discs/lines.

Muscle contraction

How do muscles contract?

1. When a muscle is relaxed, the myosin-binding sites on the actin molecules are covered by a tropomyosin-troponin complex and the myosin heads are in an energized state.
2. A nerve impulse triggers the release of acetylcholine, which triggers a muscle action potential, which causes the release of calcium.
3. Calcium binds with the tropomyosin-troponin complex to free up the myosin-binding sites.
4. The myosin heads bind to actin with a power stroke, which draws the thin filaments inward toward the H-zone. The thick filaments remain in the same place.
5. The muscle shortens (contracts).
6. The myosin heads detach from the actin and attach to another myosin-binding site further along the thin filament.
7. The cycle continues as long as ATP and calcium are present.

How do muscles relax?

1. Acetylcholine is broken down by an enzyme. This stops further muscle action potentials and therefore stops the release of calcium and leads to a decrease in calcium levels.
2. When there is not enough calcium available to bind with the tropomyosin-troponin complex, it moves back over the myosin-binding sites and blocks the myosin heads from binding with the actin.
3. Thus, the thin filaments slip back into their relaxed position and no more contraction takes place.

Types of muscular contraction

1. Muscle tone is the constant, partial contraction of a muscle. It gives muscles their firmness and tension and is necessary for maintaining posture.
2. There are two types of muscle contraction: isotonic contractions and isometric contractions.
3. In isotonic contractions, muscles contract, shorten, and create movement. Isotonic contractions include concentric contractions, which are always toward the center and involve the shortening of a muscle, and eccentric contractions, which are

always away from the center and involve the lengthening of a muscle.

4. In isometric contractions, muscles contract but there is no shortening of the muscle and no movement is generated.

Muscle metabolism

1. Muscles need energy in the form of ATP to contract. They obtain this through the phosphagen system or glycolysis.

2. In the phosphagen system, muscles use the small amount of ATP that they store in their own fibers.

3. In glycolysis, muscles break down glucose and convert it into pyruvic acid and ATP. The ATP is used by the muscles while the pyruvic acid (pyruvate) still needs to be broken down.

4. In anaerobic glycolysis, there is not enough oxygen to completely break down the pyruvic acid so it is converted into lactic acid.

5. In aerobic respiration, there is enough oxygen to completely break down the pyruvic acid into carbon dioxide, water, ATP, and heat. This process is called cellular respiration or biological oxidation.

6. Muscle fatigue occurs when a muscle can no longer respond to stimulus or maintain its contractions.

Types of skeletal muscle fibers

1. There are three types of skeletal muscle fibers: slow oxidative, fast oxidative, and fast glycolytic.

2. Slow oxidative fibers are red and small, have a good oxygen supply, and produce ATP aerobically and split it slowly. They are also very resistant to fatigue and are plentiful in muscles of endurance or those that maintain posture.

3. Fast oxidative fibers are red and medium sized, have a good oxygen supply, and produce ATP aerobically and split it quickly. They are less

resistant to fatigue than slow oxidative fibers and are plentiful in muscles used for walking and running.

4. Fast glycolytic fibers are white and large, have a poor oxygen supply, and produce ATP anaerobically and split it very fast. They fatigue easily and are plentiful in muscles used for fast movements such as throwing a ball.

Skeletal muscles and movement

How skeletal muscles produce movement

1. A muscle is usually attached to two articulating bones.

2. The point where the muscle inserts in the stationary bone is called the origin. The point where it inserts in the moving bone is the insertion. When muscles contract they shorten and usually move the moving bone toward the stationary bone.

3. Muscles work in pairs: the prime mover (agonist) causes a movement and the antagonist opposes the movement by relaxing and lengthening in a controlled way to ensure the movement is performed smoothly by the prime mover.

4. Prime movers are supported by synergists and fixators.

> Olives Sell In Markets
> Origin stays Still, Insertion Moves

Photographs of principal skeletal muscles

The photographs following will help you to recognize some of the principal muscles of the body, as will the images of the anterior and posterior muscle chains. These colorful images will hopefully help you to see "muscles in action."

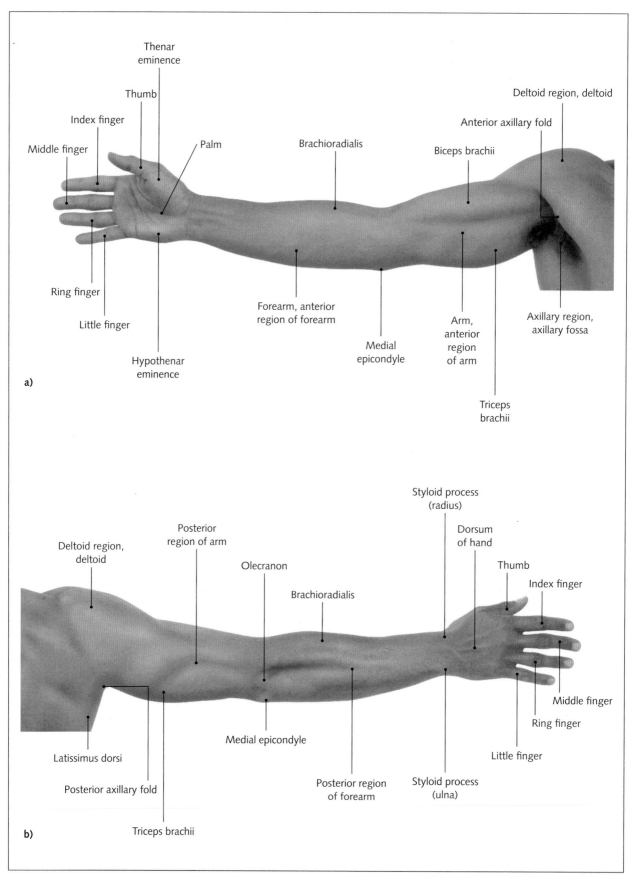

Figure 5.29 *Upper limb*

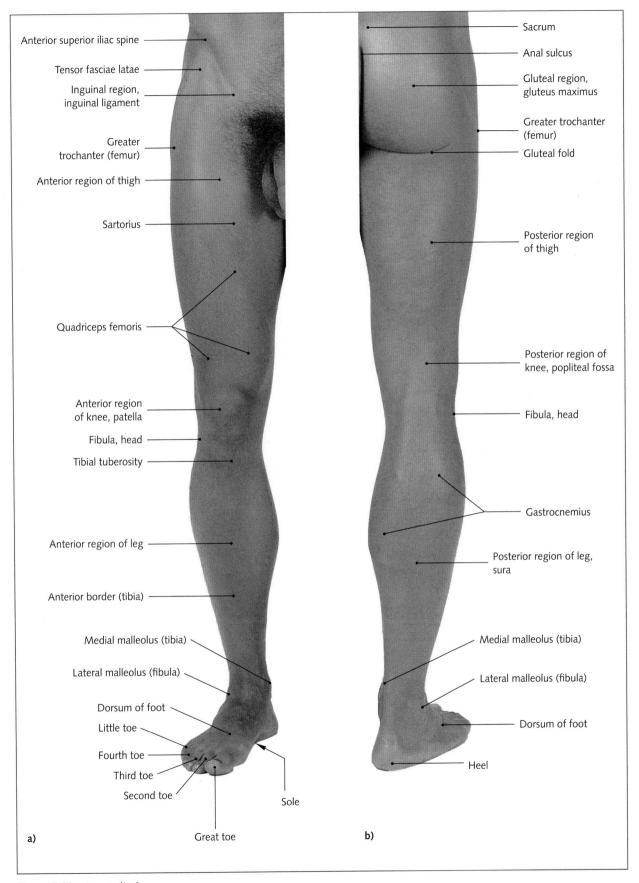

Figure 5.30 *Lower limb*

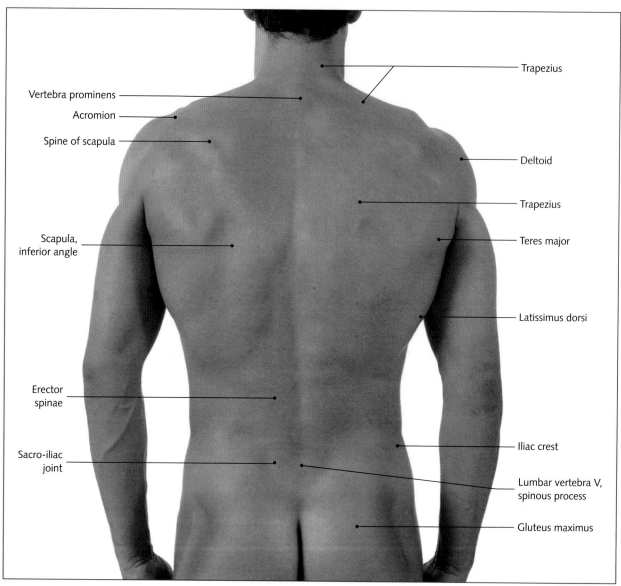

Figure 5.31 *The back*

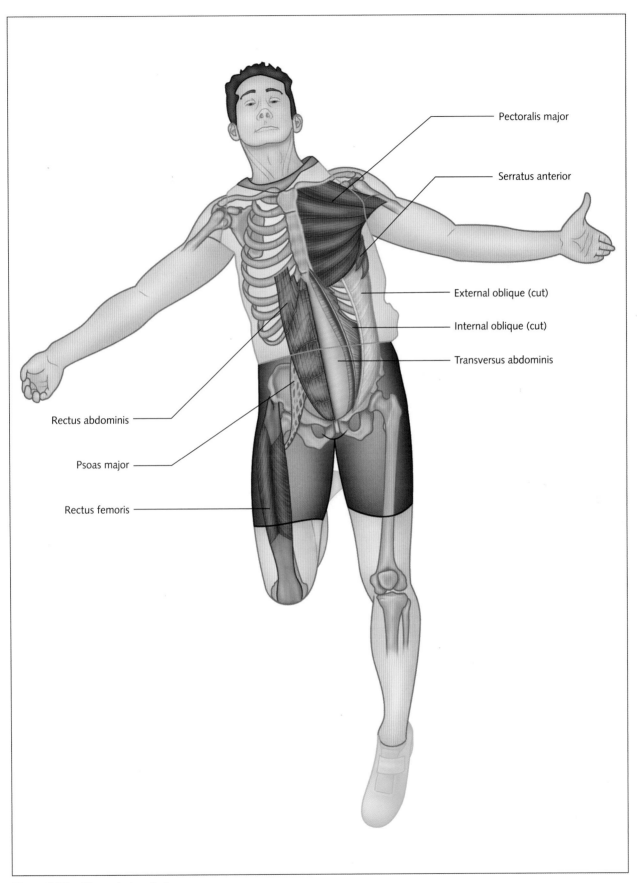

Figure 5.32   *The anterior chain*

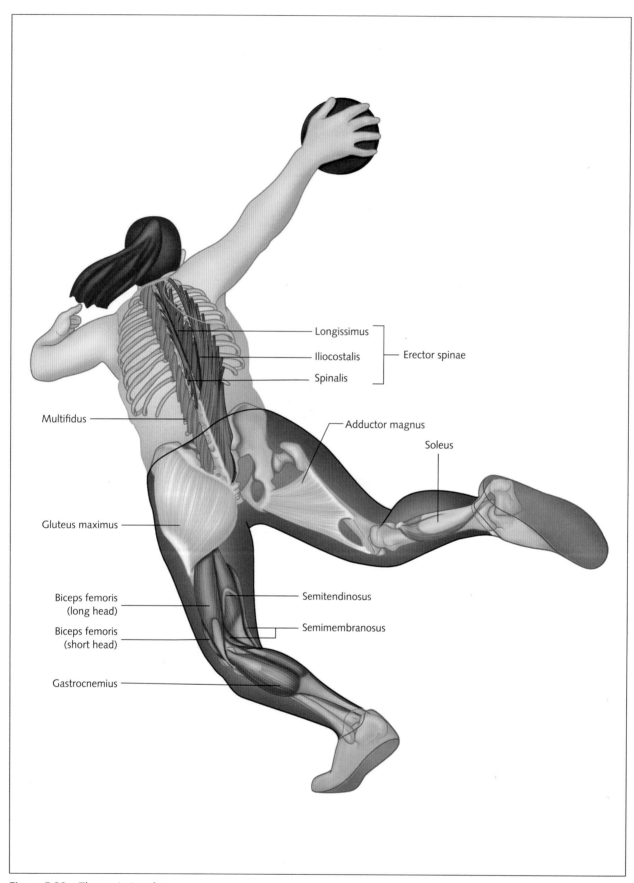

Figure 5.33 *The posterior chain*

Review

1. Describe the functions of the muscular system.
2. Identify the three different types of muscular tissue.
3. Discuss the differences between the three types of muscular tissue.
4. Describe the different connective tissues associated with muscles.
5. What is a muscle fiber?
6. Describe a sarcomere and identify the different filaments and proteins within it.
7. Describe how a muscle contracts.
8. Describe how a muscle relaxes.
9. Define muscle tone.
10. Identify the two different types of muscular contraction.
11. Identify the differences between concentric and eccentric contractions.
12. Describe how muscles obtain their energy to contract.
13. Identify the difference between aerobic and anaerobic processes.
14. Describe how lactic acid is produced and what its effects on the muscles are.
15. Define muscle fatigue.
16. Describe the three types of muscle fibers.
17. Describe how muscles produce movements at joints.
18. Define the following terms: origin, insertion, prime mover, antagonist, synergist, fixator.
19. Write a list of at least five different muscle characteristics that are often reflected in a muscle's name. For example, a muscle's origin and insertion can be reflected in its name (e.g., sternocleidomastoid).
20. List the characteristics of the following common pathologies:
    • Carpal tunnel syndrome
    • Rupture
    • Cramp.

Multiple-Choice Questions

1. Thermogenesis is:
   a. The process by which glucose is broken down in the body
   b. The process by which heat is generated in the body
   c. The process by which organ volumes are controlled in the body
   d. None of the above

2. Tendons attach:
   a. Muscles to bones
   b. Bones to bones
   c. Aponeuroses to bones
   d. Fascia to bones

3. Which of the following statements is correct?
   a. Smooth muscle contracts to pump blood around the body
   b. Skeletal muscle contracts to pump blood around the body
   c. Cardiac muscle contracts to pump blood around the body
   d. None of the above

4. Which of the following statements is correct?
   a. Skeletal muscle is striated, voluntary, and pumps blood around the body
   b. All muscles are striated, involuntary, and help move substances through the body
   c. Cardiac muscle is non-striated, involuntary, and helps regulate blood pressure
   d. Smooth muscle is non-striated, involuntary, and helps regulate organ volume

5. Elasticity is the ability of muscles to:
   a. Respond to stimuli
   b. Return to their original shape after contracting or extending
   c. Extend or stretch
   d. Shorten or thicken

6. The orbicularis oculi muscle functions in:
   a. Opening the eye
   b. Opening the mouth
   c. Closing the eye
   d. Closing the mouth

7. The perimysium is a connective tissue membrane that:
   a. Surrounds each individual muscle fiber
   b. Separates muscles into functional groups
   c. Encircles the entire muscle
   d. Surrounds bundles of muscle fibers

8. Which of the following structures contains the filaments that move to overlap one another and cause a muscle to shorten?
   a. Sarcoplasm
   b. Sarcolemma
   c. Sarcomere
   d. Sarcoplasmic reticulum

9. The pterygoideus lateralis originates on the:
   a. Sphenoid
   b. Humerus
   c. Tibia
   d. Triquetrum

10. Which mineral is necessary for the contraction of muscles?
    a. Iron
    b. Calcium
    c. Zinc
    d. Boron

11. Muscle tone is necessary for:
    a. Relaxing muscles
    b. Contracting muscles
    c. Maintaining posture
    d. Moving substances around the body

12. Which of the following muscles form the rotator cuff?
    a. Trapezius, rhomboids, levator scapulae
    b. Biceps femoris, semitendinosus, semimembranosus
    c. Rectus femoris, vastus lateralis, vastus medialis, vastus intermedius
    d. Subscapularis, supraspinatus, infraspinatus, teres minor

13. Which of the following muscles form the quads?
    a. Trapezius, rhomboids, levator scapulae
    b. Biceps femoris, semitendinosus, semimembranosus
    c. Rectus femoris, vastus lateralis, vastus medialis, vastus intermedius
    d. Subscapularis, supraspinatus, infraspinatus, teres minor

14. Which of the following can cause muscle fatigue?
    a. A build-up of lactic acid
    b. A sufficient supply of oxygen
    c. A sufficient supply of glycogen
    d. A lack of lactic acid

15. Which type of muscle fiber is plentiful in the muscles used for throwing a ball?
    a. Slow oxidative
    b. Fast oxidative
    c. Fast glycolytic
    d. None of the above

6

The Nervous System

Introduction

Air particles vibrate and we hear words, poetry, even music. Waves of light bend to form colors, shapes, and images. Simple molecules are transformed into smells or tastes that remind us of our childhood—that can make us laugh or cry.

All of these sensations, thoughts, and emotions are created in one system of our bodies—the nervous system. It is a system that not only gives us a sense of who, what, and where we are, but also enables us to survive and to change the environment in which we live.

The study of the nervous system is called **neurology**, and in this chapter we will take a look at how this system is able to control all the other systems of our body and help us control our environment.

Student objectives

By the end of this chapter you will be able to:

- Describe the functions of the nervous system
- Describe the organization of the nervous system
- Identify the different types of neurons
- Describe the structure of a motor neuron
- Describe the structure and function of the brain
- Identify the cranial nerves
- Describe the structure and function of the spinal cord
- Identify the spinal nerves and plexuses
- Describe the structure and function of the sense organs: eyes, ears, nose, and mouth
- Identify the common pathologies of the nervous system.

Functions of the Nervous System

The nervous system is made up of millions of nerve cells that all communicate with one another to control the body and maintain homeostasis. These cells detect what is happening both inside and outside the body, interpret these happenings, and cause a response. Basically, the nervous system has three functions: sensory, integrative, and motor.

Infobox

Anatomy and physiology in perspective

Your nervous system is not alone in controlling your body and maintaining homeostasis. It works closely with a second control system called the endocrine system, which secretes hormones. One of the main differences between the two systems is that the nervous system can respond rapidly to stimuli and works faster than the endocrine system. You will learn more about the endocrine system in chapter 7.

Sensory function

A stimulus is something that provokes a response, be it a change in the temperature of the air or a pin prick to a finger. **Sensory receptors** pick up stimuli from both inside and outside the body. All the information gathered by these sensory receptors is called **sensory input**.

Integrative function

Once the nervous system has new sensory input, it **analyzes, processes,** and *interprets* this information in the brain and spinal cord. It is also able to store the information and make decisions regarding it.

Motor function

Having picked up a change in the environment and decided what to do about it, the final function of the nervous system is the ability to **act**, or **respond** to a stimulus, by glandular secretions or muscular contractions. This is called **motor output**.

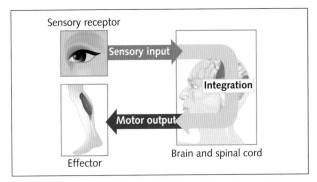

Figure 6.1 *Functions of the nervous system*

Organization of the Nervous System

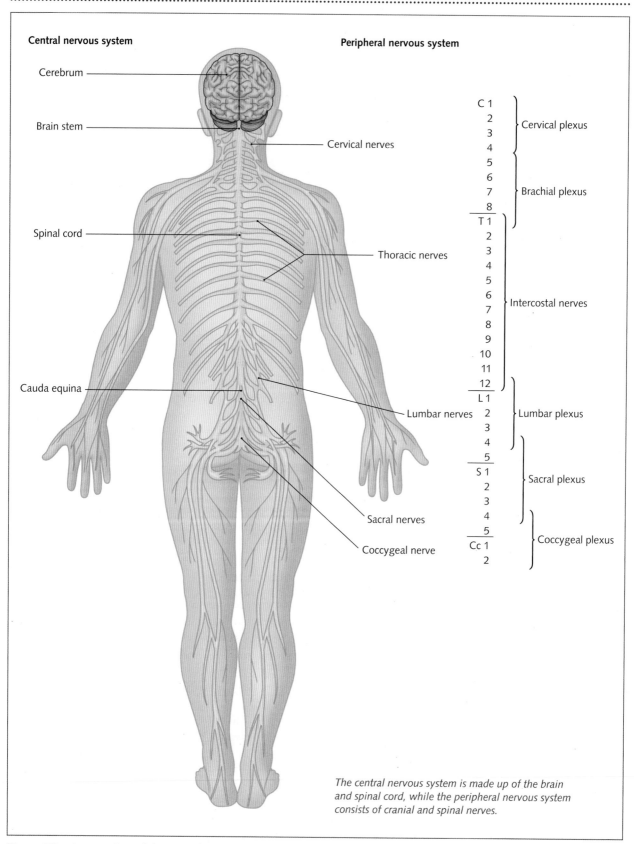

Figure 6.2 *An overview of the central and peripheral nervous systems*

You may have heard people talking about the "central nervous system" or the "autonomic nervous system" or the "parasympathetic nervous system" and wondered what exactly is going on. In fact, you may be wondering exactly how many nervous systems you really have. The answer is simple: you only have one nervous system. But, because it is such a complex system, it is divided into a number of different parts. What is important here, before we go any further, is that you understand that all these different parts function together as one coordinated system.

Now let us look at all these divisions. To begin with, the nervous system is divided into the **central nervous system (CNS)** and the **peripheral nervous system (PNS)**. The PNS is then subdivided into the **somatic** and **autonomic nervous systems**. The autonomic nervous system is then divided into the **sympathetic** and **parasympathetic nervous systems**.

Central nervous system

The CNS is made up of the brain and spinal cord. It functions in analyzing and storing information, making decisions, and issuing orders. It is where memories are made and stored, emotions generated, and thoughts conceived. We will study the brain and spinal cord in detail later in this chapter.

Peripheral nervous system

The PNS is made up of nerve cells that reach every part of the body, and consists of:

- **Cranial nerves:** Cranial nerves arise from the brain and carry impulses to and from the brain.
- **Spinal nerves:** Spinal nerves emerge from the spinal cord to carry impulses to and from the rest of the body. Spinal nerves contain two types of nerve cells (neurons):
  - **Sensory (afferent) neurons:** Sensory, or afferent, neurons conduct impulses from sensory receptors to the CNS
  - **Motor (efferent) neurons:** Motor, or efferent, neurons conduct impulses from the CNS to muscles and glands

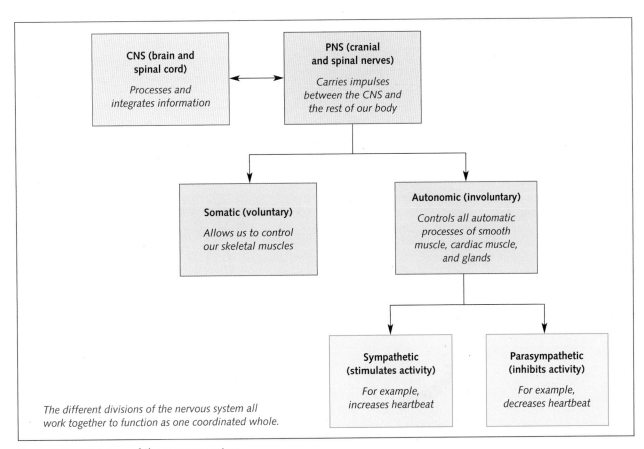

The different divisions of the nervous system all work together to function as one coordinated whole.

Figure 6.3 *Divisions of the nervous system*

The PNS is subdivided into the somatic nervous system (SNS) and the autonomic nervous system (ANS).

Somatic nervous system

The word *soma* means "body," and the SNS allows us to control our skeletal muscles. Thus, it is sometimes also called the **voluntary nervous system**. It contains:

- Sensory neurons that convey information from the **cutaneous** and **special sense receptors** to the CNS
- Motor neurons that conduct impulses from the CNS to the **skeletal muscles** only.

We do not always control our skeletal muscles voluntarily. Sometimes they contract involuntarily through what is called a **reflex arc**.

Autonomic nervous system

The ANS controls all processes that are automatic or involuntary. Thus, it is sometimes also called the **involuntary nervous system**. It contains:

- Sensory neurons that convey information from the **viscera** to the CNS
- Motor neurons that convey information from the CNS to **smooth muscle**, **cardiac muscle**, and **glands**. The motor portion of the ANS has two branches that help the body adapt to changing

> ### Did you know?
>
> Have you ever had a doctor (or even a friend) tap you just below your kneecap and your lower leg has jerked up? This is called the **knee-jerk** and is a reflex-arc response to a stimulus. In other words, it is a response over which you have no control because no message is sent to the brain. Instead, the sensory nerve impulse is transmitted from the knee to the spinal cord where it is then immediately transmitted to motor neurons and back into the knee.

circumstances. They work in opposition to one another and so are able to counterbalance each other to maintain homeostasis. They are the:

- **Sympathetic nervous system:** The sympathetic nervous system reacts to changes in the environment by stimulating activity and therefore using energy. For example, the sympathetic nervous system increases the heartbeat
- **Parasympathetic nervous system:** The parasympathetic nervous system opposes the actions of the sympathetic nervous system by inhibiting activity and therefore conserving energy. For example, the parasympathetic nervous system decreases the heartbeat

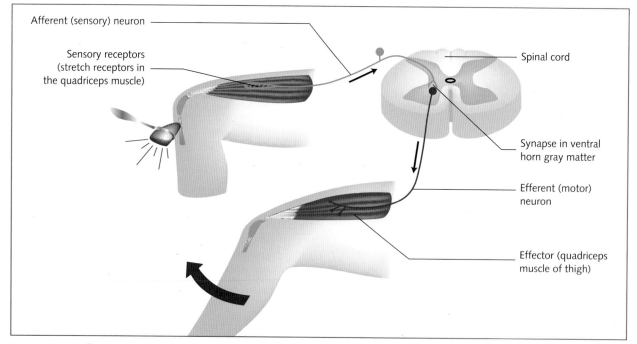

Figure 6.4 *Reflex arc*

EFFECTS OF THE SYMPATHETIC AND PARASYMPATHETIC NERVOUS SYSTEMS

Sympathetic stimulation	Structure	Parasympathetic
Pupil dilated	Iris muscle	Pupil constricted
Vasoconstriction	Blood vessels in head	No effect
Secretion inhibited	Salivary glands	Secretion increased
Rate and force of contraction increased	Heart	Rate and force of contraction decreased
Vasodilation	Coronary arteries	Vasoconstriction
Bronchodilation	Trachea and bronchi	Bronchoconstriction
Peristalsis reduced, sphincters closed	Stomach	Secretion of gastric juice increased
Glycogen to glucose conversion increased	Liver	Blood vessels dilated, secretion of bile increased
Epinephrine and norepinephrine secreted into blood	Adrenal medulla	No effect
Peristalsis reduced, sphincters closed	Large and small intestines	Secretions and peristalsis increased, sphincter relaxed
Smooth muscle wall relaxed, sphincter closed	Bladder	Smooth muscle wall contracted, sphincter relaxed

Nervous Tissue

The nervous system contains only two types of cells: **neuroglia** and **neurons.**

Neuroglia

Neuroglia, or glia, are smaller and more numerous than neurons and are the "glue," or supporting cells, of nervous tissue. They insulate, nurture, and protect neurons and maintain homeostasis of the fluid surrounding neurons. There are six different types of neuroglia, but they all have two things in common: they cannot transmit nerve impulses and they can divide by mitosis. Of the six different types of neuroglia, four of them are present only in the CNS. These are astrocytes, oligodendrocytes, microglia, and ependymal cells. The remaining two are present in the PNS and are Schwann cells and satellite cells.

Infobox

Anatomy and physiology in perspective

Brain tumors called **gliomas** are made out of neuroglia. This is because, unlike neurons, neuroglia can divide by mitosis.

Neurons

Neurons are the cells responsible for the sensory, integrative, and motor functions of the nervous system. They can differ in size and shape, but they all share one essential characteristic: they transmit impulses or electrical signals to, from, or within the brain.

Types of neurons

Neurons can be functionally classified according to the type of information they carry and the direction in which they carry that information. The chart below shows this classification.

Did you know?

Neurons can vary from a millimeter to a meter in length and can conduct impulses at speeds ranging from one to more than a hundred meters per second.

Structure of a motor neuron

All neurons have three parts: a **cell body, dendrites,** and an **axon.** Here we will look at the structure of a *typical* motor neuron.

Cell body

The cell body is the metabolic center of the neuron and is quite similar to a generalized animal cell in that it consists of a nucleus, cytoplasm, and organelles such as mitochondria, Golgi complex, and lysosomes. However, the cell body of a motor neuron does not include centrioles and therefore division via mitosis is

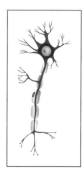

CLASSIFICATION OF NEURONS			
Neuron	Information carried	Direction	
		From:	To:
Sensory/afferent	Sensory nerve impulse	Skin, sense organs, muscle, joints, viscera	CNS
Motor/efferent	Motor nerve impulse	CNS	Muscles or glands (called effectors)
Association/interneurons	These are not specifically sensory or motor neurons; rather, they connect sensory and motor neurons in neural pathways		

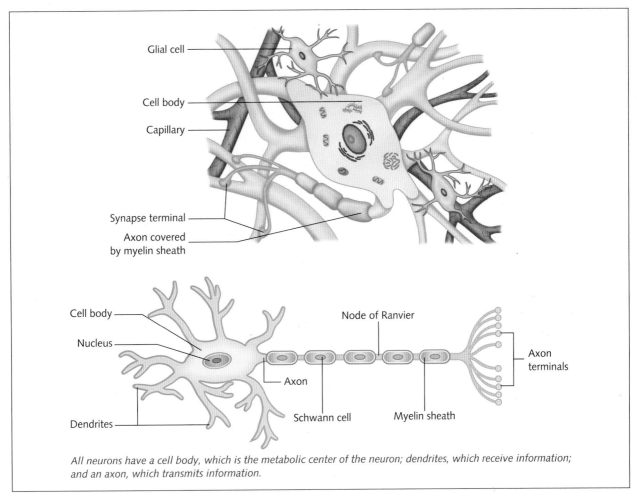

Glial cell

Cell body

Capillary

Synapse terminal

Axon covered
by myelin sheath

Cell body

Nucleus

Axon

Dendrites

Node of Ranvier

Schwann cell

Myelin sheath

Axon
terminals

All neurons have a cell body, which is the metabolic center of the neuron; dendrites, which receive information; and an axon, which transmits information.

Figure 6.5 *Structure of a motor neuron*

not possible. The cell body also includes organelles that are specific to neurons only:

- **Nissl bodies:** These are made of rough endoplasmic reticulum and are the site of protein synthesis.
- **Neurofibrils:** These form the cytoskeleton of the cell to maintain its shape.

Infobox

Anatomy and physiology in perspective

Most neurons cannot divide by mitosis, so once they die they cannot be replaced. Thus, you are born with all your neurons and if they die through aging, or are killed by head injuries, alcohol, or drugs, the damage is permanent.

Dendrites

Dendrites are the receiving or input portion of the cell. The word *dendro* means "tree," and dendrites are branching processes that project from the cell body. They are short and unmyelinated (this will be discussed shortly). Neurons can have many dendrites projecting from their cell body.

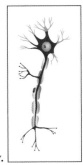

Axon

The axon is the transmitting portion of a cell. It transmits nerve impulses away from the cell body and toward another neuron, a muscle fiber, or a gland cell. An axon looks like a long tail, and the end of it divides into many fine processes called axon terminals.

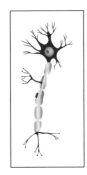

- **Axon terminals:** These are found at the end of the axon and contain membrane-enclosed sacs called **synaptic vesicles.**
- **Synaptic vesicles:** These sacs store chemical substances that influence other neurons, muscle fibers, or gland cells. These substances are called **neurotransmitters** and they are released into an extracellular space called the **synaptic cleft.**

Some axons are **myelinated.** This means they are covered in a **myelin sheath,** which protects and insulates the axon. This insulation speeds up the conduction of the nerve impulse. Myelin sheaths are created by neuroglia as follows:

- **Schwann cells (neurolemmocytes)** are neuroglia found in the PNS. They wrap themselves around small segments of a single axon so that the segment becomes completely enclosed by multiple layers of Schwann cell membrane. The cytoplasm and nucleus of the Schwann cells forms the outermost layer and is called the **neurilemma (neurolemma).** The membrane of the Schwann cells forms the innermost layer and is known simply as the myelin sheath.
- Between each Schwann-cell-enclosed segment is a small gap that is not covered. These gaps are called **nodes of Ranvier (neurofibril nodes).** They are found at intervals along the sheath.
- **Oligodendrocytes** are neuroglia found in the CNS. They myelinate parts of many axons together, and myelinated neurons in the CNS do not have a neurilemma.

> **Did you know?**
>
> The amount of myelin surrounding our neurons is responsible for the speed of the conduction of nerve impulses. It increases from birth to maturity and this is why infants respond more slowly to stimuli than adults do.

> **Infobox**
>
> **Anatomy and physiology in perspective**
>
> Multiple sclerosis (MS) is a disorder in which myelin sheaths are destroyed. This slows down the conduction of nerve impulses and can eventually lead to the short-circuiting of impulses. This is why symptoms of MS can include muscular weakness, abnormal sensations, and double vision (MS is discussed in more detail in the pathology section at the end of this chapter).

> **Did you know?**
>
> Myelin is a whitish color and it is what gives the white matter found in the brain and spinal cord its appearance. White matter consists of the myelinated processes of neurons, while gray matter contains unmyelinated structures such as neuroglia, cell bodies, axon terminals, and unmyelinated axons and dendrites.

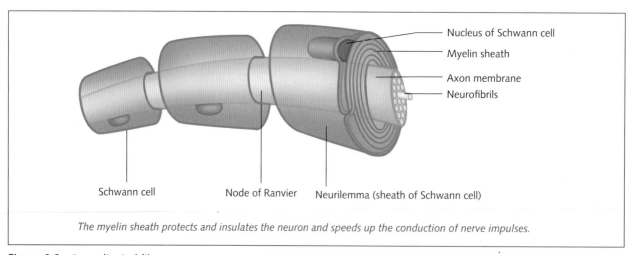

Nucleus of Schwann cell
Myelin sheath
Axon membrane
Neurofibrils

Schwann cell   Node of Ranvier   Neurilemma (sheath of Schwann cell)

The myelin sheath protects and insulates the neuron and speeds up the conduction of nerve impulses.

Figure 6.6 *A myelinated fiber*

Transmission of a Nerve Impulse

A neuron has two main characteristics:

- **Irritability:** This is the ability to respond to a stimulus and convert it into an impulse.
- **Conductivity:** This is the ability to transmit an impulse from a neuron to another neuron, muscle, or gland.

A neuron responds to a stimulus and converts it into an impulse via electrical means. It then conducts the impulse chemically to another neuron. Thus, nerve impulses are transmitted **electrochemically**. We will firstly look at the electrical transmission and then at the chemical transmission.

Electrical transmission across the plasma membrane

A nerve impulse is transmitted across the plasma membrane of an unmyelinated axon or across the nodes of Ranvier on a myelinated axon. For ease of learning, we will consider transmission across the plasma membrane only, but before we look at exactly what happens, here is some basic information that will help you understand the process:

- **Ion:** This is an electrically charged molecule.
- **Sodium ions (Na^+):** These are the chief extracellular ions and are therefore usually found outside the plasma membrane.

- **Potassium ions (K^+):** These are the chief intracellular ions and are therefore usually found on the inside.

A nerve impulse is generated and propagated as follows:

- An inactive plasma membrane has a resting membrane potential that is **polarized**. This means that there is an electrical voltage difference across the membrane, with the external voltage being positive and the internal one being negative. Remember that the main external ions are sodium, while the main internal ones are potassium.
- The dendrites of the neuron are **stimulated**.
- This stimulus causes ion channels in a small segment of the plasma membrane to open and allow the movement of sodium ions into the cell. This causes the inside of the cell to become positive and the outside negative. This is called **depolarization**.
- Depolarization causes the membrane potential to be reversed and this initiates an **action potential (impulse)**.
- When one segment of the membrane becomes depolarized, it causes the segment next to it to be depolarized, and so a wave of depolarization is propagated down the length of the plasma membrane.
- This is how the action potential travels to the end of the neuron, from where it is chemically transmitted.

Did you know?

Have you ever wondered how local anesthetics work? They block the sodium channels of the plasma membrane of an area. Therefore, nerve impulses cannot pass and the area anesthetized is sensation-free.

Speed of nerve transmission

The speed of propagation of an impulse is not related to the strength of the stimulus. It is proportional to the diameter of the fiber, the thickness of the myelin sheath, and the temperature. The larger the diameter, the more myelin present, and the warmer the temperature, the faster the impulse will be propagated.

This means that the fibers in our body that let us know about potential danger have the largest diameter and therefore the quickest rate of conduction (between 12 and 130 meters per second). These include fibers that relay impulses associated with touch, pressure, position of joints, heat, cold, and skeletal muscles.

The fibers in our body that are related to the autonomic system and therefore the involuntary, automatic functioning of the body have the slowest rate of conduction (between 0.5 and 2 meters per second). They have the smallest diameters and are usually unmyelinated, and include fibers that relay impulses to the heart, smooth muscles, and glands.

> ## Infobox
> ....
> ### Anatomy and physiology in perspective
>
> Propagation of an impulse can be slowed down or even partially blocked by low temperatures. This is why applying ice to a painful area reduces the sensation of pain.

Chemical transmission across the synapse

Transmission between nerves can be either electrical or chemical. Electrical transmission is very fast and allows for the two-way transmission of an impulse across a gap junction. It takes place between neurons in the CNS, viscera, smooth muscle, and cardiac muscles.

Chemical transmission, on the other hand, is slower and only allows for one-way transmission of an impulse. It occurs across a **synapse**, which is a small space filled with extracellular fluid between the end of a neuron and another neuron, muscle, or gland.

When the action potential reaches the end of the neuron it causes vesicles containing neurotransmitters to open up and release a neurotransmitter into the synaptic cleft.

- Two to three different neurotransmitters can be present in a single neuron. Neurotransmitters can be excitatory or inhibitory and their action depends on the receptors to which they bind. Examples of neurotransmitters include:
  - **Acetylcholine**
  - **Dopamine**
  - **Norepinephrine (norepinephrine)**—this is both a neurotransmitter and a hormone

- The neurotransmitter diffuses across the synaptic cleft and binds to the receptors of the next neuron, muscle, or gland, where it now acts as a stimulus.
- The neurotransmitter in the synaptic cleft is then quickly removed by diffusion, enzyme degradation, or being actively transported back into the cells, where it is recycled.

> ## Did you know?
> ....
> Synapses are the site of action for many drugs that affect the brain—these can be either therapeutic or addictive drugs.

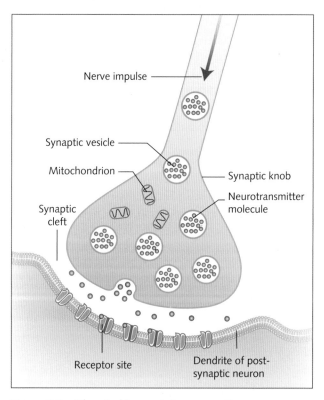

Figure 6.7 *Chemical transmission across the synapse*

> ## Infobox
> ....
> ### Anatomy and physiology in perspective
>
> The drug cocaine blocks the transporters that cause the removal of the neurotransmitter dopamine from the synaptic cleft. Therefore, dopamine remains in the synaptic cleft and causes an excess stimulation of certain regions of the brain. This results in what is described as a sense of euphoria.

Nerves

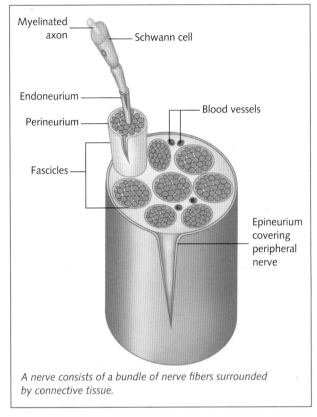

Myelinated axon
Schwann cell
Endoneurium
Perineurium
Blood vessels
Fascicles
Epineurium covering peripheral nerve

A nerve consists of a bundle of nerve fibers surrounded by connective tissue.

Figure 6.8 *Structure of a nerve*

A neuron is a single nerve cell consisting of dendrites, a cell body, and an axon. A nerve is composed of the axons and dendrites of a group or bundle of neurons, bound together by connective tissue. The structure of a nerve is very similar to that of a muscle. It consists of a bundle of nerve fibers surrounded by connective tissue.

- The **endoneurium** surrounds each individual nerve fiber.
- The **perineurium** surrounds groups of nerve fibers, called **fascicles**.
- The **epineurium** binds the fascicles together and is the outer covering of the nerve.

Nerves are classified into three different types:

- **Sensory or afferent nerves:** These contain sensory fibers that carry sensory impulses toward the CNS.
- **Motor or efferent nerves:** These contain motor fibers that carry motor impulses away from the CNS.
- **Mixed nerves:** These contain both sensory and motor fibers. All spinal nerves are mixed nerves.

Some important vocabulary associated with nerves includes:

- **Nerve fiber:** The term "fiber" refers to the processes that project from a nerve body, these being dendrites and axons. However, the term is usually used to refer to the axon and its sheath only.
- **Ganglion (plural = ganglia):** A bundle or knot of nerve cell bodies.
- **Tract:** Tracts are bundles of fibers that are not surrounded by connective tissue. They are found in the CNS and some of them interconnect regions of the brain.

Brain

What is it that makes us so different from other mammals? Physically, we are generally one of the weaker mammals: our skin is thin and tears easily; our jaws are relatively small and weak; and our senses of smell, hearing, and sight are not as powerful as those of many other mammals. However, we are able to light fires to warm us when we are cold, build homes to protect us from the environment, and even create objects with which to kill animals that are stronger and faster than us. How is this so?

What makes humans so unique is our large brain, which is approximately six times heavier than that of a dog of the same weight (Barnard, 1981, p. 50). This brain gives us the ability to not simply adapt to the changes in our environment, but also to adapt our environment to suit us. This is what makes us different from other mammals: thanks to our incredible brains we can sense changes, think about them, make decisions, and act on them.

An overview of the brain

An adult brain weighs approximately 2.9 lb (1.3 kg) and consists of a hundred billion neurons and a thousand billion neuroglia (Tortora and Grabowski, 1996, p. 391). It lies in the cranial cavity and is composed of four regions:

- **Brain stem:** This is continuous with the spinal cord and consists of the:
  - **Medulla oblongata**
  - **Pons (pons Varolii)**
  - **Midbrain**

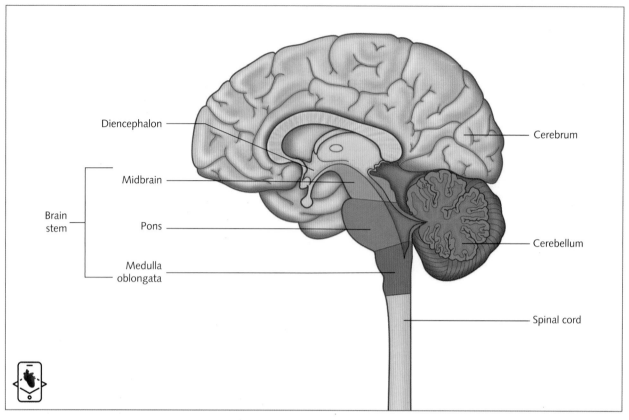

Figure 6.9 *The human brain*

- **Cerebellum:** This cauliflower-shaped region is found at the back of the head, behind the brain stem.
- **Diencephalon:** This lies above the brain stem and includes the:
  - **Epithalamus**
  - **Thalamus**
  - **Hypothalamus**
- **Cerebrum:** This appears as a cap over the diencephalon and fills most of the cranium. It is divided into two halves—namely, the right and left **cerebral hemispheres**. The outer, most superficial layer of the cerebrum is called the **cerebral cortex**. The inner layer consists of **white matter** and **basal ganglia**. The **limbic system** is located between the cerebrum and diencephalon.

Protection of the brain

The brain is a vital and sensitive organ and therefore needs maximum protection. The body provides this in a number of ways:

- The hard bones of the **cranium** form a nearly impenetrable wall against the external environment.

- Three layers of connective tissue cover the brain and provide further barriers to the external environment. These are called the **meninges**.
- The brain itself floats in a fluid called **cerebrospinal fluid**. This acts as a shock absorber so that the brain does not knock against the hard walls of the cranium. It also provides a barrier against any substances trying to enter the brain from the internal environment.

Did you know?

Meningitis is inflammation of the meninges.

Cranial meninges
Three layers of connective tissue encircle and protect the brain and spinal cord. They are called the cranial and spinal meninges and are continuous with one another, sharing the same basic structure and names. The meninges are:

- **Dura mater:** This is the outer covering of the brain, continuous with the periosteum of the

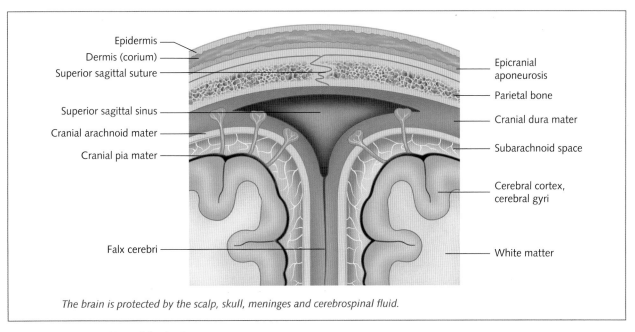

Epidermis
Dermis (corium)
Superior sagittal suture
Superior sagittal sinus
Cranial arachnoid mater
Cranial pia mater
Falx cerebri

Epicranial aponeurosis
Parietal bone
Cranial dura mater
Subarachnoid space
Cerebral cortex, cerebral gyri
White matter

The brain is protected by the scalp, skull, meninges and cerebrospinal fluid.

Figure 6.10   *Protection of the brain*

cranial bones. It does not leave the skull apart from at the following three folds:

- **Falx cerebri** separates the two hemispheres of the cerebrum
- **Falx cerebelli** separates the two hemispheres of the cerebellum
- **Tentorium cerebelli** separates the cerebrum from the cerebellum
- **Arachnoid mater:** This is the middle covering of the brain, separated from the other two meninges by spaces:
  - The **subdural space** lies between the dura mater and arachnoid
  - The **subarachnoid space** lies between the arachnoid and pia mater and contains cerebrospinal fluid
- **Pia mater:** This is the thin inner covering of the brain. It dips into all the folds and spaces of the brain tissue.

Cerebrospinal fluid (CSF)

This is a clear, colorless liquid that circles the CNS, protecting it and helping to maintain homeostasis. It contains glucose, proteins, lactic acid, urea, cations, anions, and a few white blood cells.

Functions of CSF

Cerebrospinal fluid is crucial not only in protecting the CNS, but also in maintaining homeostasis:

- It acts as a **shock absorber** for the brain and spinal cord.
- It provides the correct **chemical environment** in which neurons can function.
- It acts as a medium for the **exchange of nutrients and waste** between the blood and the nervous tissue and provides a constant supply of oxygen and glucose for nerve cells.

Did you know?

The adult brain comprises only 2% of the weight of the entire body but it uses 20% of the body's resting oxygen consumption. It therefore needs a constant supply of oxygen, and even a short interruption of only one to two minutes can impair brain cells. Permanent damage of brain cells will result from a lack of oxygen supply for four minutes (Tortora and Grabowksi, 1996, p. 396).

Infobox

Anatomy and physiology in perspective

The brain needs a constant supply of glucose because it is unable to store large amounts of it. If there is a low level of glucose in the blood going to the brain, then symptoms such as mental confusion, dizziness, or even loss of consciousness can result.

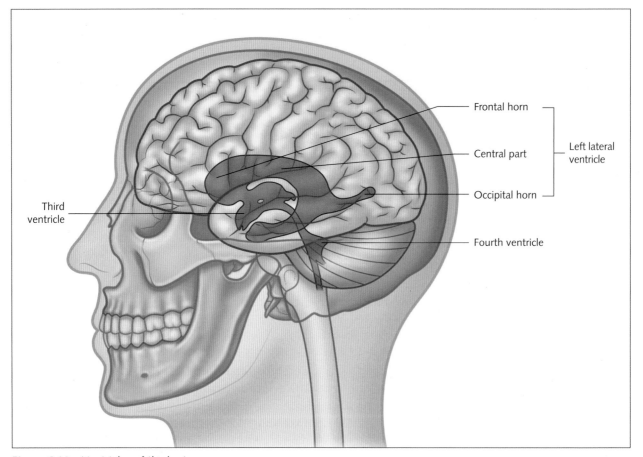

Figure 6.11 *Ventricles of the brain*

Ventricles

CSF flows through and fills cavities in the brain called **ventricles**. There are four of them:

- **Left and right lateral ventricles:** These two lateral ventricles are found in the hemispheres of the cerebrum, either side of the midline.
- **The third ventricle:** This narrow ventricle is found at the midline below the lateral ventricles.
- **The fourth ventricle:** This ventricle lies below and behind the third ventricle and is found between the brain stem and the cerebellum.

Did you know?

Although the function of the blood–brain barrier is to protect the brain from harmful substances, it does also keep out potentially beneficial or therapeutic substances such as drugs that could be used to treat brain tumors or disorders of the CNS.

Formation of CSF

CSF is formed from blood plasma at networks of capillaries on the walls of the ventricles. These networks are called the **choroid plexuses** and they contain specialized cells called **ependymal cells,** which are found on the capillaries. These cells filter the blood plasma and remove any potentially harmful substances from it. Thus, the CNS is protected from many harmful substances that can be found in the blood, and this barrier is referred to as the **blood–brain barrier.**

Absorption of CSF

CSF is formed at the choroid plexuses in the ventricles, circulates through the ventricles into the subarachnoid space, and it then circulates in the central canal of the spinal cord and the subarachnoid space around the brain and spinal cord. It is finally reabsorbed back into the blood through arachnoid villi. CSF is absorbed as quickly as it is formed and this ensures that its pressure remains constant.

Infobox

···

Anatomy and physiology in perspective

The blood–brain barrier is a selective barrier that protects the brain. However, some substances are helped across it by transporters such as lipids. Thus, lipid-soluble substances—like alcohol, caffeine, nicotine, and anesthetics—can pass directly into the brain cells.

Regions of the Brain

The charts following take a more detailed look at the regions of the brain.

Brain stem

The brain stem is a continuation of the spinal cord and connects the spinal cord to the diencephalon. It consists of the medulla oblongata, pons, and midbrain, and its main function is to relay motor and sensory impulses between the spinal cord and the other parts of the brain. Running along the length of the brain stem is a mass of gray matter called the **reticular formation**.

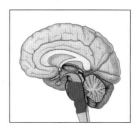

Region	Description	Functions
Medulla oblongata (often referred to as the **medulla**)	• Found at the top of the spinal cord • Approximately 1⅕ in (3 cm) long	The medulla oblongata contains: • All sensory and motor white matter **tracts that connect the brain with the spinal cord;** most of these tracts cross over from the left to the right and vice versa, so the left side of the brain controls the muscles of the right side of the body and vice versa • A cardiovascular center, which regulates the **heartbeat** and **diameter of blood vessels** • A medullary rhythmicity area, which regulates **breathing** • Centers for the coordination of **swallowing, vomiting, coughing, sneezing,** and **hiccupping** • Nuclei of origin for **cranial nerves VIII–XII;** cranial nerves will be discussed later in this chapter • Neurons that function in **precise voluntary movements, posture,** and **balance**
Pons Varolii (pons)	• Lies above the medulla oblongata and in front of the cerebellum • Approximately 1 in (2.5 cm) long	*Pons* means "bridge" and the pons acts as a bridge between the spinal cord and brain as well as between different parts of the brain itself; the pons also contains: • Nuclei of origin for **cranial nerves V–VIII** (**note**: cranial nerve VIII has its origins in both the medulla oblongata and the pons) • Areas that function with the medullary rhythmicity area to help control **respiration**

Region	Description	Functions
Midbrain (mesencephalon)	• Lies between the pons and the diencephalon • Approximately 1 in (2.5 cm) long	The midbrain contains white matter tracts and gray matter nuclei that function as: • Reflex centers for **movements of the eyes, head, and neck** in response to **visual and other stimuli** • Reflex centers for **movements of the head and trunk** in response to **auditory stimuli** • Areas that control **subconscious muscle activities** • Areas that function with the basal ganglia and cerebellum to help coordinate **muscular movements** • Nuclei of origin for **cranial nerves III and IV**
Reticular formation	This is a mass of gray matter that extends the entire length of the brain stem	The reticular formation functions in: • The **motor control of visceral organs and in muscle tone** • **Consciousness and awakening from sleep**

Infobox

Anatomy and physiology in perspective

The brain stem plays a vital role in many activities, and injuries to it can be fatal or, at the least, very serious. Injuries can result from a hard blow to the back of the head or upper neck. If the medulla oblongata is injured then paralysis, loss of sensation, irregular breathing, or irregular heart functioning may occur. On the other hand, if the reticular formation is injured a coma may result.

Infobox

Anatomy and physiology in perspective

Damage to the cerebellum causes clumsy and uncoordinated movements and people who have damaged it can sometimes appear drunk: they are unable to keep their balance or perform simple coordinated movements such as touching their finger to their nose with their eyes closed. The cerebellum can be damaged by a tumor, stroke, or blow to the head.

Cerebellum

The cerebellum is the second largest portion of the brain and it looks like a piece of cauliflower. It functions in producing smooth, coordinated movements as well as in posture and balance, and is what gives us the ability to perform complex movements like somersaulting, dancing, or throwing a ball.

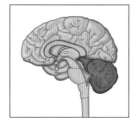

Diencephalon (interbrain)

The diencephalon is also called the interbrain, and it lies above the brain stem, where it is enclosed by the cerebral hemispheres. It contains the **epithalamus, thalamus,** and **hypothalamus,** and has a number of different functions, including housing the pituitary and pineal endocrine glands.

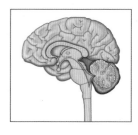

Region	Description	Functions

Cerebellum	Found at the back of the head, behind the medulla oblongata and pons and beneath the cerebrum	Its main functions include:
		
		• **Coordinating and smoothing complex sequences of skeletal muscular contraction**
		  – It receives input from **proprioceptors** in muscles, tendons, and joints as well as from receptors for equilibrium and visual receptors in the eye
		  – It takes this information and compares the intended movement that has been programmed in the cerebrum with what is actually happening and so is able to smooth and coordinate movements
		• **Regulating posture and balance**

Epithalamus	Forms the roof of the third ventricle and is found above the thalamus	The epithalamus contains: • The **pineal gland**, part of the endocrine system (see chapter 7) • The **choroid plexus**, which is the group of capillaries that forms cerebrospinal fluid
Thalamus	• The word *thalamus* means "inner chamber" • It is approximately 1⅕ in (3 cm) long and makes up about 80% of the diencephalon • It encloses the third ventricle of the brain	Functions of the thalamus include: • It is the main **relay station** for **sensory impulses to the cerebral cortex**; sensory impulses include those of **hearing, vision, taste, touch, pressure, vibration, heat, cold,** and **pain** • It contains an area for the **crude appreciation of sensations** such as pain, temperature, and pressure before they are relayed to the cerebral cortex, where the sensations are refined • It contains nuclei that play a role in **voluntary motor actions** and **arousal** • It contains nuclei for certain **emotions** and **memory**, as well as for **cognition**, which is the ability to acquire knowledge
Hypothalamus	Found below the thalamus	The hypothalamus is one of the main **regulators of homeostasis**; sensory input from either the internal or external environment eventually comes to the hypothalamus It also contains receptors that monitor **osmotic pressure, hormone concentrations,** and **blood temperature** In addition, the hypothalamus is connected to the endocrine system Its functions include: • **Regulating the ANS:** By controlling the contraction of smooth and cardiac muscle and the secretions of many glands, the hypothalamus regulates visceral activities such as heart rate and the movement of food through the gastrointestinal tract

Region	Description	Functions
		• **Controlling the pituitary gland:** – It releases hormones that control the secretions of the pituitary gland – It also synthesizes two hormones that are transported to, and stored in, the posterior pituitary gland until they are released; these are **oxytocin** and **antidiuretic hormone (vasopressin)** • **Regulating emotional behavior:** Working together with the limbic system (to be discussed shortly), the hypothalamus functions in regulating emotional behavior such as rage, aggression, pain, pleasure, and sexual arousal • **Regulating eating and drinking:** The hypothalamus controls sensations of hunger, fullness, and thirst • **Controlling body temperature** • **Regulating sleeping patterns**

Cerebrum

The cerebrum sits like a large cap covering and basically obscuring the rest of the brain, and it is often referred to as the "seat of intelligence." It is this area that gives us the ability to read, write, speak, remember, create, and imagine.

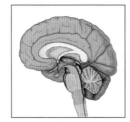

The cerebrum's outer, most superficial layer is made up of ridges and grooves that look like deep wrinkles. This layer is called the **cerebral cortex** (the word *cortex* means "rind") and it consists of **gray matter**. Beneath the gray matter of the cerebral cortex is an inner layer of **white matter**, the **limbic system,** and the **basal ganglia**.

The ridges of the cortex are called **gyri** or **convolutions**, its shallow grooves are **sulci**, and its deep grooves are **fissures**. A deep fissure called the **longitudinal fissure** separates the cerebrum into two halves: the right and left hemisphere. Although they appear to be separate, these hemispheres are still connected internally by the **corpus callosum**, which is a large bundle of white-matter transverse fibers. Each hemisphere is subdivided into four lobes named after the bones that cover them: the **frontal, parietal, temporal,** and **occipital** lobes.

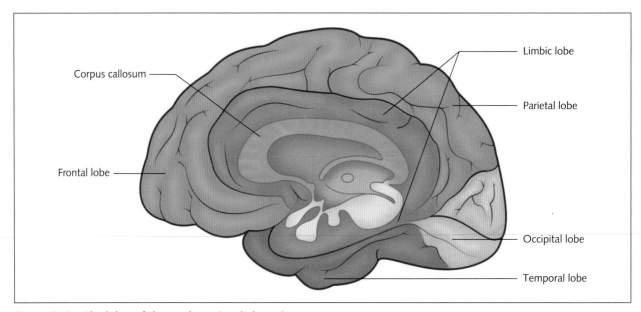

Figure 6.12 *The lobes of the cerebrum (medial view)*

Region	Description	Functions

Cerebral cortex	• Approximately the size and shape of two closed fists held together
	• It consists of gray matter, ridged and grooved and separated into two hemispheres
		The cerebral cortex is large and has many areas related to different functions—a simplistic view of it is that it receives almost all the sensory impulses of the body and interprets them into meaningful patterns of recognition and awarenes. It has:
		
		• **Sensory areas** that receive and process information; these are mainly found in the posterior half of the hemispheres:
		  – **General sensory area** for receiving impulses related to touch, proprioception, pain, and temperature; the body can be mapped onto this sensory area and the exact part of the body where the sensation is originating can be pinpointed
		  – **Visual area** for receiving information regarding characteristics of visual stimuli, such as shape, color, and movement
		  – **Auditory area** for receiving information regarding characteristics of sound, such as rhythm and pitch
		  – **Gustatory area** for taste
		  – **Olfactory area** for smell
		• **Motor areas** that output information; these are mainly found in the anterior portion of each hemisphere:
		  – **Area for the voluntary contraction of specific muscles or muscle groups**
		  – **Speech area** that translates spoken or written words into thoughts and then into speech
		• **Association areas** that consist of both sensory and motor areas; these are found mainly on the lateral surfaces of the cerebral cortex:
		  – The **somatosensory association area** receives, integrates, and interprets physical sensations; it also stores memories of past experiences for comparison with new information, enabling you to interpret complicated sensations, such as being able to determine the shape and texture of an object without actually looking at it
		  – The **visual association area** enables you to relate present sensations to past experiences and therefore be able to recognize objects
		  – The **auditory association area** enables you to relate present sensations to past experiences and therefore be able to recognize a sound and determine whether it is speech, music, or simply a noise
		  – The **gnostic area** integrates information and enables you to develop thoughts from a variety of sensory inputs, such as smell, taste, etc.

Region	Description	Functions
		– The **premotor area** enables you to perform complicated learned motor activities such as writing – The **frontal eye field area** controls scanning movements of the eye, enabling you to perform activities such as scanning a paragraph of writing for a specific word – The **language areas** coordinate the muscles associated with speech and breathing so that you can speak
White matter	Lies beneath the cerebral cortex	The white matter consists of axons that transmit nerve impulses around the cortex and between the brain and spinal cord
Limbic system	Found on the inner border of the cerebrum, the floor of the diencephalon and encircling the brain stem	The limbic system is often called the "emotional brain" because it controls the emotional and involuntary aspects of behavior; it is the area associated with **pain, pleasure, anger, rage, fear, sorrow, sexual feelings,** and **affection**; it also functions in **memory**
Basal ganglia	These are groups of nuclei found in the cerebral hemispheres; they are interconnected by many nerve fibers	The basal ganglia receive information from, and provide output to, the cerebral cortex, thalamus, and hypothalamus They control large **automatic movements of the skeletal muscles** and also help regulate muscle tone

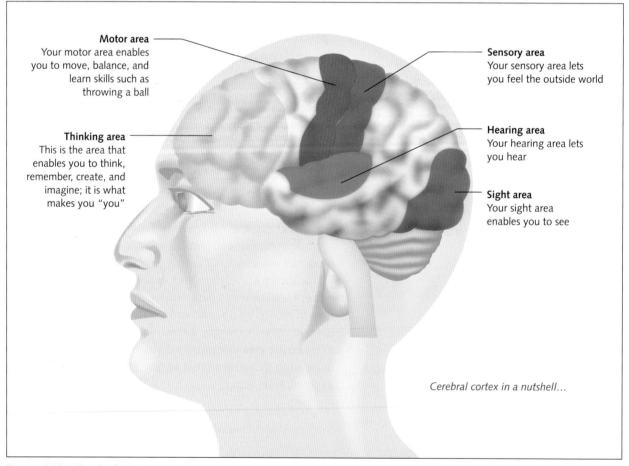

Motor area
Your motor area enables you to move, balance, and learn skills such as throwing a ball

Thinking area
This is the area that enables you to think, remember, create, and imagine; it is what makes you "you"

Sensory area
Your sensory area lets you feel the outside world

Hearing area
Your hearing area lets you hear

Sight area
Your sight area enables you to see

Cerebral cortex in a nutshell...

Figure 6.13 *Cerebral cortex*

The brain in a nutshell

Note: This is a very simplified version of the brain.

Brain stem (medulla oblongata, pons, midbrain)

- Link between the brain and spinal cord
- Autonomic control

Cerebellum

- Movement, posture, and balance

Diencephalon (epithalamus, thalamus, hypothalamus)

- Relays sensory impulses to the cerebral cortex
- Regulates homeostasis

Cerebrum (cerebral cortex/gray matter, white matter, limbic system, basal ganglia)

- Emotions and intelligence

Cranial Nerves

The cranial nerves are considered part of the PNS. There are 12 pairs of them, 10 which originate from the brain stem and 2 originate from inside the brain. They are named according to their distribution or function and numbered according to where they arise in the brain (in order from anterior to posterior).

Most of the cranial nerves contain both motor and sensory fibers and so are mixed nerves. Only three are purely sensory: the olfactory, optic, and vestibulocochlear nerves.

CRANIAL NERVES		
Number	Name	Function
I	Olfactory	Smell
II	Optic	Vision
III	Oculomotor	Movement of eyelid and eyeball; control of lens shape and pupil size; carries autonomic nerves
IV	Trochlear	Movement of eyeball
V	Trigeminal *Three branches: Ophthalmic, maxillary, and mandibular*	**Motor function (mandibular branch only):** Chewing **Sensory function:** Sensations of touch, pain, and temperature from the skin of the face and the mucosa of the nose and mouth, and sensations supplied by proprioceptors in the muscles of mastication
VI	Abducens	Movement of eyeball
VII	Facial *Five branches: Temporal, zygomatic, buccal, mandibular, and cervical*	Facial expression; carries autonomic fibers for secretion of saliva and tears

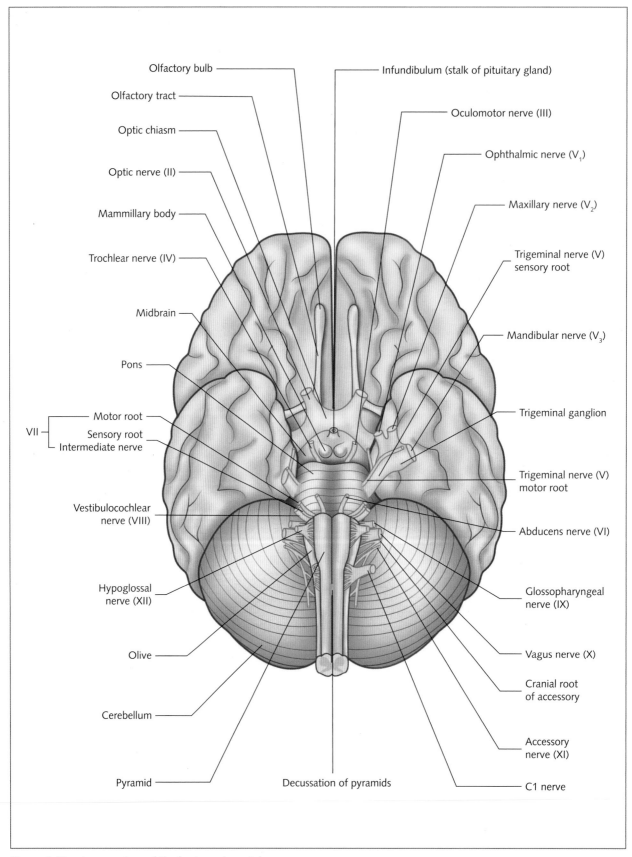

Figure 6.14 *An overview of the brain and cranial nerves*

CRANIAL NERVES		
Number	Name	Function
VIII	Vestibulocochlear *Two branches: Vestibular and cochlear*	**Vestibular branch:** Balance **Cochlear branch:** Hearing
IX	Glossopharyngeal	Sensory to oropharynx; carries autonomic supply for secretion of saliva and sensory from carotid body and sinus
X	Vagus	**Motor function:** Secretion of digestive fluids and contraction of smooth muscle of organs of the thoracic and abdominal cavities **Sensory function:** Sensory input from the organs of the thoracic and abdominal cavities
XI	Accessory *Two portions: Cranial and spinal*	**Cranial portion:** Joins the vagus nerve to supply motor to pharyngeal muscles **Spinal portion:** Movement of head, sternocleidomastoid and trapezius muscles
XII	Hypoglossal	Movement of tongue when talking and swallowing

Spinal Cord

Approximately 16½ in (42 cm) long and on average ¾ in (2 cm) in diameter, the spinal cord is continuous with the brain stem and ends just above the second lumbar vertebra (L2).

Functions of the spinal cord

The spinal cord has two main functions that help maintain homeostasis:

- The spinal cord transports **nerve impulses** from the periphery of the body to the brain and from the brain to the periphery.
- The spinal cord receives and integrates information and produces **reflex actions**, which are predictable, automatic responses to specific changes in the environment.

Anatomy of the spinal cord

Spinal meninges

Like the brain, the spinal cord is protected by meninges: the **spinal meninges**. These meninges are continuous with the cranial meninges, and are the:

- **Dura mater**—the outer covering of the spinal cord. Between it and the wall of the vertebral column is a space filled with fat and connective tissue. This is the **epidural space**.
- **Arachnoid (mater)**—the middle covering, which is separated from the other two meninges by:
  - The **subdural space**, which is filled with interstitial fluid
  - The **subarachnoid space**, which contains CSF
- **Pia mater**—the thin, inner covering that adheres to the tissue of the spinal cord.

Cauda equina

In an adult the spinal cord extends from the medulla oblongata of the brain to the second lumbar vertebra only. However, some of the nerves that arise in the spine do not exit the vertebral column where they arise. Instead, they angle downward in the canal and only exit the column lower down. These nerves look almost like wisps of hair coming off the end of the spinal cord, and so the area is called the **cauda equina**, which means "horse's tail."

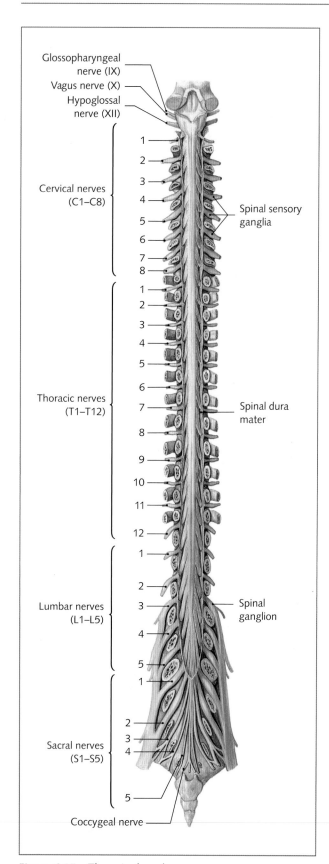

Glossopharyngeal nerve (IX)

Vagus nerve (X)

Hypoglossal nerve (XII)

Cervical nerves (C1–C8)

Spinal sensory ganglia

Thoracic nerves (T1–T12)

Spinal dura mater

Lumbar nerves (L1–L5)

Spinal ganglion

Sacral nerves (S1–S5)

Coccygeal nerve

Figure 6.15 *The spinal cord*

Internal anatomy of the spinal cord

If you take a cross-section of the spinal cord, you will see that it consists of gray H-shaped (butterfly-shaped) matter surrounded by white matter.

- The **gray matter** receives and integrates information and consists of cell bodies and unmyelinated axons and dendrites of association and motor neurons. Gray matter also contains nuclei where some nerve impulses are processed.
- The **white matter** contains tracts of myelinated fibers that transport impulses between the brain and the periphery.
  - **Ascending tracts** consist of sensory axons that conduct nerve impulses to the brain
  - **Descending tracts** consist of motor axons that conduct nerve impulses to the body

Did you know?

....

The sciatic nerve is the largest nerve in the body. It reaches from your lumbar spine right down into your feet and contains nerve fibers up to a meter long.

Spinal nerves

There are 31 pairs of nerves that originate in the spinal cord and emerge through the intervertebral foramina. These nerves form part of the PNS and connect the CNS to receptors in the muscles and glands.

Roots

Each nerve has two points of attachment to the spinal cord. These attachments are called **roots** and are the:

- **Posterior (dorsal) root:** This consists of sensory axons. The dorsal root contains a ganglion of sensory neuron cell bodies.
- **Anterior (ventral) root:** This consists of motor axons.

Because spinal nerves have both sensory and motor axons they are classified as mixed nerves.

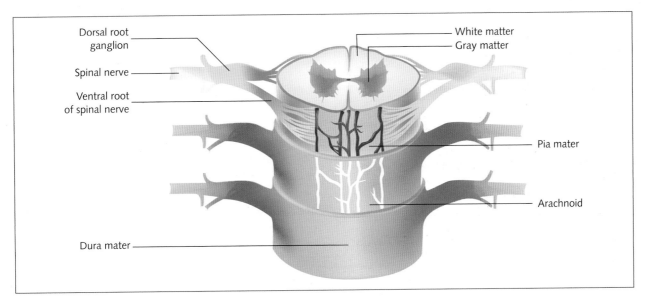

Figure 6.16 *Cross-section through the spinal cord*

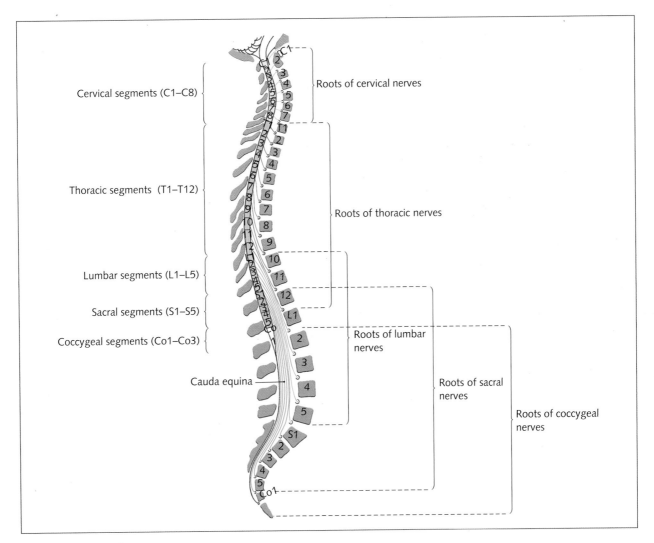

Figure 6.17 *Spinal nerves*

The nervous system in a nutshell
....

- The brain is the control center.
- The spinal cord links the brain to the body and processes reflex actions.
- Nerves connect the brain and spinal cord to the rest of the body.

Naming of the nerves

The spinal nerves are named and numbered according to where in the vertebral column they emerge.
The first spinal nerve starts between the occipital and the first cervical vertebra. There are:

- Eight pairs of cervical nerves
- Twelve pairs of thoracic nerves
- Five pairs of lumbar nerves
- Five pairs of sacral nerves
- One pair of coccygeal nerves.

Note that the lower lumbar, sacral, and coccygeal roots are not in line with their origins or corresponding vertebrae because they descend in the form of the cauda equina.

Spinal plexuses

Branches of some of the spinal nerves form networks of nerves on both sides of the body. These networks are called **plexuses** and all the nerves emerging from a particular plexus will innervate specific structures.

The table below discusses these plexuses in more detail. Please note, nerves T2–T12 do not form a plexus. These are the **intercostal nerves** that serve the muscles between the ribs, and the skin and the muscles of the anterior and lateral trunk.

Plexus	Body areas served	Important nerves
Cervical	Skin and muscles of the head, neck, and top of the shoulders	**Phrenic nerve** supplies motor fibers to the diaphragm
Brachial	Shoulder and upper limb	**Axillary nerve** supplies the deltoid and teres minor muscles **Musculocutaneous nerve** supplies the flexors of the arm **Radial nerve** supplies the muscles on the posterior aspect of the arm and forearm **Median nerve** supplies the muscles on the anterior aspect of the forearm and some muscles of the hand **Ulnar nerve** supplies some of the muscles of the forearm and most of the muscles of the hand
Lumbar	Abdominal wall, external genitals, and part of the lower limb	**Femoral nerve** supplies the flexor muscles of the thigh and extensor muscles of the leg, as well as the skin over parts of the thigh, leg, and foot **Obturator nerve** supplies the adductor muscles of the leg as well as the skin over the medial aspect of the thigh
Sacral	Buttocks, perineum, and lower limbs	**Sciatic nerve** descends through the thigh and splits into the tibial and common fibular nerves

Special Sense Organs

Eyes

Our eyes are one of the brain's vital contacts with the outside world. They enable us to know where we are, what is around us, and where we are going. The eyes are thought to contain over a million nerve fibers and more than 70% of the body's total sensory receptors. The information they gather for us is not simply one dimensional—it is far deeper than that—giving us a sense of space, color, shape, texture, and movement.

Accessory structures

Surrounding the eyes are the eyelids, eyebrows, eyelashes, and eye muscles. All of these work together to protect the eyes from foreign objects, the sun's rays, and perspiration. In addition, there are **lacrimal glands** that release tears on to the surface of the eye to clean and lubricate the eyeball. The tears are then spread by blinking. Lining the eyelids and covering part of the outer surface of the eyeball is a very thin mucous membrane that helps protect the eyeball. It is called the **conjunctiva**.

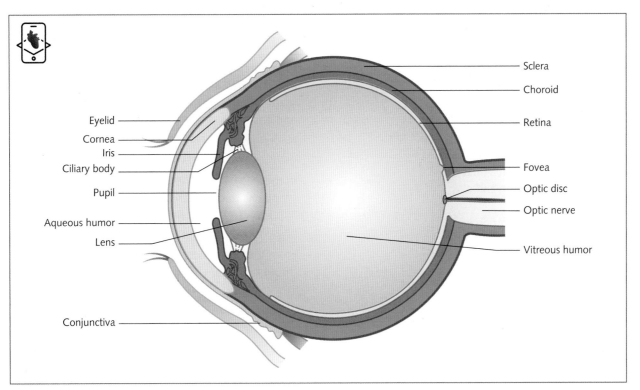

Figure 6.18 *The eye*

Anatomy of the eyeball

The eyeball is approximately 1 in (2.5 cm) in diameter. However, we only see one-sixth of it as the rest is protected by the orbit into which it fits.

The eyeball consists of a strong, protective wall and a large inner space that is divided into cavities filled with different substances.

EXTERIOR OF THE EYEBALL

The wall of the eyeball is divided into three layers: the outer fibrous tunic, the middle vascular tunic, and the inner nervous tunic (the retina)

Structure	Diagram	Details
Fibrous tunic • The outermost covering of the eyeball • The front of the fibrous tunic is the cornea and the back of it is the sclera		**Cornea:** The cornea is an avascular, transparent coat that covers the iris; it is curved and helps focus light **Sclera:** The sclera is the white of the eye and is made up of dense connective tissue; it protects the eyeball and gives it shape and rigidity
Vascular tunic • The middle layer of the wall of the eyeball • The front of the vascular tunic is the colored iris, which is surrounded by the ciliary body, which then becomes the choroid		**Iris:** This is suspended between the cornea and lens and is the colored portion of the eye; it is shaped like a flattened doughnut and the hole in the center of it is the **pupil**, which regulates the amount of light entering the eyeball; the iris consists of circular and radial smooth muscle fibers **Ciliary body:** This contains processes that secrete aqueous humor and muscles that alter the shape of the lens for near or far vision **Choroid:** This lines most of the internal surface of the sclera, is highly vascularized, and provides nutrients to the retina; it also absorbs scattered light
Nervous tunic (retina) • The innermost layer of the wall of the eyeball • It lines the posterior three-quarters of the eyeball • It consists of a non-visual pigmented portion and a neural portion • The pigmented portion lies between the choroid and the neural portion		**Pigmented portion:** This contains melanin and it absorbs stray light rays; it therefore prevents any scattering or reflection of light within the eyeball and ensures a clear, sharp image **Neural portion:** This contains three layers of neurons that process visual input. In these layers are the **photoreceptors**, which are specialized cells that convert light into nerve impulses; **rods**, which respond to different shades of gray only; and **cones**, which respond to color. From the photoreceptors, the information passes through bipolar cells into ganglion cells. The axons of the ganglion cells then extend into the **optic nerve**

INTERIOR OF THE EYEBALL

The interior of the eyeball consists of a large space that is divided into two cavities by the lens

Structure	Diagram	Details
Lens: Behind the colored iris and the dark pupil is the transparent, avascular lens		The lens is responsible for fine-tuning of focusing and it is made up of protein
Anterior cavity: In front of the lens is the anterior cavity, filled with aqueous humor		**Aqueous humor** is a watery fluid that nourishes the lens and cornea and helps produce intraocular pressure; the aqueous humor is constantly replaced
Posterior cavity (vitreous chamber): This is the largest cavity in the eyeball and lies behind the lens; it contains the vitreous body (humor)		**Vitreous body (humor)** is a jelly-like substance that helps produce intraocular pressure, which helps maintain the shape of the eyeball and keeps the retina pressed firmly against the choroid; unlike the aqueous humor, the vitreous humor is not constantly replaced

Infobox

Anatomy and physiology in perspective

Excessive intraocular pressure is called **glaucoma**. It can eventually lead to degeneration of the retina and consequent blindness.

How do we see?

If light passes through substances of different density its speed will change and its rays will bend. This is called **refraction** and it takes place as light passes through the differing densities of the cornea, aqueous humor, lens, and vitreous humor. By the time the light rays reach the retina they have bent to such an extent that the image is reversed from left to right and turned upside down. The photoreceptors on the retina then convert the light into nerve impulses, which are transported by the optic nerve to the visual cortex of the brain. Here the impulses are integrated and interpreted into visual images.

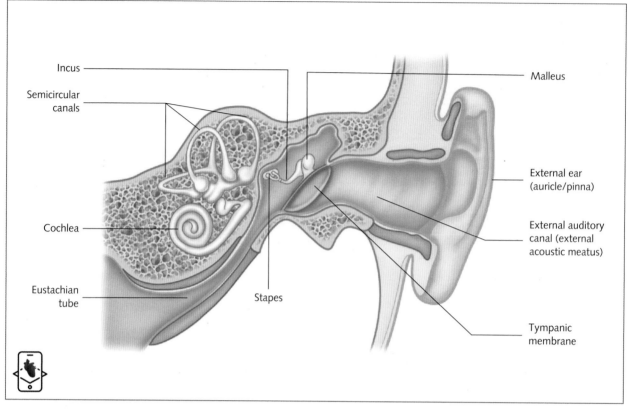

Figure 6.19   *The ear*

Ears

Our ears do not only enable us to hear and locate a sound, they also help us to balance and thus have a sense of equilibrium. Just as we only see one-sixth of the eye, we also only see a portion of the ear. What we see is only part of the external or outer ear, the rest of the ear extends to just below and behind the eye and includes the middle ear and the internal or inner ear.

The following chart gives a brief overview of the anatomy of the ear.

STRUCTURE OF THE OUTER EAR		
The outer, or external, ear collects and channels sound waves inward. It is composed of the auricle, external auditory canal, and eardrum. It also contains **ceruminous glands**, which secrete **cerumen** (earwax), which, along with hairs that are also found in the outer ear, cleans and protects the ear and prevents dust and foreign objects from entering it.		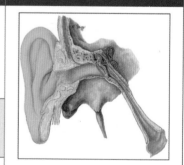
Auricle (pinna)	The part of the ear we see, composed of elastic cartilage covered by skin; the upper rim is called the **helix**, while the lower lobe is called the **lobule**	
External auditory canal (meatus)	A curved tube approximately 1 in (2.5 cm) long, it carries sound waves from the auricle to the eardrum	
Eardrum (tympanic membrane)	A very thin, semi-transparent membrane between the auditory canal and the middle ear; when sound waves hit it, it vibrates, passing them on to the middle ear	

STRUCTURE OF THE MIDDLE EAR

The middle ear is a small, air-filled cavity found between the outer ear and the inner ear. It is partitioned from the outer ear by the eardrum and from the inner ear by a bony partition containing two windows: the **oval window** and the **round window**. It contains the three auditory ossicles and is connected to the throat via the Eustachian tube.

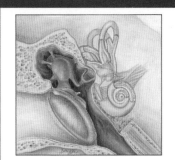

Auditory ossicles	These are three tiny bones extending across the middle ear, and each one is named after its shape: • **Hammer** (**malleus**) • **Anvil** (**incus**) • **Stirrup** (**stapes**) The handle of the hammer is attached to the inner surface of the eardrum and when the eardrum vibrates it causes the hammer to move; the hammer hits the anvil, which in turn hits the stirrup, which is attached to the oval window, a membrane-covered opening which then transmits the sound wave into the inner ear
Eustachian tube (auditory tube)	The Eustachian tube connects the middle ear with the upper portion of the throat (nasopharynx) and it functions in equalizing the middle-ear-cavity pressure with the external atmospheric pressure

STRUCTURE OF THE INNER EAR (LABYRINTH)

The inner, or internal, ear is sometimes also called the labyrinth. It consists of a bony labyrinth filled with a fluid called **perilymph** enclosing a membranous labyrinth filled with a fluid called **endolymph**. This labyrinth is divided into the **vestibule**, three **semicircular canals,** and the **cochlea**. Inside the cochlea lies the actual organ of hearing itself: the **organ of Corti**.

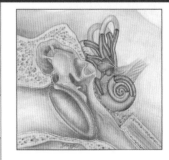

Vestibule	This is the central portion of the bony labyrinth, and contains receptors for equilibrium
Semicircular canals	These project from the vestibule and also contain receptors for equilibrium
Cochlea	• The cochlea is a bony, spiral canal that resembles a snail's shell • It is divided into three channels, one of which is the **cochlear duct**, which is separated from another channel by the **basilar membrane** • Resting on the basilar membrane is the organ of hearing, which is called the organ of Corti or the **spiral organ**
Organ of Corti	• The organ of Corti is a coiled sheet of epithelial cells containing thousands of hair cells • Extensions from these hair cells extend into the endolymph of the cochlear duct and are the receptors for auditory sensations • Over the hair cells is a very thin, flexible membrane called the **tectorial membrane**

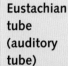

Did you know?

The stirrup (stapes) is the smallest bone in the body and is no longer than a grain of rice. Yet, despite its tiny size, it is essential to our ability to hear. Without this rice-sized bone, sound waves could not be transmitted to the inner ear.

Infobox

Anatomy and physiology in perspective

Have you ever flown in an airplane and found your ears begin to ache or felt as if you had a bubble in your ear and all sounds seemed to be coming from far away? This is because the pressure within your middle ear is unequal to the external pressure and so your eardrum is bulging inward or outward. To normalize the pressure you can either swallow or cover your mouth and nose and try to blow out at the same time.

How do we hear?

What happens when you drop a stone into a pond of water? It causes ripples to travel over the surface of the water. Sound travels in a similar way. An object vibrates and creates alternating compressions and decompressions of air molecules. These are sound waves.

Sound waves travel through the air from their source to the auricle of our ears. The auricle then directs the sound waves into the auditory canal, where they are channelled toward the eardrum. Once they hit the eardrum they cause it to vibrate, and this sets up a chain reaction of vibrations that eventually causes changes in the pressure of the endolymph in the cochlear duct. As this pressure rises and falls it moves the basilar membrane, which vibrates and causes the hair cells of the organ of Corti to move against the tectorial membrane.

The hair cells are mechanoreceptors and they convert this mechanical stimulus into an electrical one. The hair cells synapse with neurons of cranial nerve VIII, the vestibulocochlear nerve, which sends the impulses to the medulla oblongata. The fibers then extend into the thalamus, from where the auditory signals are projected to the primary auditory area of the temporal lobe of the cerebral cortex.

Did you know?

If you are listening to music through earphones and it is loud enough to be heard by the person standing next to you, then you are damaging the hair cells of your inner ear. This can lead to progressive hearing loss, which is often not noticed until extensive damage has been done.

Mouth

The mouth houses the receptors of taste. These are called **gustatory receptors** and are found in **taste buds**, which are located mainly on the tongue, the back of the roof of the mouth, and in the pharynx and larynx.

A taste bud is an oval body that contains gustatory receptor cells. Each of these cells has a single hairlike projection that projects from the receptor cell and through a small opening in the taste bud called the **taste pore**.

Once inside the mouth, food is dissolved in saliva, and the hairs of gustatory receptors dip into this saliva and are stimulated by the taste chemical within it. Thus, gustatory receptors are chemoreceptors.

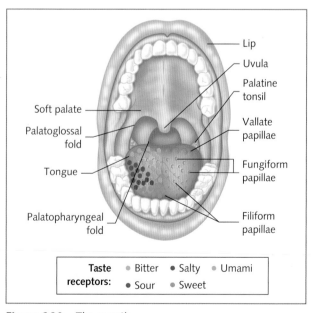

Figure 6.20 *The mouth*

The taste receptors then send messages to the areas of the brain responsible for taste, appetite, and saliva production. On the tongue, taste buds are found in elevations called **papillae**. These elevations give the tongue its rough surface.

Infobox

Anatomy and physiology in perspective

Are we born with a "sweet tooth?" Most of us do prefer sweet flavors over bitter ones, and studies have found that even newborn babies prefer sweet to bitter flavors. This may be because most natural poisons are bitter tasting, and the sense of taste may act as a protective mechanism, not allowing something that might be dangerous to enter into the body. On the other hand, a lot of non-poisonous berries and fruits are generally sweet tasting.

Nose

At the top of the nasal cavity is a small patch about the size of a postage stamp that contains olfactory receptors. Olfactory receptors are neurons that have many hairlike projections extending from their dendrites.

In the connective tissue that supports the olfactory epithelium are **olfactory glands (Bowman's glands)** that produce mucus. When you breathe in, airborne particles dissolve in this mucus and so come into contact with the hairlike cilia of the olfactory receptors. The olfactory cells are chemoreceptors and convert the chemical stimulus found dissolved in the mucus into nerve impulses. These impulses are then sent to the frontal lobe via the limbic system of the brain.

The sensory experience of eating involves both our senses of smell and taste, and what we know as

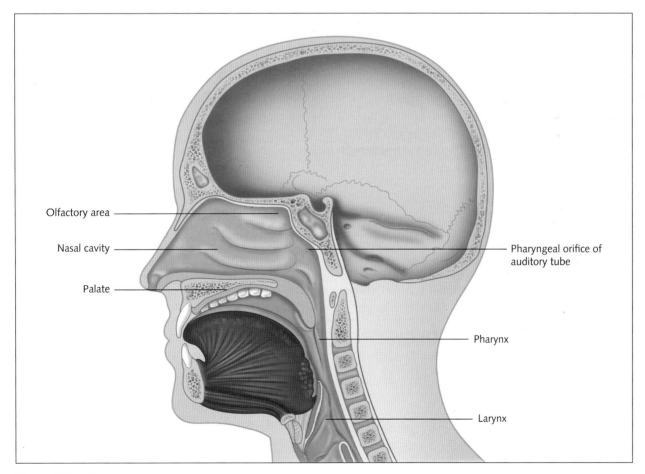

Figure 6.21 *The nose*

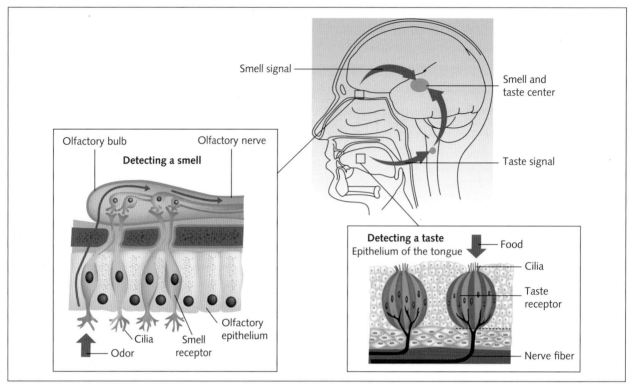

Figure 6.22 *Smell and taste*

"flavor" is actually the perception of smell and taste together. Interestingly, we can only distinguish five primary tastes (sour, sweet, bitter, salty, and umami) and combinations of them; yet we can smell over 400 different odors. This is why you often cannot taste foods if you have a blocked nose from a cold. This is also the reason that wine tasters always smell the bouquet of the wine before tasting it.

The senses of smell and taste are also unique in that their impulses travel via the limbic system to the cerebral cortex. This means that they are closely connected to our emotions and memories. For example, the smell of a certain perfume can remind you of someone you have not thought about for years.

Did you know?

Olfactory receptors are unique neurons in that they are continually being replaced. While most mature neurons in the body cannot be replaced, olfactory receptors live for approximately one month before being replaced.

Did you know?

When you sneeze, a jet of mucus droplets travels through your nose at approximately 100 mph. It is not surprising that sneezing clears your nose!

Common Pathologies of the Nervous System

Because the nervous system controls the entire body, disorders of this system can affect the body in many different ways. Possible indications of nervous system diseases or disorders can include pain, muscle malfunction, changes in sensation, sleep problems, and changes in consciousness such as dizziness, fainting, confusion, or even dementia.

Red flags

- Dizziness or vertigo with loss of consciousness
- Fainting (syncope), especially if
  - During exertion
  - Recurring
  - Accompanied by heart disease or chest pain
  - In the elderly

- Headaches if:
  - Accompanied by other neurological symptoms such as visual disturbances, altered mental status, or weakness
  - Onset begins after the age of 50 years
  - Beginning suddenly and rapidly peaking in unbearable pain ("thunderclap headaches")
  - Accompanied by reddening of the eyes and visual disturbances
- Meningitis:
  - Sudden high fever
  - Stiff neck
  - Severe headache
  - Headache with nausea or vomiting
  - Sensitivity to light
  - Skin rash
- Stroke (CVA)—remember **FAST**:
  - Face drooping
  - Arm weakness
  - Speech difficulty
  - Time to call
- Tremors, especially if accompanied by other neurological symptoms, tachycardia, or agitation
- Visual disturbances, especially if sudden loss or blurring of vision
- Weakness:
  - That becomes progressively severe
  - Accompanied by dyspnea
  - Accompanied by difficulty holding head up, chewing, talking, or swallowing
  - Accompanied by difficulty in walking or incontinence

Pathologies of the nervous system

Alzheimer's disease
Progressive degeneration of brain tissue and is one of the most common causes of dementia. It usually affects elderly people and initial symptoms are memory loss and forgetfulness. Confusion and disorientation then develop and as the disease progresses there can be episodes of paranoia, hallucination, and mood change. The cause of Alzheimer's disease is unknown, but it involves a loss of some neurons, the development of plaques on some neurons, and the entanglement of the protein filaments within neurons.

Anosmia
Loss of the sense of smell. Generally, one's ability to smell degenerates with age but it can also be affected by blocked nasal passages accompanying colds. Anosmia can also be due to problems with the nerves that transmit the sensation of smell to the brain. A loss of the sense of smell also affects one's ability to taste.

Brain tumor
Abnormal growth in the brain that can be benign or malignant. The symptoms will differ according to the area of the brain in which it is found. Possible early signs and symptoms can include constant headaches, changes in personality, drowsiness, confusion, and unusual behavior. These can develop to include dizziness, loss of balance, incoordination, nausea, and vomiting, among other signs and symptoms, such as a loss of function of the area controlled by the part of the brain affected.

Cerebral palsy
Disorder characterized by muscular incoordination and loss of muscle control that results in a lack of balance, abnormal posture, muscle spasticity, and speech impairment. It can sometimes also result in mental retardation. It is caused by damage to the motor areas of the brain during fetal life, birth, or infancy. It is not a progressive disease.

Chronic fatigue syndrome or myalgic encephalomyelitis (ME)
Condition characterized by extreme, disabling fatigue that is not relieved by rest. It is usually accompanied by symptoms such as poor memory, reduced concentration, sore throats, muscle and joint pain, headaches, and a persistent feeling of illness after exercise. A cause is not always identifiable.

Dementia
Impairment of cognitive function affecting a person's thinking, behavior, memory, or ability to perform normal, everyday tasks. It is a collection of symptoms and not a disease, and it can be caused by many underlying neurodegenerative and vascular diseases. It is most common in the elderly.

Depression
Characterized by an excessive feeling of sadness that can affect sleeping patterns, appetite, and one's ability to concentrate. It can have a number of causes, such as an illness, certain drugs, or distressing events such as

the loss of a friend or loved one, and it can tend to run in families. **Postpartum (postnatal) depression** occurs in women after childbirth and can interfere with the mother's ability to care for herself or her child.

Epilepsy

The term epilepsy refers to a group of disorders of the brain characterized by seizures. Seizures are short, recurrent, periodic attacks of motor, sensory, or psychological malfunction. The cause of epilepsy can be unknown or it can result from a head injury, brain tumor, or stroke, and seizures are often aggravated by physical or emotional stress or a lack of sleep. Other triggers can be certain drugs, infections, fever, and low blood sugar. In rare cases, repetitive sounds, flashing lights, or video games can trigger seizures.

Fainting (syncope)

Sudden loss of consciousness that is temporary and brief and usually caused by an inadequate supply of oxygen and nutrients to the brain due to a decrease in blood flow.

Headaches

Pain felt within the skull that can vary in intensity, frequency, and cause. For example, headaches can be related to stress and emotions; can be caused by other disorders of the eyes, nose, throat, sinuses, teeth, jaws, ears, or neck; or can be a symptom of a more serious disease.

Cluster headaches are severe, piercing headaches that usually affect the temples or areas around the eye on one side of the head. They don't usually last more than four hours and are not accompanied by nausea or vomiting. However, the pain is so severe that it can cause a person to pace up and down and even bang their head. After the headache the person can sometimes have a droopy eyelid, constricted pupil, runny nose, or watery eye on the side that was affected.

Migraines are severe, throbbing headaches that usually affect one side of the head. They can be accompanied by pain, nausea, vomiting, and changes in mood and behavior. Some people may experience disturbed vision and sensations, and most migraines are worsened by movement, light, sounds, and smells. Migraines can last from a few hours to a few days.

Tension headaches are generally mild to moderate headaches that affect the whole head. They are not accompanied by other signs or symptoms such as

nausea and vomiting. They can be caused by stress or emotional tension.

Insomnia

Disorder in which a person either cannot fall asleep, or cannot stay asleep for an adequate amount of time. Although it is not a disease, it can be a symptom of many different disorders ranging from stress and anxiety to extreme fatigue or even drug use or withdrawal.

Meningitis

Inflammation of the meninges that cover the brain and spinal cord. It is usually caused by a bacterial or viral infection, although it can also be caused by other conditions such as allergic reactions to certain drugs. Signs and symptoms of meningitis generally include fever, headache, vomiting, weakness, and a stiff neck.

Motor neurone disease (MND)

Degeneration of the motor system that leads to the progressive weakness and wasting away of muscles and eventual paralysis. Both skeletal and smooth muscles, such as those involved in breathing and swallowing, are affected. However, it does not affect the senses. Therefore, people with MND can still lead intellectually active lives. MND is an umbrella term for conditions involving degeneration of the motor system and includes amyotrophic lateral sclerosis (ALS), progressive muscular atrophy (PMA), progressive bulbar palsy (PBP), and primary lateral sclerosis (PLS).

Infobox

The world-renowned physicist Professor Stephen Hawking had ALS. When diagnosed with it at the age of 21, he was not expected to live longer than another two years. Yet he lived to the age of 76 years, got married, had three children, wrote international-best-selling books, produced award-winning work in theoretical physics, traveled and lectured extensively (The Stephen Hawking Foundation, n.d.). Hawking is known to have said: "Remember to look up at the stars and not down at your feet. ... And however difficult life may seem, there is always something you can do and succeed at. It matters that you don't just give up" (*Telegraph* reporters, 2018).

Pain and referred pain (synalgia)

Pain is usually a reaction to a stimulus such as heat or an injury. Pain receptors are found throughout the body and they transmit pain sensations to the CNS, where they are integrated and responded to. Pain also can produce reflex actions in which the impulse does not reach the brain as it is dealt with in the spinal cord. For example, touching a hot oven causes you to immediately withdraw your hand from the oven. This is a reflex reaction. In addition to sensory stimulus, pain can also be caused by a nerve abnormality or a psychological disorder.

Referred pain, synalgia, is pain that is felt in a different part of the body to where it is produced. For example, pain produced from a heart attack is often felt as if it is coming from the arm. Referred pain arises because sensory nerves from different parts of the body often share nerve pathways in the spinal cord.

Parkinson's disease (PD)

Progressive disorder of the CNS with an unknown cause, but its signs and symptoms—including involuntary skeletal muscle contractions such as a tremor or rigidity, impaired motor performance, and slow muscular movements—are thought to be due to an imbalance in neurotransmitter activity.

Spina bifida

Birth defect in which the spinal vertebrae do not form normally. It can vary in severity from a newborn having one or two vertebrae abnormally formed to having his or her spinal cord protruding through the skin. In such severe cases the infant will be disabled.

Stress

Any influence that causes an imbalance in one's internal environment. It is part of everyone's life and in itself it is neither good nor bad. However, it becomes a problem when people fail to manage it adequately. It can break down the body's defenses, making it more susceptible to illness and disease.

Nerve disorders

Disorders of the peripheral nerves result in muscular weakness or paralysis if motor nerves are affected, or abnormal sensations if sensory nerves are affected.

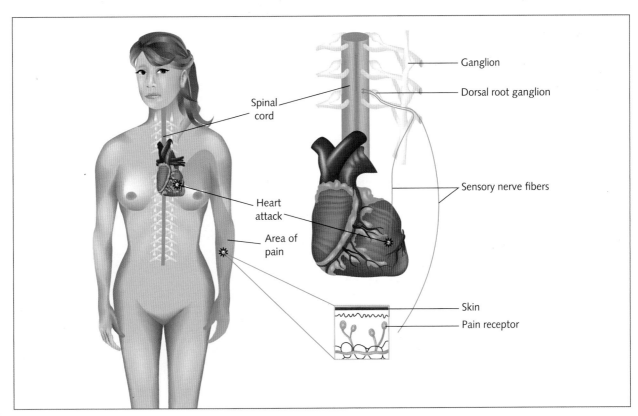

Figure 6.23   *Referred pain*

Bell's palsy

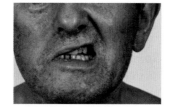

Bell's palsy

Sudden weakness or paralysis of the muscles on one side of the face. It is the result of the malfunction of the facial nerve (cranial nerve VII) and although its cause is often unknown, it may be caused by an infection. Signs and symptoms of Bell's palsy include pain behind the ear, weakening or paralysis of the facial muscles on one side of the face, and a sense of numbness.

Multiple sclerosis (MS)

Disorder in which patches of myelin and underlying nerve fibers in the eyes, brain, and spinal cord are damaged or destroyed. Plaques form on the myelin sheath of nerves in the brain and spinal cord and disrupt nerve transmission. This causes weakness, numbness, tremors, loss of vision, pain, fatigue, paralysis, loss of balance, and loss of bladder and bowel function. It is most common among women between the ages of 20 and 40 years and affects them in periods of relapses and remissions. Multiple sclerosis is thought to be an autoimmune disorder.

Neuritis

Inflammation of a nerve or group of nerves that may result from irritation to the nerve produced by injuries, vitamin deficiency (usually thiamine), or poisons. **Sciatica** is a form of neuritis characterized by severe pain along the path of the sciatic nerve (which runs down the back of the leg). It can be caused by lower-back tension, a herniated disc, or osteoarthritis, or it can result from conditions such as diabetes or pregnancy. It usually only affects one side and symptoms can include pins and needles, pain, or numbness.

Trigeminal neuralgia

Neuralgia is pain originating in a nerve, and the trigeminal nerve (cranial nerve V) carries sensations from the skin of the face and the mucosa of the nose and mouth to the brain. It is also involved in chewing. Thus, trigeminal neuralgia results in severe, stabbing pain and sensitivity on the face, lips, and tongue as well as sensitivity brought on by movements such as chewing. In most cases, its cause is unknown.

Head injuries

Although the brain is protected by the skull and meninges, it can still be injured by car accidents, sports injuries, or other falls or accidents. Head injuries can be fatal, and their effects differ depending on their severity and where in the brain the injury is.

Concussion is the temporary loss of consciousness following a head injury. It is not accompanied by external injuries, but can sometimes produce memory loss, headaches, dizziness, nausea, and vomiting.

A **contusion** is the bruising of the brain resulting from a direct blow to the head. If the swelling or bleeding is severe, signs and symptoms can include severe headaches, nausea, and vomiting, as well as impairments of the area affected.

A **laceration** is the tearing of the brain and is usually caused by skull fractures. Signs and symptoms include those of contusions. Severe lacerations can lead to further tissue damage due to the swelling of the brain.

Infobox

....

Neurogenesis versus neuroplasticity

For nearly one hundred years, scientists have been debating whether or not the adult brain can grow new neurons through the process of neurogenesis. In 1928 Cajal declared that the adult human brain cannot make new neurons, but then studies done in both 1998 and 2013 suggested that new neurons are produced daily in the adult hippocampus. However, in 2018 a new study led by Alvarez-Buylla studied 59 human brains and declared that no new neurons were found in the adult brains (Shen, 2018). So the topic of neurogenesis is still open to debate and there are no clear-cut answers. However, what is emerging with a lot of scientific evidence behind it is the idea of neuroplasticity. Neuroplasticity is the brain's ability to change, adapt, or reorganize its neural pathways and synapses. This enables it to adjust to new environments and compensate for injuries and disease, and is an important factor in recovery from brain injuries.

Cerebrovascular accident (CVA, stroke)

This occurs when the arteries to the brain become blocked or rupture and brain tissue consequently dies. Signs and symptoms of strokes depend on the area affected by the stroke, but general early signs and symptoms include a sudden weakness or paralysis of the face and leg on one side of the body, slurred speech, confusion, loss of balance and coordination, and sudden severe headaches. Strokes can be caused by a number of things and those at risk are the aged; people with atherosclerosis (the narrowing or blockage of arteries), high blood pressure, or diabetes; and smokers. There are three types of stroke:

- **Hemorrhagic attack:** Hemorrhagic strokes are caused by a ruptured blood vessel.
- **Ischemic attack:** Ischemic strokes are caused by a blocked artery.
- **Transient ischemic attack (TIA):** This is a mini-stroke caused by a temporary inadequate blood supply to the brain.

Spinal cord injuries

Although the spinal cord is well protected by the spinal column, meninges, and cerebrospinal fluid, it can still be injured. Injuries can result from accidents such as car accidents or falls, or they can be caused by internal infections, poor blood supply, cord compression, or diseases such as multiple sclerosis. Signs and symptoms of spinal cord injury differ according to the area injured, and different patterns of numbness, weakness, and loss of function will indicate which areas are damaged.

Eye disorders

Disorders of the eye includes changes in vision, loss of vision, changes in the appearance of the eye, and changes in eye sensations.

Cataract

Clouding over of the lens of the eye known as opacity leading to a loss of vision. Cataracts are common in elderly

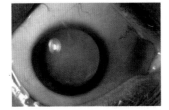
Cataract

people but can also be congenital or result from disease or injury to the lens.

Conjunctivitis (pink-eye)

Inflammation of the conjunctiva and can be caused by viral, bacterial, or fungal infections. Signs and symptoms usually include redness, irritation, light sensitivity, and a watery discharge from the eye.

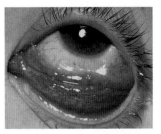
Conjunctivitis

Corneal ulcers

Sore on the cornea that can be caused by injury to or irritation of the cornea and can easily become infected. Signs and symptoms include pain, the sense of

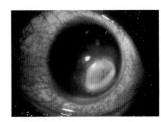
Corneal ulcers

something being in the eye, sensitivity to bright light, and increased tear production.

Glaucoma

Loss of vision due to abnormally high pressure in the eye. It results from the inability of the eye to drain aqueous humor as quickly as it produces it. The aqueous humor

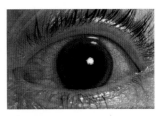
Glaucoma

then builds up, and the excess pressure damages the optic nerve and causes vision loss. People most at risk of glaucoma are those whose relatives have glaucoma, people with significant far- or nearsightedness, diabetics, and people who have had an eye injury.

Sty (hordeolum)

Infection of the sebaceous glands at the base of the eyelashes. It usually lasts only two to four days and is characterized by inflammation,

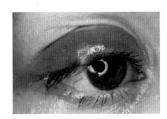
Sty (hordeolum)

tenderness, and pain that then develops into a pus-filled cyst.

Ear disorders

Disorders of the ears, such as hearing loss, are most common in elderly people as the ears are negatively affected by aging, wear and tear, and the cumulative effects of infections and noise. However, young children commonly suffer from ear infections.

Deafness
Partial or total loss of hearing that can affect one ear or both ears. It has many causes, such as a mechanical problem in the ear that blocks the sound waves or damage to the hair cells or auditory nerve by infections or injuries. Hearing loss can also be age related.

Earache
Pain in the ear caused by an ear infection or the result of a blocked Eustachian tube that affects the equalizing of ear pressure. Earache can sometimes be referred pain from infections in the nose, throat, sinuses, or mouth.

Glue ear (secretory or serous otitis media)
Accumulation of fluid in the middle ear usually caused by otitis media or a blocked Eustachian tube. Symptoms include a feeling of fullness in the ear and a popping or crackling sound on swallowing, and is usually accompanied by temporary hearing loss.

Otitis media
Infection of the middle ear that can be caused by a bacterium or virus and is often a complication of colds or allergies. Signs and symptoms of otitis media can include fever; pain; and a red, bulging eardrum.

Tinnitus
The sensation of hearing sounds in the ear that have not originated from the external environment. It is most common in elderly people owing to age-related hair-cell loss but it can also be a symptom of other ear disorders such as injury to the ear, infections, or a blocked ear canal or Eustachian tube.

Vertigo
Sensation of one's self or one's surroundings constantly moving or spinning, and is usually accompanied by nausea and a loss of balance. Vertigo can be a symptom of many diseases or caused by a variety of conditions of the inner ear or the vestibular nerve.

NEW WORDS	
Afferent	Nerves or neurons that transmit impulses to the CNS
Conductivity	The ability to transmit an impulse from a neuron to another neuron, muscle, or gland
Efferent	Nerves or neurons that transmit impulses from the CNS to the muscles and glands
Ganglion	A bundle or knot of nerve cell bodies
Ion	An electrically charged molecule
Irritability	The ability to respond to a stimulus and convert it into an impulse
Meninges	The three connective tissue membranes that enclose the brain and spinal cord
Nerve fibers	The processes that project from a nerve body, i.e., dendrites and axons
Neurology	The study of the nervous system
Neurotransmitter	A chemical that transmits impulses across synapses from one nerve to another
Plexus	A network of nerves (or blood vessels)
Proprioceptor	A specialized nerve receptor located in muscles, joints, and tendons that provides sensory information regarding body position and movements
Tract	A bundle of fibers that is not surrounded by connective tissue
Viscera	The organs of the abdominal body cavity

Study Outline

Functions of the nervous system

These include sensory, integrative, and motor functions.

Organization of the nervous system

1. The nervous system is divided into the:
   - Central nervous system (CNS), which is composed of the brain and spinal cord
   - Peripheral nervous system (PNS), which is composed of the cranial and spinal nerves.
2. The PNS is then divided into the:
   - Somatic nervous system, which is the voluntary nervous system that controls the skeletal muscles
   - Autonomic nervous system, which is the involuntary nervous system that controls the smooth and cardiac muscles and glands.
3. The autonomic nervous system is subdivided into the:
   - Sympathetic nervous system, which reacts to changes by stimulating activity
   - Parasympathetic nervous system, which opposes the sympathetic nervous system and inhibits activity.

Nervous tissue

1. The nervous system contains only two types of cells: neuroglia and neurons.
2. Neuroglia (glia) insulate, nurture, and protect neurons.

Neurons

Neurons transmit impulses to, from, and within the brain. There are three types of neurons:

- Sensory/afferent: These carry sensory nerve impulses from the skin, sense organs, muscles, joints, and viscera to the CNS.
- Motor/efferent: These carry motor nerve impulses from the CNS to the muscles or glands.
- Association/interneurons: These connect sensory and motor neurons in neural pathways.

Structure of a motor neuron
1. Neurons are made up of three parts:
   - Dendrites, which receive impulses
   - A cell body, which contains the nucleus
   - An axon, which transmits the impulses.
2. Axon terminals are found at the end of axons and contain synaptic vesicles that store neurotransmitters.
3. Some axons are myelinated. This means they are covered in a myelin sheath:
   - A myelin sheath protects and insulates the neuron and speeds up the conduction of the impulse.
   - Myelin is produced by Schwann cells in the PNS.
   - The outermost layer of the myelin sheath is called the neurilemma.
   - At intervals along the myelin sheath are gaps called nodes of Ranvier.

Transmission of a nerve impulse

1. Nerve impulses are transmitted electrochemically.
2. Nerve impulses are transmitted across the plasma membrane of an unmyelinated axon or across the nodes of Ranvier of a myelinated axon.
3. An inactive membrane has an electrical voltage across its membrane, with mainly sodium ions on the outside of the membrane and potassium ions on the inside. This means it is polarized.
4. The dendrites of the neuron are stimulated and this causes the movement of sodium ions into a segment of the cell.
5. The cell therefore becomes depolarized, and this initiates an impulse.
6. The impulse then travels along the membrane in a wave of depolarization.
7. When the impulse reaches the end of the axon it is chemically transmitted across the synapse by neurotransmitters.

Brain

1. The brain lies in the cranial cavity and is protected by the bones of the cranium, the meninges, and cerebrospinal fluid.
2. The three meninges are the outer dura mater, middle arachnoid (mater), and inner pia mater.
3. Cerebrospinal fluid functions as a shock absorber, provides the correct chemical environment for neurons, and acts as a medium for the exchange of nutrients and waste.
4. The brain has four major regions:
   - The brain stem consists of the medulla oblongata, pons, and midbrain. It is the link

between the brain and spinal cord and plays an important role in autonomic functioning.

- The cerebellum functions in movement, posture, and balance.
- The diencephalon contains the epithalamus, thalamus, and hypothalamus and functions in relaying sensory impulses to the cerebral cortex and regulating homeostasis. It also houses the pituitary and pineal glands.
- The cerebrum consists of the cerebral cortex (gray matter), white matter, the limbic system, and basal ganglia. It functions in emotions and intelligence.

SCDC
Stem, Cerebellum, Diencephalon, Cerebrum

Cranial nerves

The 12 pairs of cranial nerves are as follows:

1. Olfactory—nose, smell
2. Optic—eyes, vision
3. Oculomotor—eyes, movement
4. Trochlear—eyes, movement
5. Trigeminal (ophthalmic, maxillary, and mandibular branches)—eyes, jaw movement, facial skin sensations
6. Abducens—eyes, movement
7. Facial (temporal, zygomatic, buccal, mandibular, and cervical branches)—facial expression, taste, saliva, tears
8. Vestibulocochlear (vestibular and cochlear branches)—ears, hearing, balance
9. Glossopharyngeal—tongue, pharynx, saliva
10. Vagus—thorax, abdomen
11. Accessory (cranial and spinal portions)—head, pharynx, and larynx
12. Hypoglossal—tongue, talking, swallowing.

Oh, Oh, Oh, To Touch And Feel Very Good Velvet And Hair*
Olfactory, Optic, Oculomotor, Trochlear, Trigeminal, Abducens, Facial, Vestibulocochlear, Glossopharyngeal, Vagus, Accessory, Hypoglossal

---

*The author would like to thank the Anatomy Department at the Durban University of Technology for the above memorable saying.

Spinal cord

1. The spinal cord is continuous with the brain stem and ends just above L2.
2. The spinal cord functions in transporting nerve impulses between the brain and the rest of the body and in producing reflex actions.
3. The spinal cord is protected by the vertebral column, cerebrospinal fluid, and the spinal meninges, which are continuous with the cranial meninges.
4. Internally, the spinal cord contains gray matter—which consists of cell bodies that integrate impulses—and white matter, which consists of myelinated fibers that transport impulses.
5. There are 31 pairs of spinal nerves as follows:
   - 8 pairs of cervical nerves
   - 12 pairs of thoracic nerves
   - 5 pairs of lumbar nerves
   - 5 pairs of sacral nerves
   - 1 pair of coccygeal nerves.
6. Spinal nerves connect the CNS to the rest of the body.
7. Spinal nerves are mixed nerves. They have a posterior/dorsal root consisting of sensory axons and an anterior/ventral root consisting of motor axons.
8. Branches of spinal nerves form networks called plexuses. All nerves emerging from a specific plexus will innervate specific structures.
9. The spinal plexuses are:
   - The cervical plexus—serves the head, neck, and top of shoulders
   - The brachial plexus—serves the shoulder and upper limb
   - The lumbar plexus—serves the abdominal wall, external genitals, and part of the lower limb
   - The sacral plexus—serves the buttocks, perineum, and lower limbs.
10. There is no thoracic plexus. These nerves form the intercostal nerves that serve the thorax.

Special sense organs

Eyes

1. The eyeball consists of a strong protective wall and a large inner space.
2. The wall of the eyeball is divided into three layers:
   - The outer fibrous tunic contains the cornea, which helps focus light, and the sclera, which is the white of the eye.

- The middle vascular tunic contains the colored iris and its pupil, the ciliary body that secretes aqueous humor, and the choroid, which provides nutrients to the retina.
- The inner nervous tunic, also called the retina, consists of a non-visual pigmented portion that absorbs stray light rays and a neural portion that contains photoreceptors, which convert light into nerve impulses.

3. The interior of the eyeball contains the lens, which is responsible for the fine-tuning of focusing; the anterior cavity, which is filled with aqueous humor that nourishes the lens and helps produce intraocular pressure; and the posterior cavity (vitreous chamber), which contains the vitreous body, which helps produce intraocular pressure and maintain the shape of the eyeball.
4. Waves of light are bent as they pass through the structures of the eyeball. They then hit the retina where they are converted into nerve impulses and transported by the optic nerve to the brain.

Ears

1. The ear is divided into three regions: the outer, middle, and inner ear.
2. The outer ear is composed of the auricle, external auditory canal, and eardrum. It channels air waves in toward the middle ear.
3. The middle ear contains the auditory ossicles, which are the hammer, anvil, and stirrup (malleus, incus, and stapes). These bones transmit sound waves to the inner ear.
4. The inner ear is a labyrinth containing the vestibule and semicircular canals, which are responsible for the sense of equilibrium, and the cochlea, which contains the organ of Corti. The organ of Corti (spiral organ) is the organ of hearing.
5. Sound waves are transmitted as vibrations through the ear until they reach hair cells in the organ of Corti, where they are converted into nerve impulses and transported by the vestibulocochlear nerve to the brain.

Mouth

1. The mouth contains taste buds, which house gustatory receptors (receptors of taste).
2. Taste buds are located mainly in the elevations on the tongue called papillae.
3. Gustatory receptors are cells that have a hairlike projection that makes contact with the stimulus (taste), which has been dissolved in saliva. As tastes are chemicals, gustatory receptors are chemoreceptors.
4. The hairs come into contact with the stimulus and convert it into a nerve impulse, which is transported to the brain.
5. The five primary taste sensations are sour, salty, bitter, sweet, and umami.

Nose

1. Olfactory epithelium is located at the top of the nasal cavity. It contains olfactory receptors.
2. Olfactory receptors are cells with hairlike projections that make contact with the odor, which has dissolved in the mucus that covers the inside of the nose. As odors are chemicals, olfactory receptors are chemoreceptors.
3. The hairs come into contact with the stimulus and convert it into a nerve impulse, which is then transported to the brain.

Review

1. Describe the functions of the nervous system.
2. Identify the divisions/organization of the nervous system.
3. Describe the central nervous system.
4. Describe the peripheral nervous system.
5. Identify the functions of the somatic nervous system.
6. Identify the functions of the autonomic nervous system.
7. Describe the divisions of the autonomic nervous system.
8. Identify the two types of cells found in the nervous system and explain their differences.
9. Describe the three different types of neuron.
10. Describe the structure of a motor neuron.
11. Explain how an impulse is transmitted across a nerve and from nerve to nerve.
12. Identify the four major regions of the brain.
13. Name the three meninges.
14. Describe the functions of cerebrospinal fluid.
15. Describe the main function of each of the following cranial nerves:
    - Optic, II
    - Trigeminal, V
    - Facial, VII
    - Vagus, X
    - Hypoglossal, XII.

16. Explain what the cauda equina is.
17. How many pairs of spinal nerves are there?
18. Name and describe the four spinal plexuses.
19. Outline how the eye functions.
20. Outline how the ear functions.
21. Outline how the mouth functions.
22. Outline how the nose functions.

Multiple-Choice Questions

1. Functions of the spinal cord include:
   a. Controlling the somatic nervous system
   b. Processing and storing memories
   c. Producing reflex actions
   d. Transporting sensory information regarding taste and smell

2. How many pairs of cranial nerves are there?
   a. 8
   b. 10
   c. 12
   d. 14

3. Which of the following functions of the cerebrum is correct?
   a. Gives us the ability to read, write, and speak
   b. Controls homeostasis in the body
   c. Controls skeletal muscles and helps regulate posture and balance
   d. Transports all sensory and motor information from the spinal cord to the rest of the brain

4. The Eustachian tube is found in the:
   a. Ears
   b. Eyes
   c. Mouth
   d. Nose

5. Which of the following statements is correct?
   a. The sympathetic nervous system generally inhibits all activity
   b. The sympathetic nervous system generally conserves energy in the body
   c. The sympathetic nervous system always conserves energy in the body
   d. The sympathetic nervous system generally stimulates activity

6. Which part of a motor neuron is the receiving or input portion of the cell?
   a. Cell body
   b. Axon
   c. Dendrite
   d. None of the above

7. What are myelin sheaths produced by?
   a. Neurolemma
   b. Nodes of Ranvier
   c. Neurilemma
   d. Schwann cells

8. Which cranial nerves function in swallowing movements?
   a. Accessory
   b. Abducens
   c. Oculomotor
   d. Vestibulocochlear

9. Cranial nerves are part of the:
   a. Central nervous system
   b. Peripheral nervous system
   c. Sense of smell
   d. Sense of taste

10. What type of cells are olfactory receptors?
    a. Chemoreceptors
    b. Mechanoreceptors
    c. Vascular receptors
    d. None of the above

7

The Endocrine System

Introduction

Why is it that some people are exceptionally tall while others are small? Or some people can have children while others can't? What is it that controls such processes in our bodies? It is the same system that controls our blood pressure, immune system, metabolism, and even our response to danger. It is the endocrine system.

The study of the glands and hormones of the endocrine system is **endocrinology**. In this chapter you will learn about the endocrine system and discover how it works together with your nervous system to control all the other systems of your body.

Student objectives

By the end of this chapter you will be able to:

- Describe the functions of the endocrine system
- Describe the organization of the endocrine system
- Explain what a hormone is and how it works
- Identify the differences between the nervous and endocrine systems
- Describe the endocrine glands and the hormones they produce
- Identify the common pathologies of the endocrine system.

Did you know?

The endocrine glands are not the only tissues in the body that secrete hormones. The kidneys, stomach, liver, small intestine, skin, heart, and placenta also contain cells that secrete small amounts of hormones.

Before looking at the functions of the endocrine system, it helps to understand exactly what endocrine glands and hormones are. There are two types of glands in the body: exocrine and endocrine.

- **Exocrine glands:** These secrete substances into ducts that carry the substances into body cavities or to the outer surface of the body. Examples of exocrine glands include sudoriferous (sweat), sebaceous (oil), mucous, and digestive glands.
- **Endocrine glands:** These secrete substances into the extracellular space around their cells. The secretions then diffuse into blood capillaries and are transported by the blood to target cells located throughout the body. Substances secreted by endocrine glands are called **hormones**.

Hormones are chemical messengers that regulate cellular activity. They are:

- Secreted by endocrine glands
- Transported in the blood.

Functions of the Endocrine System

The endocrine system has many functions as it affects a variety of cells and tissues in the body. A simplistic view of its functions is that it coordinates body functions such as:

- Growth
- Development
- Reproduction
- Metabolism
- Homeostasis.

It also helps regulate activities of the immune system and the process of **apoptosis**. This is the normal, ordered death and removal of cells as part of the body's development, maintenance, and renewal.

Hormones

Types of hormones

Hormones are synthesized from either steroids or amino acids:

- The sex hormones and those of the adrenal cortex are **steroid** hormones.
- Hormones such as insulin and oxytocin are **amino-acid-based** hormones.

Some molecules, such as norepinephrine, are both hormones and neurotransmitters, depending on their action.

Action of hormones

Hormones are transported by the blood to target cells that contain receptors to which the hormones bind. These receptors are very specific and will only bind to a specific hormone, much like two pieces of a jigsaw puzzle slotting together. Once the hormones have bound to the receptors they act like switches that turn on chemical and metabolic processes within the cell.

General processes stimulated by hormones include:

- Synthesis of new molecules
- Changes in the permeability of the plasma membrane
- Transportation of substances into or out of cells
- Changes in the rates of metabolic reactions
- Contraction of smooth or cardiac muscle.

Control of hormone release

The secretion of hormones into the bloodstream needs to be controlled as underproduction or overproduction of a hormone can result in disease. Hormone secretion is controlled by signals from the nervous system, chemical changes in the blood, and other hormones.

- **Neural stimulation:** Signals from the nervous system can stimulate the release of hormones into the bloodstream. For example, sympathetic nervous stimulation causes the release of epinephrine.
- **Chemical changes in the blood:** Changes in the levels of certain ions—for example, calcium—or nutrients can stimulate the release of hormones. For example, blood calcium levels regulate the secretions of the parathyroid glands.
- **Hormonal stimulation:** The presence of a hormone can stimulate the release of another hormone. For example, hormones secreted by the anterior pituitary gland stimulate the release of other hormones into the bloodstream.

Once hormones have been released into the body, their levels are controlled by a negative feedback mechanism. This is a system in which rising levels of a hormone will inhibit the further release of that hormone.

Together, the nervous and endocrine systems control all the processes that take place in the body, and to a certain extent they control one another. For example, the nervous system can stimulate or inhibit the release of hormones, while the endocrine system can promote or inhibit nerve impulses. However, there are some key differences between these two systems as demonstrated in the following chart.

Study tip

When comparing the nervous system with the endocrine system, think of phoning a friend for a quick chat (nervous system) compared with going around for a leisurely dinner (endocrine system).

COMPARISON OF THE NERVOUS AND ENDOCRINE SYSTEMS		
Characteristic	**Nervous system**	**Endocrine system**
Messenger	Nerve impulse	Hormone
Transportation	Nerve axons	Blood
Cells affected	Mainly muscles, glands, and other neurons	All types of cells
Action	Muscular contractions and glandular secretions	All types of changes in metabolic activities, growth, development, and reproduction
Time to act	Very quick (milliseconds)	Slower (from seconds to days)
Duration of effects	Brief	Longer

Did you know?

The pituitary gland is the size and shape of a large pea, yet it is the "master gland" of the body. Despite its small size, its hormones control most of the other glands of the body. The pituitary gland does, however, have its own master—the hypothalamus.

Endocrine Glands and Their Hormones

The endocrine system coordinates growth, development, reproduction, metabolism, and homeostasis.

Hypothalamus

The hypothalamus is not always considered an endocrine gland as it is part of the nervous system. However, it is included in this chapter because of its vital connection to the pituitary gland. The hypothalamus:

- Releases a number of hormones that control the secretions of the pituitary gland

- Synthesizes two hormones that are then transported to, and stored in, the posterior pituitary gland. These hormones are oxytocin and antidiuretic hormone (vasopressin).

Pituitary gland

The pituitary gland is located in the hypophyseal fossa of the sphenoid bone, and is found behind the nose and between the eyes. It is attached to the hypothalamus by a stalk and comprises an anterior and a posterior portion.

Study tip

The charts on the following pages discuss the endocrine glands, their hormones, and their functions. They also list examples of what can go wrong if the gland is not functioning properly. Most of these disorders are due to either overproduction (**hypersecretion**) or underproduction (**hyposecretion**) of hormones. Some of these disorders are discussed in more detail at the end of this chapter. However, they have been included here to help you understand the functions of the glands.

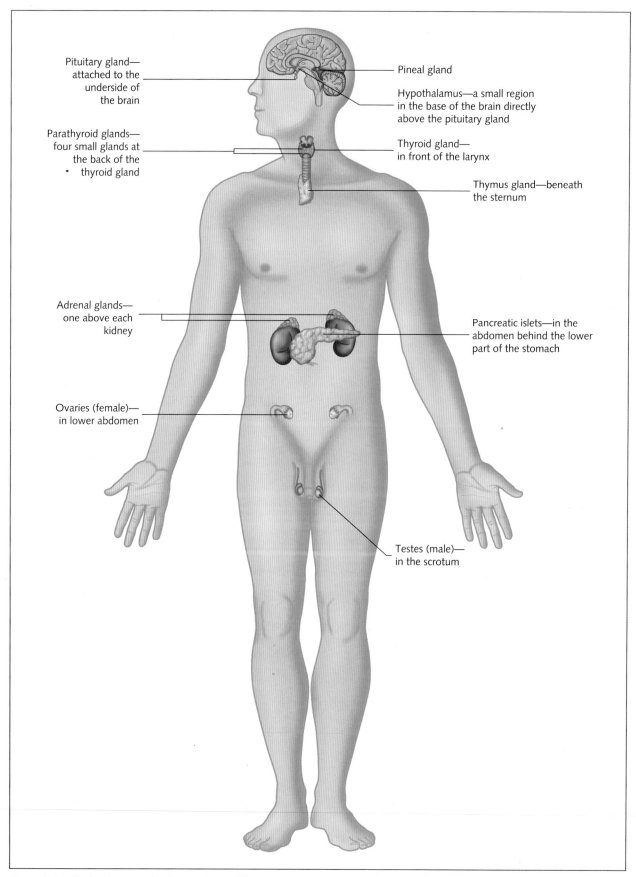

Pituitary gland—
attached to the
underside of
the brain

Pineal gland

Hypothalamus—a small region
in the base of the brain directly
above the pituitary gland

Parathyroid glands—
four small glands at
the back of the
thyroid gland

Thyroid gland—
in front of the larynx

Thymus gland—beneath
the sternum

Adrenal glands—
one above each
kidney

Pancreatic islets—in the
abdomen behind the lower
part of the stomach

Ovaries (female)—
in lower abdomen

Testes (male)—
in the scrotum

Figure 7.1 *Endocrine glands of the male and female*

HORMONES OF THE PITUITARY GLAND

Hormone	Target tissue	Actions	Disorders and diseases
Anterior pituitary gland			
All the hormones released by the anterior pituitary gland, except for human growth hormone, regulate other endocrine glands:			
Human growth hormone (hGH), or somatotropin	Bone, muscle, cartilage, and other tissue	Stimulates growth and regulates metabolism	**Hyposecretion:** Pituitary dwarfism **Hypersecretion:** Gigantism, acromegaly
Thyroid-stimulating hormone (TSH), or thyrotropin	Thyroid gland	Controls the thyroid gland	**Hyposecretion:** Myxedema **Hypersecretion:** Graves' disease (**Note:** These diseases are more commonly caused by a problem with the thyroid gland itself)
Follicle-stimulating hormone (FSH)	Ovaries and testes	**In females:** Stimulates the development of oocytes (egg cells or immature ova) **In males:** Stimulates the production of sperm	**Hyposecretion:** Sterility
Luteinizing hormone (LH)	Ovaries and testes	**In females:** Stimulates ovulation, the formation of the corpus luteum, and secretion of estrogens and progesterone **In males:** Stimulates the production of testosterone	**Hyposecretion:** Sterility **Hypersecretion:** Stein–Leventhal syndrome (polycystic ovary syndrome)
Prolactin (PRL), or lactogenic hormone	Mammary glands	**In females:** Stimulates the secretion of milk from the breasts **In males:** Action is unknown	**Hypersecretion in females:** Galactorrhea (abnormal lactation), amenorrhea (absence of menstrual cycles)
Adrenocorticotropic hormone (ACTH), or corticotropin	Adrenal cortex	Stimulates and controls the adrenal cortex	**Hyposecretion:** Addison's disease **Hypersecretion:** Cushing's syndrome

HORMONES OF THE PITUITARY GLAND			
Hormone	**Target tissue**	**Actions**	**Disorders and diseases**
Melanocyte-stimulating hormone (MSH)	Skin	Exact actions are unknown, but can cause darkening of the skin	No known disorders
Posterior pituitary gland			
The posterior pituitary gland does not synthesize hormones. Instead, it stores and releases hormones synthesized by the hypothalamus			
Oxytocin (OT)	Uterus, mammary glands	Stimulates contraction of uterus during labor and stimulates the "milk let-down" reflex during lactation	No known disorders
Antidiuretic hormone (ADH), or vasopressin	Kidneys, sudoriferous glands, blood vessels	Antidiuretic effect (i.e., conserves water by decreasing urine volume and perspiration), raises blood pressure	**Hyposecretion:** Diabetes insipidus

---

Infobox

··

Anatomy and physiology in perspective

A deficiency of human growth hormone results in dwarfism. One of the world's most famous dwarfs was Tom Thumb (Charles Sherwood Stratton, 1838–1883), who was less than 35 in (90 cm) tall. Gigantism, on the other hand, results from an over-secretion of human growth hormone. Robert Wadlow (1918–40) had this condition and reached 8 feet 9 in (2.7 m) tall and weighed 485 lb (220 kg).

Pineal gland

The pineal gland is located in the epithalamus (part of the diencephalon) of the brain, where it is attached to the roof of the third ventricle. It is made of neuroglia and secretory cells.

HORMONES OF THE PINEAL GLAND			
Hormone	**Target tissue**	**Actions**	**Disorders and diseases**
Pineal gland			
The pineal gland produces the hormone melatonin, which is thought to be involved in the sleep/wake cycle (circadian rhythm) as well as the onset of puberty. Melatonin's release is stimulated by darkness and inhibited by light			

HORMONES OF THE PINEAL GLAND			
Hormone	**Target tissue**	**Actions**	**Disorders and diseases**
Melatonin	Body's biological clock	Causes sleepiness	**Hyposecretion:** Insomnia **Hypersecretion:** Seasonal affective disorder (SAD)

In the classroom

Melatonin is called the "Dracula of hormones" because it only comes out at night (National Sleep Foundation, n.d.). Knowing that high levels of melatonin induce sleepiness and low levels keep a person awake, have a class discussion around the following:

- SAD (seasonal affective disorder): Why is SAD most common during winter? What role do melatonin levels play in this disorder?
- Insomnia: What is happening to your melatonin levels when you stay up late at night watching television or using technology?
- Jet lag: Why does traveling across multiple time zones affect your sleep?
- If you wake up in the middle of the night, why should you avoid turning the lights on?

Thyroid gland

The thyroid gland is a butterfly-shaped gland found wrapped around the trachea just below the larynx.

HORMONES OF THE THYROID GLAND			
Hormone	**Target tissue**	**Actions**	**Disorders and diseases**
Thyroid gland The thyroid secretes two hormones that play a vital role in the body's metabolism. These are **thyroxine (T_4)** and **tri-iodothyronine (T_3)**. T_4 circulates in the body and is converted into T_3, the more biologically active hormone, in the tissues. Together they are often referred to as thyroid hormone. The thyroid also secretes **calcitonin**			
Thyroid hormone (tri-iodothyronine and thyroxine)	Cells and tissues throughout the body	Controls oxygen use and the basal metabolic rate (the minimum amount of energy used by the body to maintain vital processes), cellular metabolism, and growth and development	**Hyposecretion:** Cretinism, myxedema **Hypersecretion:** Graves' disease, thyrotoxicosis **Thyroid enlargement:** Goiter
Calcitonin (CT), or thyrocalcitonin	Bone	Lowers blood calcium levels	No known disorders

Parathyroid glands

The parathyroids are small, round masses of tissue found on the posterior surfaces of the thyroid gland.

HORMONES OF THE PARATHYROID GLAND			
Hormone	Target tissue	Actions	Disorders and diseases
Parathyroid glands			
The parathyroid glands release only one hormone, **parathormone**. It works together with calcitonin from the thyroid gland and **calcitriol** from the kidneys to control blood calcium levels			
Parathormone (PTH), or parathyroid hormone	Bone	Increases blood calcium and magnesium levels; decreases blood phosphate levels; promotes formation of calcitriol by the kidneys	**Hyposecretion:** Tetany, hyperglycemia **Hypersecretion:** Demineralization of bones

Thymus gland

The thymus gland is located in the thorax, behind the sternum and between the lungs. It is large in infants and reaches its maximum size around puberty. Its size then begins to decrease with age.

HORMONES OF THE THYMUS GLAND			
Hormone	Target tissue	Actions	Disorders and diseases
Thymus gland			
The thymus gland plays an important role in the immune system and secretes a number of **thymic hormones** involved in immunity, including thymosin, thymic humoral factor (THF), thymic factor (TF), and thymopoietin			
Thymic hormones	T cells (found throughout the body)	Promote growth of T cells, which are a type of white blood cell	Decreased immunity

Did you know?

Some hormones, such as norepinephrine, are also neurotransmitters.

Pancreatic islets

The pancreas is a long organ, approximately 5–6 in (12.5–15 cm) in length. It is found behind and slightly below the stomach, and is both an endocrine and an exocrine gland as it also functions in digestion (its digestive functions will be discussed in chapter 11). Scattered in the pancreas are small patches of endocrine tissue called **pancreatic islets**, or **islets of Langerhans**.

HORMONES OF THE PANCREATIC ISLETS			
Hormone	Target tissue	Actions	Disorders and diseases
Pancreatic islets			
Pancreatic islets are composed of four types of hormone-secreting cells: alpha cells, beta cells, delta cells, and PP cells (F cells). These cells secrete four different hormones, which generally help regulate blood glucose levels			
Glucagon (from alpha cells)	Liver	Accelerates the breakdown of glycogen into glucose; stimulates the release of glucose into the blood—therefore, raises blood glucose levels	**Hypersecretion:** Hyperglycemia
Insulin (from beta cells)	All body cells	Accelerates the transport of glucose into cells; converts glucose into glycogen—therefore, lowers blood glucose levels	**Hyposecretion:** Diabetes mellitus **Hypersecretion:** Hyperinsulinism
Somatostatin (from delta cells)—this is identical to growth-hormone-inhibiting hormone secreted by the hypothalamus	Pancreas	Inhibits insulin and glucagon release; slows absorption of nutrients from the gastrointestinal tract	**Hypersecretion:** Diabetes mellitus
Pancreatic polypeptide (from PP cells (F cells))	Pancreas and gall bladder	Inhibits secretion of pancreatic fluid, bicarbonate, and enzymes. Inhibits contraction of gall bladder	

Adrenal glands

The adrenal glands (also called the suprarenal glands) are found above the kidneys. Although an adrenal gland looks like a single organ, it contains two regions that are structurally and functionally different. The outer **adrenal cortex** surrounds the inner **adrenal medulla**.

HORMONES OF THE ADRENAL GLANDS

Hormone	Target tissue	Actions	Disorders and diseases
Adrenal cortex			
The adrenal cortex produces steroid hormones that are essential to life, and loss of them can lead to potentially fatal dehydration or electrolyte imbalances. These hormones are grouped into mineralocorticoids, glucocorticoids, and sex hormones			
Mineralocorticoids (mainly **aldosterone**)	Kidneys	Regulate mineral content of the blood by increasing blood levels of sodium and water, and decreasing blood levels of potassium	**Hyposecretion of glucocorticoids and aldosterone:** Addison's disease **Hypersecretion of aldosterone:** Aldosteronism
Glucocorticoids (mainly **cortisol**)	All body cells	Regulate metabolism; help body resist long-term stressors; control effects of inflammation; depress immune responses	**Hyposecretion of glucocorticoids and aldosterone:** Addison's disease **Hypersecretion:** Cushing's syndrome
Sex hormones (**androgens** and **estrogens**)		Very small contribution to sex drive and libido	**Presence of feminizing hormones in males:** Gynecomastia (enlargement of breasts) **Hypersecretion:** Hirsutism
Adrenal medulla			
The adrenal medulla is innervated by neurons of the sympathetic division of the autonomic nervous system and can very quickly release hormones that are collectively referred to as **catecholamines**. These hormones are, to a large extent, responsible for the fight-or-flight response of the body and they help the body cope with stress			
Epinephrine (**adrenaline**) and **norepinephrine** (**noradrenaline**)	All body cells	Fight-or-flight response: • Increase blood pressure • Dilate airways to the lungs • Decrease rate of digestion • Increase blood glucose level • Stimulate cellular metabolism	**Hypersecretion:** Prolonged fight-or-flight response

Ovaries and testes

The female sex glands, the ovaries, and the male sex glands, the testes, are called the **gonads**. The ovaries are almond-sized organs found in the pelvic cavity. The testes are suspended in a sac, the scrotum, outside the pelvic cavity. The ovaries and testes are discussed in more detail in chapter 13.

HORMONES OF THE OVARIES AND TESTES			
Hormone	**Target tissue**	**Actions**	**Disorders and diseases**
Ovaries			
The ovaries only begin to function properly at puberty when stimulated by FSH and LH from the anterior pituitary gland. The ovaries produce **estrogens** and **progesterone**			
Estrogens (includes estriol, estrone, and estradiol)	Reproductive system	Stimulate the development of feminine secondary sex characteristics; together with progesterone, they regulate the female reproductive cycle	Imbalances in secretions can lead to a range of reproductive disorders
Progesterone	Reproductive cycle	Together with estrogens, regulates the female reproductive cycle; helps maintain pregnancy	Imbalances in secretions can lead to a range of reproductive disorders
Testes			
The testes produce both sperm and male sex hormones called **androgens**. The most important androgen is **testosterone**			
Testosterone	Reproductive system	Stimulates development of masculine secondary sex characteristics; promotes growth and maturation of male reproductive system and sperm production; stimulates sex drive	Sterility

Aging and Our Hormones

Surprisingly, our hormones are generally not negatively affected by the process of aging. However, certain changes in hormonal function do mark our journey through life.

Puberty is a significant time, in which a child becomes sexually mature. It generally occurs around the age of 12 in girls and 14 in boys and is stimulated by the gonadotropic hormones of the pituitary gland. It is characterized by the appearance of secondary sexual characteristics in both sexes and the start of menstruation in girls.

Pregnancy is a time in which a woman creates a child and becomes a mother. Many hormones are at work in a woman's body during pregnancy, especially estrogen and progesterone. Once properly developed in the uterus, the placenta also secretes hormones to help maintain the pregnancy.

Menopause is a very significant time for women as it marks the end of their ability to bear children. It generally occurs between the ages of 45 and 55 and is characterized by the cessation of ovulation and menstruation.

Stress Response in More Detail

The stress response is initiated by the hypothalamus, which stimulates both nervous and endocrine reactions that have a ripple-like effect throughout our bodies. The hypothalamus stimulates:

- **The sympathetic nervous system:** Sympathetic nerve impulses activate the short-lived but immediate fight-or-flight response. The physiology of "freezing" is not yet fully understood.
- **The endocrine system:** Hormones from the anterior pituitary gland initiate the longer-lasting resistance reaction.

Fight-or-flight response

The fight-or-flight response is our body's immediate reaction to stressors and it works via the **hypothalamic-pituitary-adrenal axis (HPA axis)**.

Nerve impulses from the hypothalamus stimulate the sympathetic division of the autonomic nervous system, which stimulates visceral effectors and the adrenal medulla. Visceral effectors act on cardiac and smooth muscle, while the adrenal medulla releases epinephrine and norepinephrine. Together, these mobilize the fight-or-flight response by inhibiting non-essential body processes, such as digestive, urinary, and reproductive functions, and stimulating the body's resources for fighting or fleeing.

The table below highlights the physiological changes that occur during the fight-or-flight response to ensure the skeletal muscles, heart, brain, and lungs can function optimally, so that the body can have the energy and strength to run away from danger or to stay and fight.

THE FIGHT-OR-FLIGHT RESPONSE	
Requirement	**Physiology**
Increased blood supply to heart, lungs, brain, and skeletal muscles	• Heart rate increases • Blood vessels to heart, lungs, brain, and skeletal muscles dilate • Blood vessels to skin and most viscera contract • Spleen contracts to release stored red blood cells into bloodstream
Increased blood pressure	Reduced blood flow to kidneys activates renin–angiotensin–aldosterone pathway causing kidneys to retain sodium; this elevates blood pressure and preserves blood volume in case of bleeding
Increased oxygen supply	Airways dilate
Increased glucose/energy supply	Liver converts stored glycogen into glucose

Resistance reaction

The resistance reaction is a longer-lasting response to stress and it involves a cascade of hormones whose release is initiated by the hypothalamus. The table below details this hormonal cascade.

THE RESISTANCE REACTION				
Hormone released by hypothalamus and acting on anterior pituitary gland	**Hormone released by anterior pituitary gland**	**Target organ for hormone from anterior pituitary gland**	**Hormone released by target organ**	**Overall effect**
Corticotropin-releasing hormone (CRH)	Adrenocorticotropic hormone (ACTH)	Adrenal cortex	Cortisol	• Increased availability of glucose, fatty acids, and amino acids for energy production and cellular repair • Reduction in inflammation
Growth-hormone-releasing hormone (GHRH)	Human growth hormone (hGH)	Liver	Insulin-like growth factors (IGFs)	Increased availability of glucose and fatty acids for energy
Thyrotropin-releasing hormone (TRH)	Thyroid-stimulating hormone (TSH)	Thyroid gland	Thyroid hormones (T_3 and T_4)	Increased use of glucose for energy production

Effects of long-term stress: Exhaustion

The stress response involves a series of neuroendocrine reactions that help us survive. These physiological reactions should be only quick and short-lived, but unfortunately many people experience stress on an on-going basis. Constantly high levels of stress hormones, especially cortisol, can lead to the following:

• Hypertension
• Hyperglycemia
• Wasting of muscle
• Suppression of the immune system.

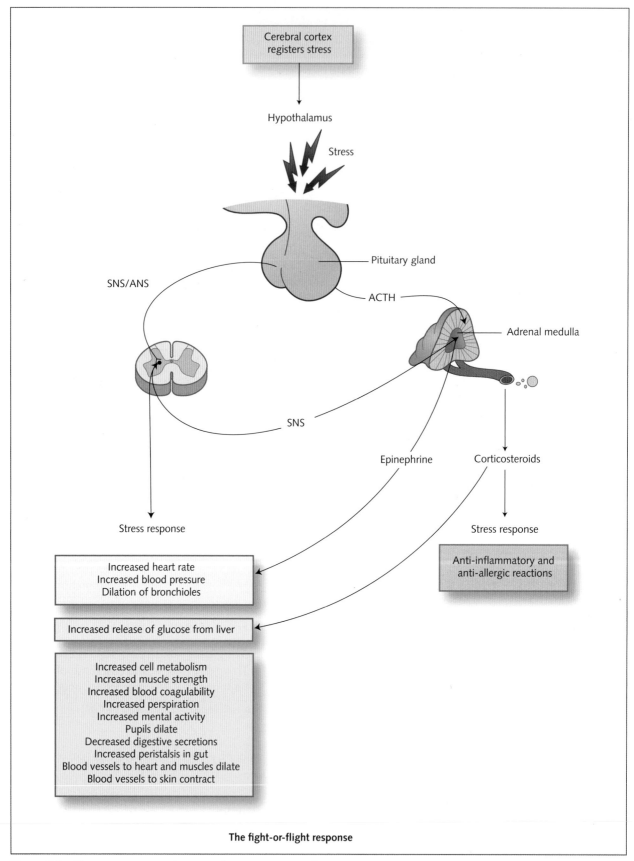

Figure 7.2 *The stress response (ACTH, adrenocorticotropic hormone; ANS, autonomic nervous system; SNS, sympathetic nervous system)*

Common Pathologies of the Endocrine System

Considering the endocrine system affects every organ and tissue in the body, it is not surprising that pathologies of this system have diverse and often non-specific signs and symptoms, such as:

- Depression
- Lethargy
- Muscle weakness
- Weight changes
- Changes in heat tolerance
- Increased urination and increased thirst
- Palpitations
- Headaches
- Coarsening of features.

Red flags

- The development of masculine physical characteristics (virilization) in women or the abrupt appearance of abnormal/masculine hair growth patterns (hirsutism) in women
- Delayed puberty
- Failure to thrive (lethargy, depression, weight loss, weakness)
- Severe headaches
- Recurring headaches accompanied by excessive sweating (diaphoresis), tachycardia, and palpitations.

Pathologies of the adrenal glands

Addison's disease

Caused by the hyposecretion of glucocorticoids and aldosterone by the adrenal cortex, this condition is characterized by patches of excessive pigmentation, low blood pressure, weakness, tiredness, and dizziness on standing. The causes of Addison's disease are not always known although it is sometimes thought to be an autoimmune disorder or due to the destruction of the adrenal cortex by cancer or infection.

Cushing's syndrome

Caused by the hypersecretion of corticosteroid hormones by the adrenal cortex and is characterized by fatigue and excessive

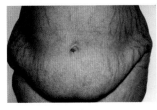

Cushing's syndrome

fat deposits on the face, torso, and back. A person with Cushing's syndrome usually has a large, round face coupled with thin skin that bruises or tears easily. The hypersecretion of corticosteroid hormones can be caused by a problem in either the adrenal glands or the pituitary gland.

Infobox

Anatomy and physiology in perspective

Corticosteroids (steroidal anti-inflammatory drugs) are a popular type of medicine because of their anti-inflammatory, anti-allergic, and immunosuppressive effects. They are used to treat a range of diseases, including asthma, arthritis, and allergies. Short-term use has few negative side effects; however, long-term use can cause symptoms of Cushing's disease such as increased appetite and weight gain, fat deposits in the face and abdomen, suppression of growth in children, thinning and bruising of skin, delayed wound healing, and muscular weakness.

Pathologies of the pancreatic islets

Diabetes mellitus

Not to be confused with diabetes insipidus, this is a disorder in which there is an elevation of glucose in the blood (hyperglycemia). Symptoms include increased thirst and urination, weight loss in spite of increased appetite, fatigue, nausea, vomiting, frequent infections, and blurred vision. There are two main types of diabetes mellitus:

- **Type 1 diabetes (insulin-dependent diabetes mellitus):** Type 1 diabetes is most common in people under the age of 20 years, and is a hereditary autoimmune disorder in which the body's immune system destroys its own insulin-producing cells.
- **Type 2 diabetes (non-insulin-dependent diabetes mellitus):** Type 2 diabetes is more common in people who are overweight and do not eat a healthy diet. In type 2 diabetes, insulin levels may be normal but body cells are resistant or less sensitive to it. Therefore, the metabolism of carbohydrates, fats, and protein is altered. During pregnancy some women develop higher than normal blood glucose levels. This is known as

gestational diabetes, and although most women's blood glucose levels return to normal after childbirth, these women are at a higher risk of developing type 2 diabetes mellitus.

> ### Did you know?
>
> According to the World Health Organization (2018), the incidence of type 2 diabetes mellitus is increasing rapidly. Although this type of diabetes is largely preventable through diet and lifestyle, it is still considered to be a major cause of blindness, kidney failure, heart attacks, strokes, and lower limb amputations.

Pathologies of the parathyroid glands

Calcium deficiency (hyperglycemia)

Calcium is an essential element in the body and is necessary for the formation of bones and teeth, muscular contraction, the normal functioning of many enzymes, blood clotting, and normal heart rhythm. Calcium deficiency, hyperglycemia, can be caused by low levels of parathormone from the parathyroid glands. This can be due to damaged parathyroid glands, low levels of magnesium, the body not responding properly to parathormone, vitamin D deficiency, kidney damage, insufficient dietary calcium, or disorders that affect calcium absorption. Signs and symptoms of calcium deficiency include confusion, memory loss, depression, muscle aches and spasms, tingling sensations, and abnormal heart rhythms. Calcium deficiency can also cause tetany, which is characterized by muscle twitches and spasms.

Pathologies of the pineal gland

Seasonal affective disorder (SAD)

Disorder that usually occurs at the onset of winter and is thought to be caused by a lack of sunlight, which is necessary for the secretion of melatonin by the pineal gland. SAD is characterized by depression, a lack of interest in one's usual activities, oversleeping, and overeating.

Pathologies of the pituitary gland

Acromegaly

Occurs in adults and is excessive growth caused by hypersecretion of human growth hormone (hGH). Because the bones of an adult have already stopped lengthening, hypersecretion of hGH does not cause a further growth in height. Instead, it causes the thickening of the bones of the hands, feet, cheeks, and jaw, as well as the tissues on the eyelids, lips, tongue, and nose. The skin also thickens; sweat glands enlarge, leading to excessive perspiration; and other tissues, such as heart tissue and nervous tissue, can also be affected.

Diabetes insipidus

Excessive production of large amounts of very dilute urine, and is characterized by excessive thirst and excessive urination, which can quickly lead to dehydration. Diabetes insipidus is caused by a lack of antidiuretic hormone (vasopressin), which is produced by the pituitary gland.

Gigantism (giantism)

Excessive growth caused by hypersecretion of hGH in children. It causes the abnormal lengthening of the long bones of the arms and legs so that the individual becomes unusually tall. Usually, the body proportions remain normal. Gigantism is the opposite of **dwarfism**, which can be caused by hyposecretion of hGH in children and results in a lack of growth.

Pathologies of the thyroid gland

Goiter

Enlarged thyroid gland that is a symptom of many different thyroid disorders. It is often caused by a lack of dietary iodine, which is necessary for the correct functioning of the thyroid gland.

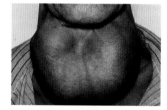

Goiter

Graves' disease

Form of hyperthyroidism that is a hereditary autoimmune disorder in which the thyroid gland is continually stimulated to produce hormones. Signs

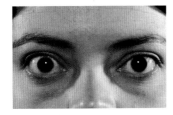

Graves' disease

include an enlarged thyroid gland and edema behind the eyes, which can cause exophthalmos (protrusion of the eyeballs).

Hashimoto's disease

Autoimmune disease in which the thyroid gland is inflamed (thyroiditis) and the secretion of thyroid hormones is sometimes affected. Hashimoto's disease occurs when the thyroid gland is attacked by its own antibodies, and it is often accompanied by other disorders such as diabetes mellitus.

Myxedema (hypothyroidism)

Hyposecretion of thyroid hormones in adults that is characterized by a swollen, puffy face due to edema of the facial tissues, a slow heart rate, low body

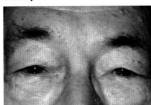

Myxedema (hypothyroidism)

temperature, sensitivity to cold, and dry hair and skin. People with myxedema also feel tired and tend to gain weight easily.

Did you know?

Postpartum thyroiditis is inflammation of the thyroid within the first year after giving birth. It has symptoms common to postpartum depression, such as tiredness and moodiness, and is therefore often misdiagnosed and incorrectly treated as the "baby blues."

Thyrotoxicosis (hyperthyroidism)

Commonly called hyperthyroidism and is the hypersecretion of thyroid hormones. It can be caused by a tumor, overgrowth of the gland, Graves' disease, or overstimulation due to an overactive pituitary gland. Thyrotoxicosis causes a speeding up of vital body functions, and signs and symptoms include a rapid heartbeat, sweating, loss of weight, anxiety, and an intolerance of heat.

NEW WORDS	
Apoptosis	The normal, ordered death and removal of cells as part of tissue development, maintenance, and renewal
Endocrine glands	Ductless glands that secrete substances into the extracellular space around their cells; these secretions then diffuse into blood capillaries and are transported by the blood to target cells located throughout the body
Endocrinology	The study of the endocrine glands and the hormones they secrete
Exocrine glands	Glands that secrete substances into ducts that carry the substances into body cavities or to the outer surface of the body
Gonads	Sex organs that produce mature sex cells
Hormone	A chemical messenger that regulates cellular activity and is produced by an endocrine gland and transported in the blood
Hypersecretion	Over- or excessive secretion
Hyposecretion	Under-secretion

Study Outline

Hormones controlled by the pituitary gland

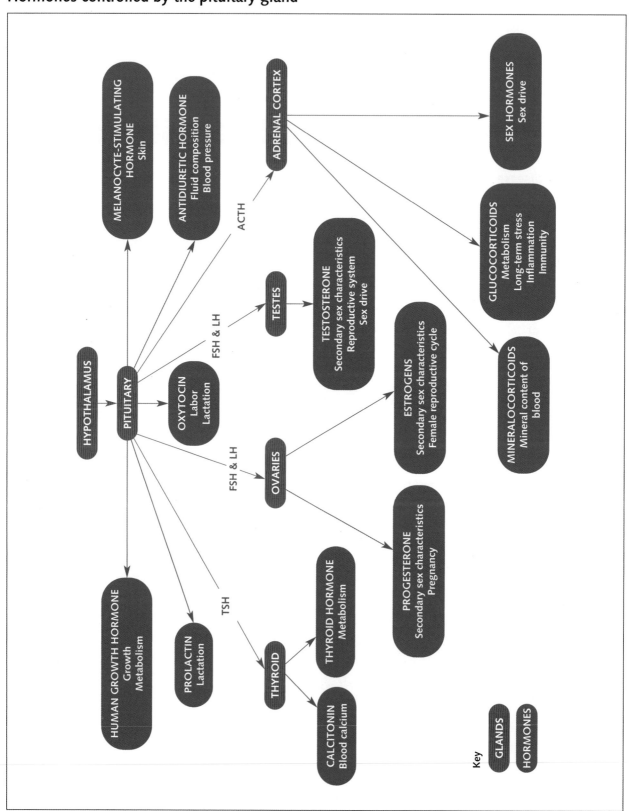

Hormones not controlled by the pituitary gland

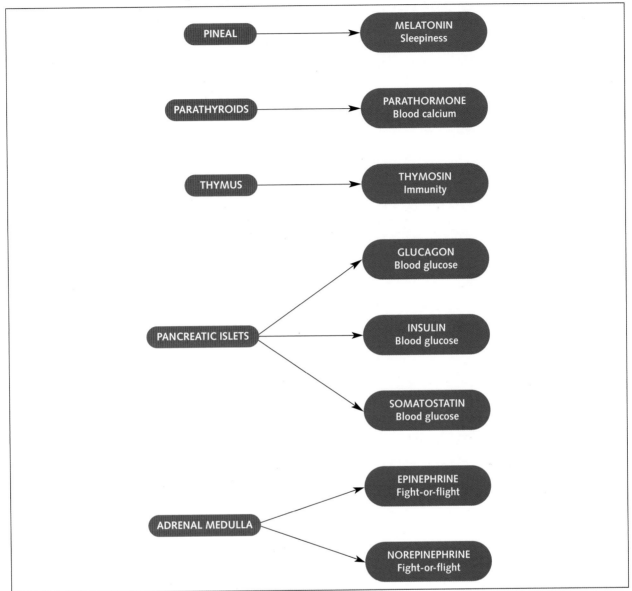

Review

1. Identify the difference between endocrine and exocrine glands.
2. Give two examples of exocrine glands.
3. Describe the functions of the endocrine system.
4. List the endocrine glands of the body.
5. Explain what a hormone is.
6. Explain how a hormone works.
7. Identify the main differences between the endocrine and nervous systems.
8. Explain the role of the hypothalamus in the endocrine system.

9. Draw up and complete a table with the following information for all the endocrine glands:
   - Name of gland
   - Location of gland
   - Hormones secreted
   - Actions of hormones.
10. Describe the following diseases:
    - Myxedema
    - Diabetes mellitus
    - Cushing's syndrome
    - Diabetes insipidus.

Multiple-Choice Questions

1. Which of the following statements is correct?
   a. The adrenal cortex secretes epinephrine
   b. The adrenal cortex secretes glucagon
   c. The adrenal cortex secretes mineralocorticoids
   d. The adrenal cortex secretes insulin

2. Goiter is a pathology of the:
   a. Ovaries
   b. Thyroid
   c. Parathyroids
   d. Adrenals

3. Where is the pituitary gland located?
   a. In the head
   b. In the neck
   c. In the pelvis
   d. None of the above

4. Which of the following statements is correct?
   a. Endocrine glands secrete substances directly into ducts
   b. Endocrine glands secrete substances directly into target cells
   c. Endocrine glands secrete substances into the lymphatic system
   d. None of the above

5. Functions of antidiuretic hormone include:
   a. Decreasing urine production
   b. Increasing urine production
   c. Decreasing stress levels
   d. Increasing stress levels

6. Addison's disease is caused by:
   a. Hypersecretion of pancreatic hormones
   b. Hyposecretion of pancreatic hormones
   c. Hypersecretion of adrenal hormones
   d. Hyposecretion of adrenal hormones

7. The hormone melatonin is secreted by which endocrine gland?
   a. Pituitary
   b. Pineal
   c. Thyroid
   d. Thymus

8. Luteinizing hormone is secreted by which endocrine gland?
   a. Ovaries
   b. Adrenals
   c. Pineal
   d. Pituitary

9. The release of which hormone is stimulated by the sympathetic nervous system?
   a. Somatostatin
   b. Melatonin
   c. Insulin
   d. Epinephrine

10. Which two hormones function in controlling blood calcium levels?
    a. Oxytocin and human growth hormone
    b. Calcitonin and oxytocin
    c. Calcitonin and parathormone
    d. Human growth hormone and parathormone

The Respiratory System

Introduction

If the surface area of your skin is approximately the size of a dining-room table, then the surface area of your lungs is the size of a tennis court; however, they are only one-fifth of the skin's weight. These unique organs play a vital role in the life of every cell in your body—without them there would be no oxygen and thus no energy.

In this chapter you will explore the respiratory system and follow the movement of air from the atmosphere into the cells of the body.

Student objectives

By the end of this chapter you will be able to:

- Describe the functions of the respiratory system
- Describe the organization of the respiratory system
- Describe the organs and structures of the respiratory system
- Explain the key stages of respiration
- Identify the common pathologies of the respiratory system.

Functions of the Respiratory System

Every cell in the body needs oxygen to produce energy in the form of adenosine triphosphate (ATP). Without oxygen cells are unable to produce energy, and will therefore die. Oxygen is vital to the survival of cells; yet, ironically, no cells have the ability to store it. They need a constant, new supply from the external environment. In addition, a by-product of cell metabolism is carbon dioxide. This is a waste product that needs to be constantly removed from the body as an accumulation of it can poison cells.

Two systems work very closely to ensure there is a continuous supply of oxygen to all the cells of the body and a continuous removal of carbon dioxide.

These are the respiratory and cardiovascular systems. The respiratory system takes in oxygen from the air we breathe and eliminates carbon dioxide, while the cardiovascular system transports these two gases between the respiratory system and the cells of the body.

Gaseous exchange

The primary function of the respiratory system is the intake of oxygen and the elimination of carbon dioxide. This exchange of gases is called **respiration** and it takes place between the atmosphere, the blood, and the cells in different phases:

- **Pulmonary ventilation:** The word *pulmo* refers to the lungs, and pulmonary ventilation is another term for breathing. Air is inspired, or breathed, into the lungs and expired, or breathed, out of the lungs.
- **External respiration (pulmonary respiration):** This is gaseous exchange between the lungs and the blood. In external respiration, the blood gains oxygen and loses carbon dioxide.
- **Internal respiration (tissue respiration):** This is gaseous exchange between the blood and tissue cells. In internal respiration the blood loses oxygen and gains carbon dioxide.

Note: Cellular respiration (oxidation) is a metabolic reaction that takes place within a cell. It uses oxygen and glucose and produces energy in the form of ATP. A by-product of cellular respiration is carbon dioxide.

Olfaction

The respiratory system also functions in olfaction, which is the sense of smell. One of its structures, the nose, houses the olfactory receptors, and olfaction is discussed in more detail in chapter 6.

Sound production

Vibrating air particles produce sound. As we breathe air out, air passes through the larynx (voice box), where there are specialized membranes called **vocal cords**. The air causes these to vibrate and produce sounds, which are converted into words by the muscles of the pharynx, face, tongue, and lips. The pharynx, mouth, nasal cavity, and paranasal sinuses also act as resonating chambers for sound.

Organization of the Respiratory System

The respiratory system is divided into two zones:

- **The conducting zone:** This is a series of interconnecting passageways that allows air to reach the lungs. No gaseous exchange occurs here. The function of the structures of this zone is to transport air to the alveoli and to filter, moisten, and warm it. Structures of the conducting zone include the nose, pharynx, larynx, trachea, and the bronchi and their smaller branches.

- **The respiratory zone:** This is where the exchange of gases occurs. The alveoli form the respiratory zone.

> ### Functions of the nose in a nutshell
>
> - Inhaling air
> - Filtering, warming, and moistening air
> - Receiving olfactory stimuli
> - Acting as a resonating chamber for sound.

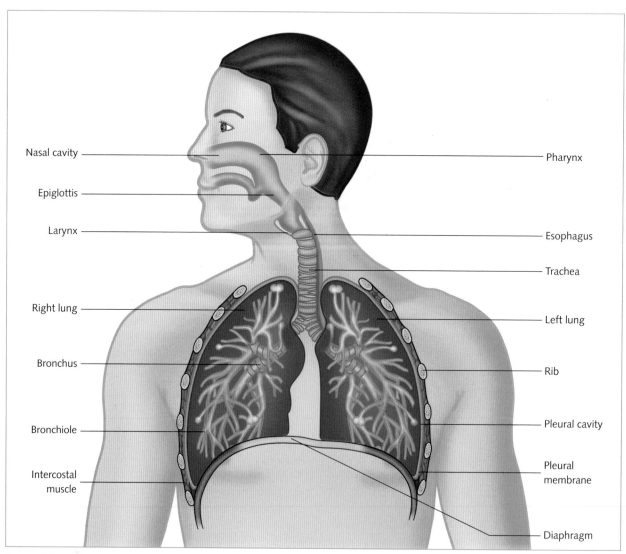

Figure 8.1 *Overview of the respiratory system*

Nose

Air enters the respiratory system through the nose, which is a framework of bone and hyaline cartilage that is covered by skin and lined internally with a mucous membrane.

The nose has the following structures:

- Two **external nares,** which are the openings to the nose and are commonly called the nostrils; inside the nares are coarse hairs that filter out large dust particles
- A large internal cavity called the **nasal cavity,** which is divided into two by the **septum**
- At the back of the nasal cavity are two **internal nares (choanae),** which are openings that connect the nasal cavity to the pharynx.

The nasal cavity contains:

- The **olfactory receptors** necessary for the sense of smell
- Duct openings from the paranasal sinuses; these allow mucus to drain from the sinuses into the nasal cavity
- The **nasal conchae (turbinate bones),** which look like shelves projecting from the lateral walls of the nasal cavity; the air whirls around them and, as it does so, it is warmed by the blood in their capillaries

The nasal cavity is lined with:

- A **mucous membrane** that secretes mucus, which moistens the air and traps dust particles
- **Cilia** that move the dust-laden mucus down toward the pharynx, where it can be swallowed or spat out

Infobox

Anatomy and physiology in perspective

If the cilia lining the respiratory system are damaged, they cannot move dust-laden mucus out of the system. The only way it can then be removed is through coughing. Substances in cigarette smoke inhibit the movement of cilia and therefore coughing, or smoker's cough, is common among people who smoke.

Infobox

Anatomy and physiology in perspective

What exactly are sinuses and why can they cause us so much discomfort? Paranasal sinuses are air-filled spaces within the cranial and facial bones. They are located near the nasal cavity and serve as resonating chambers for sound when we speak. They are also lined with a mucous membrane and have tiny openings into the nasal cavity called **ostia**.

When you have a cold or an allergic reaction to something, the mucous membranes in the sinuses can swell and the mucus will be unable to pass through the tiny ostia and drain as it should normally do. This can lead to inflammation, infection, and a great deal of pain and discomfort. There are three pairs of **paranasal sinuses**, named after the bone in which they are located: the **frontal, maxillary,** and **sphenoid sinuses**. There are also the **ethmoid sinuses**, which consist of many spaces inside the ethmoid bone.

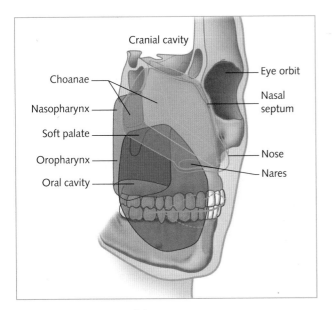

Figure 8.2 *Skeleton of the nose*

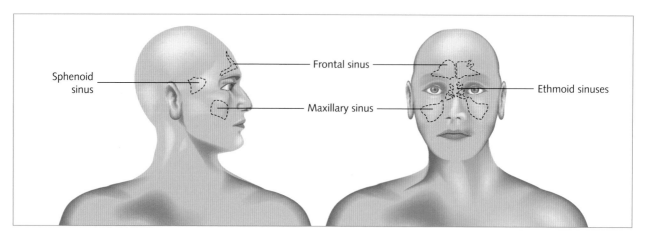

Figure 8.3 *Paranasal sinuses*

Pharynx (throat)

After being breathed in through the external nares (nostrils) and warmed, moistened, and filtered in the nasal cavity, air then passes through the internal nares and into the pharynx (throat). This is a funnel-shaped tube whose walls are made up of skeletal muscles lined by mucous membrane and cilia. The mucus traps dust particles, and cilia move the mucus downward.

The pharynx is divided into three portions, which are named after the structure to which they are closest: the **nasopharynx** (nasal cavity), **oropharynx** (oral cavity), and **laryngopharynx**, or **hypopharynx** (larynx).

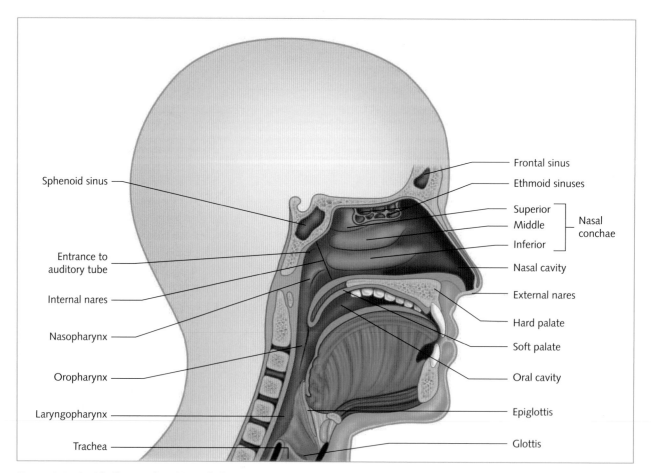

Figure 8.4 *Inside the nasal cavity and pharynx*

The nasopharynx:

- Receives air and dust-laden mucus from the nasal cavity and transports it downward toward the oropharynx
- Contains the **pharyngeal tonsil (adenoid)**, which functions in immunity
- Contains openings from the **Eustachian tubes** and exchanges small amounts of air with them to equalize the pressure between the pharynx and middle ear.

The oropharynx:

- Receives air from the nasopharynx and air, food, and drink from the mouth; it transports these downward to the laryngopharynx
- Contains the **palatine** and **lingual tonsils**, which function in immunity.

The laryngopharynx (hypopharynx):

- Receives air from the laryngopharynx and transports it into the larynx
- Receives food and drink from the laryngopharynx and transports it into the esophagus.

Functions of the pharynx in a nutshell

- Acting as a passageway for air, food, and drink
- Acting as a resonating chamber for sound
- Housing the tonsils, which function in immunity.

Larynx (voice box)

The pharynx transports air to the larynx, which is a short passageway between the laryngopharynx and the trachea. The larynx is made up of eight pieces of rigid hyaline cartilage and a leaf-shaped piece of elastic cartilage called the **epiglottis**, which protects the opening of the larynx. The first piece of cartilage in the larynx is the **thyroid cartilage**.

Did you know?

The thyroid cartilage is more commonly known as the Adam's apple and is usually larger in males owing to the influence of male sex hormones.

It gives the larynx its triangular shape. The last piece is the **cricoid cartilage**, which connects the larynx to the trachea.

Did you know?

Male hormones, called androgens, cause the vocal folds to thicken and lengthen. This means the folds vibrate more slowly than the thinner, shorter folds common in women, and so men generally have a lower pitched voice than women.

The larynx plays two important roles in the respiratory system:

- It routes air and food into their correct channels: When we swallow liquids or food, the larynx rises and the epiglottis moves downward to form a lid over the opening of the larynx. This stops any liquids or food from entering into the larynx. When we are not swallowing, the larynx is in its normal position and the epiglottis does not cover the larynx. Thus, air can move freely into it.
- **It produces sound:** Sound waves are produced by the alternating compression and decompression of air molecules. In the larynx are cords of mucous membrane called the **vocal folds (vocal cords)** that vibrate when air molecules are forced against them during exhalation. This vibration causes sound.

Infobox

Anatomy and physiology in perspective

If small particles of food, fluid, dust, or even smoke do pass into the larynx, they are immediately expelled by a cough reflex.

Infobox

Anatomy and physiology in perspective

Laryngitis is inflammation of the larynx. It is often characterized by hoarseness or voice loss because the inflammation prevents the folds from contracting properly or vibrating freely.

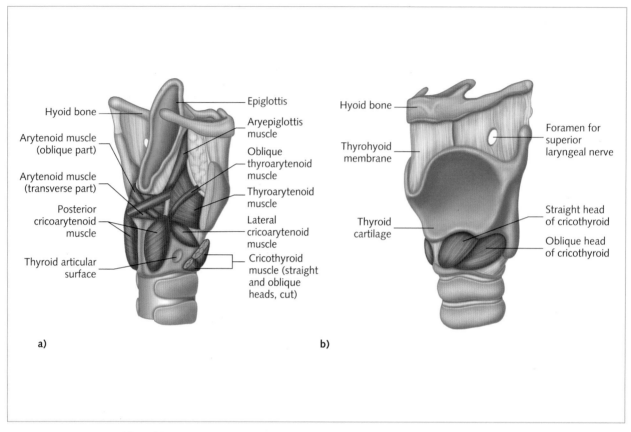

Figure 8.5 *Larynx and hyoid bone, (a) posterolateral view; (b) lateral view*

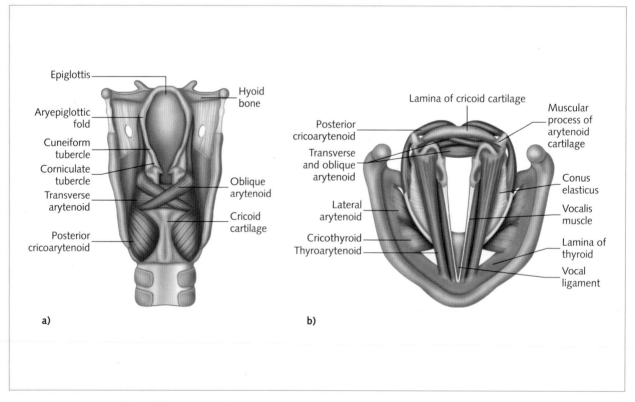

Figure 8.6 *Larynx and hyoid bone, (a) posterior view; (b) superior view*

Functions of the larynx in a nutshell

- Routing air and food into their correct channels
- Producing sound.

In the classroom

Put your hand on the middle of your throat and swallow. You will be able to feel your larynx rising as you swallow.

Trachea (windpipe)

From the larynx, air moves into the trachea, or windpipe. This is a long, tubular passageway that transports air from the larynx into the bronchi. The trachea lies in front of the esophagus and is composed of 16–20 incomplete C-shaped rings of hyaline cartilage.

Functions of the trachea in a nutshell

Transports air from the larynx into the bronchi.

The *open parts* of the C-shape are held together with transverse smooth muscle fibers and elastic connective tissue. This open area lies against the esophagus and allows for expansion of the esophagus during swallowing.

The *cartilage parts* of the C-shape are solid so that they can support the trachea and keep it open despite changes in breathing. The trachea is lined with mucous membrane and cilia that move any minute dust particles still in the respiratory system upward, away from the lungs to the throat, where they can be swallowed or spat out.

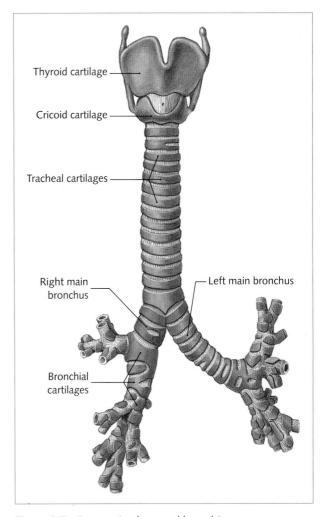

Figure 8.7 *Larynx, trachea, and bronchi*

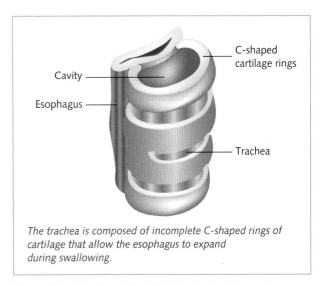

The trachea is composed of incomplete C-shaped rings of cartilage that allow the esophagus to expand during swallowing.

Figure 8.8 *Relationship of the trachea to the esophagus*

Bronchi

Having traveled down the trachea, air is split into branchlike passageways called **bronchi** (singular = **bronchus**). These bronchi repeatedly divide inside the lungs into smaller and smaller branches that finally carry the air into the alveoli. Their division is similar to the branching of a tree from a large central trunk (trachea) into branches (bronchi), twigs (bronchioles) and finally leaves (alveoli). This continual dividing of the passageways means that air can be transported to literally millions of alveoli, where gaseous exchange can finally take place.

Branching of the bronchi is as follows:

- **Primary bronchi:** The trachea divides into the right and left primary bronchi. The right primary bronchus is shorter and wider than the left and carries air into the right lung. The left primary bronchus carries air into the left lung.
- **Secondary bronchi (lobar bronchi):** The primary bronchi then divide into secondary bronchi. There is one secondary bronchus for each of the lobes of the lungs: the right lung has three lobes and therefore has three secondary bronchi, while the left lung has two lobes and therefore has two secondary bronchi.
- **Tertiary bronchi (segmental bronchi):** The secondary bronchi then divide into tertiary bronchi. Each tertiary bronchus supplies a segment of lung tissue, which in itself has many lobules. A **lobule** is a small compartment of tissue containing a lymphatic vessel, blood vessels (an arteriole and a venule), and a branch from a terminal bronchiole. Each lobule is wrapped in elastic connective tissue.
- **Bronchioles:** Tertiary bronchi divide into bronchioles:
  - The bronchioles themselves divide repeatedly until they finally become **terminal bronchioles**
  - Terminal bronchioles subdivide into microscopic branches called **respiratory bronchioles**
  - The respiratory bronchioles finally divide into **alveolar ducts**

Similar to the trachea, the bronchi are composed of incomplete rings of cartilage and are lined with mucous membrane. However, as branching takes place, gradual changes occur to the structure of the branches until the cartilage is finally replaced by spiral bands of smooth muscle and the protective mechanism of the cilia is replaced by the action of macrophages.

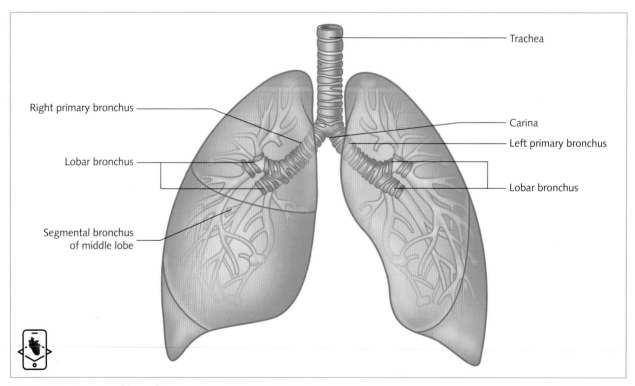

Figure 8.9   *Lungs and bronchi*

Lungs

The word *lunge* means "lightweight," and although the total surface area of the lungs is approximately 40 times the external surface area of the entire body, they weigh less than 2.2 lb (1 kg). This unique surface area is thanks to the branching of the bronchi and bronchioles as described previously.

The two lungs are cone-shaped organs that occupy most of the thoracic cavity. They extend from the diaphragm to slightly above the clavicles and are surrounded and protected by the ribs. The lungs are:

- Different in size and shape—the right lung is shorter, thicker and broader than the left; this is because the diaphragm is higher on the right side to accommodate the large liver beneath it
- Separated from one another by the heart and the **mediastinum**, which is a mass of tissue extending from the sternum to the vertebral column
- Covered with and protected by the **pleural membrane**—this is a serous membrane made up of two layers:
  - The superficial **parietal pleura**, which lines the walls of the thoracic cavity
  - The deep **visceral pleura**, which covers the lungs

The space between the two layers is called the **pleural cavity**. It contains a lubricating fluid that is secreted by the membranes to reduce friction between them. Thus, they are able to slide freely over one another.

Infobox

Anatomy and physiology in perspective

The mediastinum divides the thoracic cavity into two distinct chambers, so that if one lung collapses the other one will not be affected and will be able to continue functioning.

Alveoli

Once air has traveled through the conducting passageways of the respiratory system, it finally arrives at the air sacs, or **alveoli** (singular **alveolus**), inside the lungs.

- Alveoli are cup-shaped pouches where the exchange of gases occurs. It is estimated that there are approximately 300 million alveoli in the lungs and they provide a huge surface area for gaseous exchange.
- The walls of the alveoli are extremely thin and composed mainly of a single layer of squamous epithelial cells.
- Alveoli contain cells that secrete **alveolar fluid,** which keeps the walls moist.
- They also contain **macrophages**, which remove any fine dust particles and microorganisms that have not already been removed in the conducting passageways.
- Alveoli are surrounded by a dense network of blood vessels called **pulmonary capillaries**. The

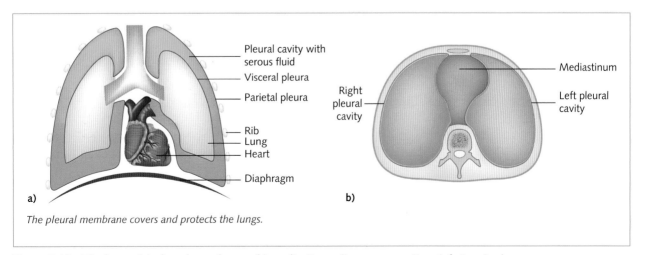

Pleural cavity with serous fluid
Visceral pleura
Parietal pleura
Rib
Lung
Heart
Diaphragm
a)

Right pleural cavity
Mediastinum
Left pleural cavity
b)

The pleural membrane covers and protects the lungs.

Figure 8.10 *The lungs, (a) pleural membrane; (b) mediastinum (transverse section, inferior view)*

thin walls of the alveoli and the thin walls of the pulmonary capillaries together form the respiratory membrane.

- The **respiratory membrane** is the site of gaseous exchange between the lungs and the blood. It is an extremely thin membrane so that the gases can diffuse rapidly across it.

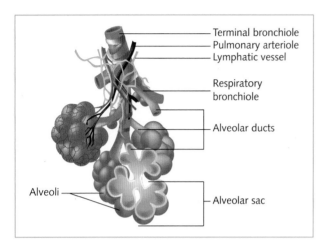

Figure 8.11　*Portion of a lobule of the lungs*

Blood supply to the lungs
The lungs actually have a double blood supply:

- **Pulmonary arteries** bring deoxygenated blood to the lungs. The blood is oxygenated by the lungs and this oxygenated blood is transported from the lungs to the heart by the **pulmonary veins**. These are the only veins in the body that carry oxygenated blood.
- **Bronchial arteries** bring oxygenated blood to the lung tissue. Most of this blood is returned to the heart by the pulmonary veins. However, some of it drains into the **bronchial veins**, which transport it to the superior vena cava and then to the heart.

Note: Blood and blood vessels will be discussed in detail in chapter 9.

> **Did you know?**
>
> The diaphragm descends approximately < ½ in (1 cm) during normal breathing. However, during strenuous breathing it can descend as much as 4 in (10 cm).

Physiology of Respiration

As mentioned earlier, respiration is the exchange of gases between the atmosphere, blood, and cells, and it occurs in pulmonary ventilation, external respiration, internal respiration, and cellular respiration. We will now look at pulmonary ventilation and external and internal respiration in more detail.

Pulmonary ventilation (breathing)

Pulmonary ventilation is the inspiration and expiration, or inhalation and exhalation, of air. In other words, it is breathing. It is a mechanical process in which air is sucked into the lungs from the atmosphere and then exhaled out, and it is dependent on the existence of a pressure gradient between the pressure inside the lungs and that outside the lungs.

Boyle's law
In order to understand the movement of air between the lungs and the atmosphere it helps if you understand Boyle's law, which states that the pressure of a gas in a closed container is inversely proportional to the volume of the container.

In other words, if a gas is put into a closed container the gas molecules will spread out to fill the container. If they have enough space around them that they rarely bump into each other or into the walls of the container, this means that the pressure in the container will be low. If the volume, or size, of the container is then reduced, the gas molecules will have less room to move about and will be closer to one another. They will, therefore, bump into each other and the walls of the container more often, and the pressure will be increased.

> **Did you know?**
>
> When resting, healthy adults move approximately 1.3 gallons (6 liters) of air in and out of their lungs every minute.

Inspiration (inhalation)
Inspiration is the movement of air from the atmosphere into the lungs. It occurs when the volume

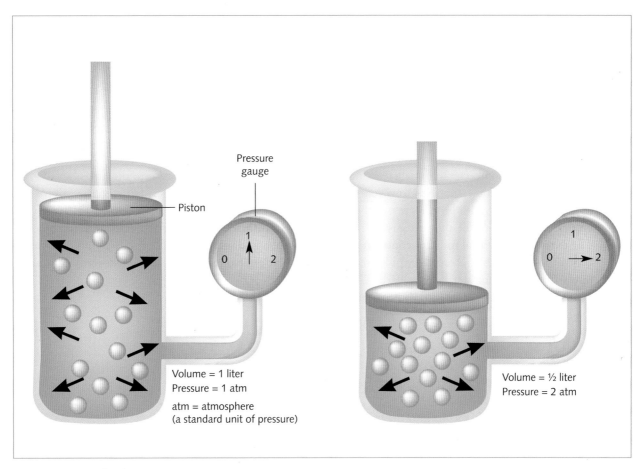

Pressure gauge

Piston

Volume = 1 liter
Pressure = 1 atm

atm = atmosphere
(a standard unit of pressure)

Volume = ½ liter
Pressure = 2 atm

Figure 8.12   *Boyle's law*

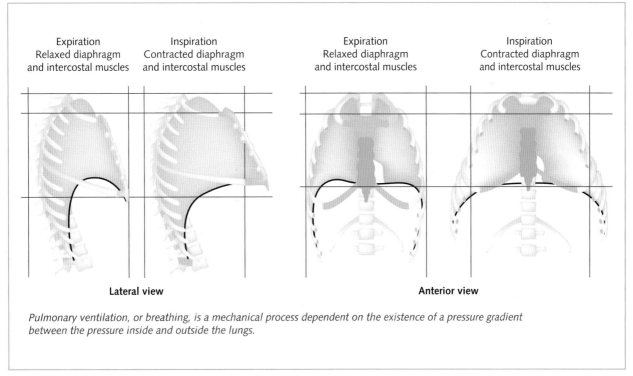

Expiration
Relaxed diaphragm
and intercostal muscles

Inspiration
Contracted diaphragm
and intercostal muscles

Expiration
Relaxed diaphragm
and intercostal muscles

Inspiration
Contracted diaphragm
and intercostal muscles

Lateral view

Anterior view

Pulmonary ventilation, or breathing, is a mechanical process dependent on the existence of a pressure gradient between the pressure inside and outside the lungs.

Figure 8.13   *Changes in the thoracic cavity during breathing*

of the lungs increases, therefore reducing the pressure within the lungs. When the pressure within the lungs is lower than the pressure outside the lungs, air is drawn in to equalize this pressure. Inspiration happens as follows:

- **The volume of the lungs (intrapulmonary volume) increases** when the size of the thoracic cavity increases. This occurs when:
  - **The diaphragm contracts:** In its relaxed state, the diaphragm is dome-shaped. However, when it contracts it flattens and this increases the vertical dimension of the thoracic cavity
  - **The external intercostal muscles contract:** When these muscles contract they pull the ribs upward and push the sternum forward. This increases the anterior–posterior dimension of the thoracic cavity
- An increased intrapulmonary volume causes a **decrease in intrapulmonary pressure.** When the pressure inside the lungs (intrapulmonary pressure) is less than the atmospheric pressure, a partial vacuum is created.
- **The partial vacuum pulls the air into the lungs.** Air flows into the lungs to equalize the pressure between the lungs and the atmosphere.

Infobox

Anatomy and physiology in perspective

Hiccups are sudden inspirations caused by spasms of the diaphragm. As the air hits the vocal folds a hiccupping sound occurs.

Expiration (exhalation)

Normal expiration: During normal, quiet breathing, expiration is a passive process that does not involve any muscular contraction. After being stretched during inspiration, the muscles of the lungs and chest recoil to their natural state and the volume of the lungs decreases. This increases the pressure within the lungs, and once the intrapulmonary pressure is greater than the atmospheric pressure, the air will move out of the lungs to the area of lowest pressure.

Active expiration: Active expiration occurs when the abdominal and internal intercostal muscles contract. These move the ribs downward and compress the abdominal viscera. This movement forces the diaphragm upward, which reduces the size of the thoracic cavity. Thus, the volume of the lungs decreases, the pressure within them increases, and expiration occurs.

External respiration (pulmonary respiration)

Once air has been breathed into the lungs, an exchange of gases takes place between the alveoli and the blood in the pulmonary capillaries. Here oxygen diffuses from the alveolar air into the blood and carbon dioxide moves out of the blood into the alveolar air, from where it is expired from the body.

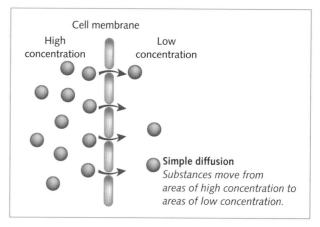

Figure 8.14 *Simple diffusion*

External respiration occurs as follows:

- The right ventricle of the heart pumps deoxygenated blood through the pulmonary arteries into the pulmonary capillaries surrounding the alveoli.
- Gaseous exchange occurs between the alveoli and the capillaries.
  - Oxygen diffuses into the blood and carbon dioxide diffuses out of the blood:
    - Because the body cells are continually removing oxygen from the blood, there is always more oxygen in the alveoli than in the blood
    - Therefore, oxygen diffuses from an area of high concentration (alveolar air) to an area of low concentration (blood)
    - Likewise, because the cells are continually releasing carbon dioxide into the blood, there is always more carbon dioxide in the

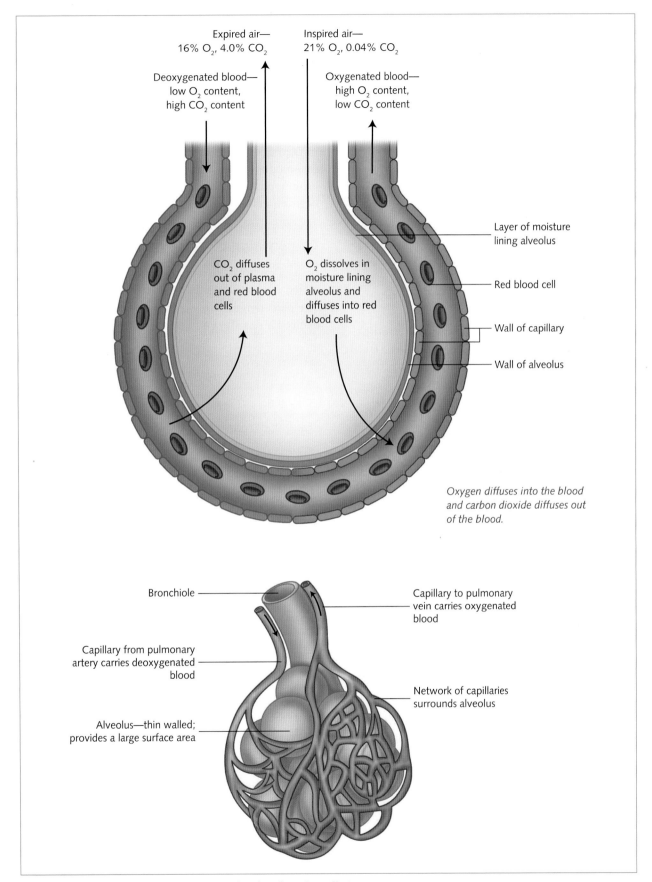

Figure 8.15 *Gaseous exchange between the alveoli and capillaries*

blood than in the alveoli. Therefore, carbon dioxide diffuses from an area of high concentration (blood) to an area of low concentration (alveolar air)
- The structure of the capillaries ensures diffusion can take place rapidly between the alveoli and the blood:
  o There are a large number of capillaries surrounding the alveoli and this provides a large surface area for the exchange of gases
  o The capillaries are also extremely narrow so that only one red blood cell can pass through them at a time. This ensures there is minimal diffusion distance between the capillaries and the alveoli, and also ensures the blood flows slowly through them so that there is sufficient time for gaseous exchange to take place
  o The respiratory membrane between the alveoli and capillaries is very thin to ensure minimal diffusion distance
- Oxygenated blood is transported to the heart, from where it is pumped into systemic circulation. Oxygen attaches to hemoglobin molecules in red blood cells and is transported in the blood as **oxyhemoglobin**. Minute amounts of oxygen are also transported in blood plasma. Carbon dioxide is transported in blood plasma as **bicarbonate ions**. Small amounts of carbon dioxide are also carried inside red blood cells.

Infobox

....

Anatomy and physiology in perspective

Carbon monoxide combines more easily and strongly to hemoglobin than oxygen does and can cause **hypoxia**, which is the inefficient delivery of oxygen to tissues, or even carbon monoxide poisoning, which can be fatal. Carbon monoxide is a colorless, odorless gas found in exhaust fumes from cars as well as fumes from burning tobacco, coal, gas, and wood.

Internal respiration (tissue respiration)

Oxygen finally enters cells and carbon dioxide leaves them through the process of internal, or tissue, respiration. This is the exchange of gases between the blood and tissue cells.

In internal respiration, oxygenated blood loses oxygen and thus becomes deoxygenated. It also gains carbon dioxide. It returns to the heart, from where it is pumped to the lungs to be oxygenated again. Thus begins a new cycle of respiration.

Composition of inspired and expired air

Air is a mixture of oxygen, carbon dioxide, nitrogen, water vapor, and a small quantity of inert gases. The percentages of these gases vary in inspired and expired air as shown in the chart below.

Gas	Inspired air (%)	Expired air (%)
Oxygen	21	16 to 17
Carbon dioxide	0.04	4 to 4.5
Nitrogen	78	78
Inert gases	0.96	0.96
Water vapor	Varies	Varies

Common Pathologies of the Respiratory System

....

Red flags

- Difficulty in breathing (**dyspnea**), shortness of breath, or rapid breathing, especially if accompanied by accessory muscle use
- A high-pitched wheezing sound when breathing (**stridor**)
- Respiratory symptoms accompanied by tachycardia, bradycardia, changes in blood pressure, confusion, sweating, pallor, anxiety, or confusion
- Severe chest pain or chest pain referred to the neck or shoulders
- Coughing up of blood (**hemoptysis**)
- Weight loss and night sweats.

What does smoking really do to your respiratory system?

Smoking decreases your respiratory efficiency in a number of ways.

- The flow of air into and out of the lungs is decreased or hindered by:
  - The constricting effect of nicotine on terminal bronchioles
  - Irritants present in smoke that increase the secretion of mucus and the swelling of the mucous membrane that lines the respiratory tract
- The amount of oxygen carried by the blood is reduced by carbon monoxide in smoke, which combines with hemoglobin more readily than oxygen does.
- The removal of dust-laden mucus and foreign debris from the system is decreased by irritants present in smoke that decrease the movement of the cilia in the lining of the respiratory tract.
- Smoking also destroys the elastic fibers of the lungs, and this can eventually lead to the collapse of small bronchioles.

Finally, smoking causes a number of respiratory disorders, including emphysema and lung cancer, and is also implicated in cardiovascular diseases such as atherosclerosis and strokes as well as the early onset of osteoporosis.

Chronic obstructive pulmonary disease (COPD)

COPD is a group of diseases and disorders that all have some degree of obstruction of the airways. It includes asthma, bronchitis, and emphysema. Coughing, wheezing, and dyspnea are common signs of COPD.

- **Coughing:** Coughs are sudden, explosive movements of air rushing upward through the respiratory passageways. They clear the passageways.
- **Wheezing:** This is a whistling sound produced when the airways are partially obstructed by, for example, a narrowing of the airways, a lodged particle, or excess mucus.
- **Dyspnea:** This is labored or difficult breathing, usually due to partially obstructed airways.
- **Sputum:** This is material coughed up from the respiratory tract.

Asthma

Chronic, inflammatory disorder in which the airways narrow in response to certain stimuli, ranging from pollen and house dust mites to cold air and emotional upsets. Asthma is characterized by periods of coughing, difficult breathing, and wheezing, and during an asthma attack the person struggles to exhale.

Red flag

Status asthmaticus is a medical emergency characterized by:

- Abnormally rapid breathing
- Wheezing—this can be present initially but may disappear as the state progresses
- Inability to speak properly
- Hyperexpansion of the chest and use of the accessory muscles (sternocleidomastoid, scalenes, and intercostals) to help breathing
- Changes in mental state and consciousness ranging from lethargy to agitation, fainting, or seizures.

Bronchitis

Inflammation of the bronchi—the airways branching off the trachea—and can be caused by infection or by exposure to irritants such as cigarette smoke. Bronchitis is characterized by excessive mucus secretion, which results in a productive cough in which sputum is raised, wheezing, and dyspnea.

Emphysema

The word *emphysema* means "blown up" or "full of air," and this is an irreversible disease in which the alveolar walls disintegrate, leaving abnormally large air spaces in the lungs. These spaces remain filled with air and the person struggles to exhale this air, and therefore is constantly exhausted from the effort of trying to breathe out. Emphysema can be caused by cigarette smoke, air pollution, or occupational exposure to industrial dust.

Infectious and environmentally related diseases and disorders

Although the respiratory system is equipped to remove many foreign particles before they reach the lungs, it is still vulnerable to infectious and environmentally related diseases because pathogens and irritants can be inhaled directly into the system.

Asbestosis

Scarring of lung tissue due to the inhalation of asbestos dust. It generally only affects people who work with asbestos that has been broken into many pieces (it is, however, illegal in many countries to install asbestos or work with it under unsafe conditions). Asbestosis is characterized by **pulmonary fibrosis**, which is scarring of the lung tissue, and the thickening of the pleural membrane. Asbestos dust is also known to cause **mesothelioma**, which is a cancer of the pleural membrane. Signs of asbestosis include shortness of breath and difficulty in breathing. It can eventually lead to respiratory failure.

Bronchiolitis

Viral infection of the bronchioles and is more common in young children than adults. It is most often caused by respiratory syncytial virus, but can be caused by other viruses. Signs include fever, respiratory distress, coryza, and congestion.

Study tip

Here is a quick reminder of the different ways in which the respiratory system defends itself from foreign particles:

- Coarse hairs inside the nostrils filter out large dust particles.
- A mucous membrane lines the respiratory passages and traps foreign particles.
- Cilia also line the respiratory passages and move dust-laden mucus toward the pharynx where it can be swallowed or spat out.
- Particles that have not been removed by the mucus and cilia are usually engulfed by macrophages in the alveoli.

Cor pulmonale

Enlargement and thickening of the right ventricle of the heart due to abnormally high blood pressure in the pulmonary arteries (pulmonary hypertension), which causes the right ventricle to work extra hard and thus thicken and enlarge. Cor pulmonale does not have many signs or symptoms until it is in its advanced stages, when they are the same as those of pulmonary hypertension: shortness of breath, light-headedness, fatigue, and chest pain. Cor pulmonale can lead to right-sided heart failure.

Coronavirus disease (COVID-19)

Viral infection caused by a coronavirus. Coronaviruses are a family of viruses, several of which affect the respiratory system. Middle East respiratory syndrome (MERS) and severe acute respiratory syndrome (SARS) are both caused by coronaviruses.

COVID-19's symptoms are similar to those of a common cold or influenza: fever, sore throat, dry cough, fatigue, nasal congestion, and general aches and pains. More severe COVID-19 symptoms include dyspnea, conjunctivitis, diarrhea, or skin eruptions, while serious COVID-19 illness includes septic shock, multiple organ dysfunction, and respiratory failure. People who are at high risk of developing serious, or even fatal, illness include the elderly and individuals who already have an underlying medical condition such as diabetes mellitus, hypertension, cancer, or pre-existing heart or lung conditions. COVID-19 is primarily spread through respiratory droplets.

Cystic fibrosis

Genetic disease that causes certain exocrine glands to produce abnormal secretions, and characterized by the production of thick mucous secretions that do not drain easily. This leads to inflammation and the replacement of healthy tissue with connective tissue. The airways, pancreas, salivary glands, and sweat glands can all be affected, and signs and symptoms can include breathing difficulty, pancreatic insufficiency, and cirrhosis of the liver.

Hay fever (seasonal allergies)

Seasonal allergy resulting from exposure to pollens and other airborne substances that only appear during certain seasons of the year. It is characterized by itching of the nose, roof of the mouth, back of the throat, and eyes, as well as sneezing.

Hyperventilation

Breathing abnormally fast when the body is at rest, and characterized by dizziness, tingling sensations, and tightness across the chest. Prolonged hyperventilation can lead to a loss of consciousness.

Influenza (flu)

Contagious viral infection of the respiratory system that is different from a common cold in that it is caused by a different virus and its symptoms are far more severe. Signs and symptoms include a runny nose, sore throat, cough, headache, fever, and muscular aches and pains.

Laryngitis

Inflammation of the larynx (voice box) and vocal folds. It is characterized by hoarseness or a loss of voice, and signs and symptoms may also include a sore throat, difficulty in breathing, and a painful or tickling cough. Laryngitis is usually caused by a viral infection of the respiratory system—for example, a common cold or bronchitis—but it can also be caused by excessive use of the voice, an allergy, or an irritation of the larynx from substances such as cigarette smoke.

Lung cancer

Cancer of the lungs that can either originate in the cells of the lungs (primary lung cancer) or metastasize to the lungs from other parts of the body. The signs and symptoms of lung cancer vary according to the type and location of the cancer, but they can include a persistent cough, blood-streaked sputum, wheezing, shortness of breath, and chronic pneumonia. Causes of lung cancer can include smoking or exposure to cigarette smoke, and occupational exposure to substances such as asbestos.

Methicillin-resistant Staphylococcus aureus (MRSA)

Common bacterium that is resistant to many types of antibiotics and is now responsible for infectious outbreaks in hospitals. The term MRSA is also used more generally to describe a number of different strains of Staphylococcus bacteria that are all resistant to one or more conventional antibiotics. Many patients in hospitals already have lowered immunity and weakened systems and so are more susceptible to infection from bacteria, which can easily be spread in a hospital environment. Some patients with MRSA show no signs of infection, while others can have swelling and tenderness at the sites affected (most commonly surgical wounds, burn sites, and catheter entry points).

Infobox

Anatomy and physiology in perspective

Antibiotic-resistant bacteria, often called "superbugs," are becoming a phenomenon of our times. It is estimated that one hundred thousand people a year get an infection while in hospital, and these infections are often extremely difficult to treat because the bacteria are resistant to so many types of antibiotics. Why has this occurred? Research shows that bacterial genes are constantly mutating. When a person takes a course of antibiotics and does not complete the course, some bacteria may not yet have been killed by the antibiotics. These bacteria then mutate and become resistant to that type of antibiotic.

Pharyngitis

Infection of the pharynx, or throat, and sometimes the tonsils. Symptoms include a sore throat, pain on swallowing, and occasionally earache. Pharyngitis can be caused by bacteria or viruses and often accompanies a common cold.

Pleurisy

Inflammation of the pleura, and common signs and symptoms include chest pain, rapid and shallow breathing, and neck and shoulder referred pain.

Did you know?

Tobacco smoking is known to be a major cause of lung cancer, which, in the UK in 2016, was considered to be the most common cause of death from cancer. It is important to be aware that lung cancer is not the only cancer associated with tobacco smoking—cancers of the larynx, esophagus, oral cavity, nasopharynx, pharynx, bladder, pancreas, kidney, liver, stomach, bowel, cervix, and ovaries are also linked to tobacco smoking. According to Cancer Research UK (2018), "Tobacco is the largest preventable cause of death in the world."

Pneumonia

Inflammation of the lungs due to the infection and inflammation of the alveoli and the tissues surrounding them. Pneumonia can be caused by a bacterium, virus, or fungus, and signs and symptoms can include a sputum-producing cough, chest pain, chills, fever, and shortness of breath. Those who are susceptible to pneumonia are the elderly, infants, immunocompromised individuals, cigarette smokers, and people with obstructive lung disease.

Pneumothorax

Condition in which there is air between the two layers of pleura. This pocket of air causes the lung to collapse. Signs and symptoms of pneumothorax depend on how much air is between the pleura and how much of the lung has collapsed, and can vary from a shortness of breath and chest pain to shock or cardiac arrest. Pneumothorax can occur spontaneously for no apparent reason, or it can be caused by lung conditions such as emphysema or cystic fibrosis. It can also be caused by trauma or injury to the lungs.

Pulmonary embolism

Blocking of the pulmonary artery by an **embolus**, which is material, such as a blood clot, carried in the blood. Pulmonary embolism is generally caused by a blood clot that has formed in a leg or pelvic vein (and occasionally by clots formed in the veins of the arms).

These clots can form in people who have been kept still for a long time—for example, those on prolonged bed rest or seated in an airplane for many hours. Signs and symptoms of pulmonary embolism will vary according to the extent of the blockage, but it is usually characterized by a sudden shortness of breath, rapid breathing, and extreme anxiety.

Pulmonary fibrosis

Thickening and scarring of the lungs developing from persistent inflammation of the lung tissue. It can be caused by a number of diseases, and it results in the shrinking and stiffening of the lungs and a decrease in their ability to transfer oxygen to the blood. Initial signs and symptoms can include a shortness of breath on exertion, loss of stamina, fatigue, and weight loss. As the disease develops it can cause cor pulmonale.

Rhinitis

Inflammation of the mucous membrane lining the nose. It is characterized by a runny or stuffy nose and often accompanies a common cold or an allergic reaction.

Sarcoidosis

Disease that affects many organs of the body, but primarily the lungs. It is characterized by the presence of **granulomas** (collections of inflammatory cells) in the lungs, lymph nodes, liver, eyes, and skin, as well as other organs. Sarcoidosis may have no signs or symptoms, or fever, fatigue, chest pain, malaise, weight loss, and aching joints may be present. The lymph nodes may also enlarge and night sweats can occur. The cause of sarcoidosis is unknown.

Severe acute respiratory syndrome (SARS)

Viral infection with flu-like signs and symptoms, such as a fever, headache, sore throat, and cough. SARS is believed to be spread through airborne droplets of fluid—for example, through coughing and sneezing. SARS is difficult to treat and because it has an incubation period of approximately ten days, infected people and those who have been in contact with an infected person need to be isolated to ensure it does not spread.

Sinusitis

Inflammation of the sinuses and is usually caused by an allergy or infection. Signs and symptoms include pain, tenderness, and swelling over the affected sinus, as well as nasal congestion and post-nasal drip.

Tuberculosis (TB)

Contagious infectious disease caused by an airborne bacterium. It can affect almost any organ in the body, but usually affects the lungs because the airborne bacterium is inhaled. The bacteria destroy parts of the lung tissue, which are replaced by fibrous connective tissue or nodular lesions called **tubercles**. Signs and symptoms can include coughing, night sweats, a sense of malaise, decreased energy, loss of appetite, and weight loss.

Whooping cough (pertussis)

Contagious bacterial infection that begins with mild cold-like symptoms and then develops into severe coughing fits. These coughing fits are characterized by a prolonged, high-pitched indrawn breath, or "whoop," at the end of them. They also usually produce large amounts of thick mucus. Although the severity of the fits soon subsides, a persistent cough can linger for many weeks or even months.

NEW WORDS	
Cough	A sudden, explosive movement of air rushing upward through the respiratory passages
Dyspnea	Labored or difficult breathing
Hypoxia	The inefficient delivery of oxygen to tissues
Mediastinum	A space in the thorax containing the aorta, heart, trachea, esophagus and thymus gland; it is found between the two pleural sacs
Olfaction	The sense of smell
Oxidation	Cellular respiration
Respiration	The exchange of gases between the atmosphere, blood, and cells
Sputum	Material coughed up from the respiratory tract
Wheezing	A whistling sound produced when the airways are partially obstructed

Study Outline

Functions of the respiratory system

Functions of the respiratory system include gaseous exchange, olfaction, and sound production.

Structure of the respiratory system

The respiratory system is divided into:

1. The conducting zone that allows air to reach the lungs
2. The respiratory zone where gaseous exchange occurs.

Nose

1. Air enters the system through the nose, where it is filtered, warmed, and moistened.

2. The nose also receives olfactory stimuli and acts as a resonating chamber for sound.

Pharynx

1. Air then goes into the pharynx (throat), which is divided into the nasopharynx, oropharynx, and laryngopharynx.
2. The pharynx is a passageway for air, food, and drink and acts as a resonating chamber for sound.

Larynx

1. From the pharynx air goes into the larynx (voice box), which routes air and food into their correct channels and produces sound.
2. The opening of the larynx is protected by the epiglottis.

Trachea

1. From the larynx, air goes into the trachea (windpipe), which is made of incomplete C-shaped rings of cartilage and which lies in front of the esophagus.
2. The trachea transports air into the bronchi.

Bronchi

The bronchi divide repeatedly to form the bronchial tree.

The bronchial tree

Trachea

⇓

Primary bronchi

⇓

Secondary bronchi

⇓

Tertiary bronchi

⇓

Bronchioles

⇓

Terminal bronchioles

⇓

Respiratory bronchioles

⇓

Alveolar ducts

Lungs

1. The lungs are cone-shaped organs that occupy most of the thoracic cavity. They are separated by the mediastinum and protected by the ribs.
2. The right lung is shorter, thicker, and broader than the left.
3. The lungs are covered and protected by the pleural membrane, which consists of the parietal pleura and visceral pleura.

Alveoli

1. Having traveled through the conducting passageways, air arrives at the alveoli (air sacs), where gaseous exchange takes place.
2. The alveoli are surrounded by a dense network of pulmonary capillaries.
3. The respiratory membrane is made up of the thin walls of the alveoli and pulmonary capillaries, and it is the site of gaseous exchange between the lungs and the blood.

Blood supply to the lungs

1. Pulmonary arteries bring deoxygenated blood to the lungs, where it is oxygenated and then transported to the heart by the pulmonary veins.
2. Bronchial arteries bring oxygenated blood to the lung tissue.

The physiology of respiration

Pulmonary ventilation (breathing)

1. Pulmonary ventilation is breathing, and it includes inspiration and expiration.
2. Pulmonary ventilation is a mechanical process dependent on the existence of a pressure gradient.
3. During inspiration, the diaphragm and external intercostal muscles contract and increase the thoracic cavity.
4. Thus, the volume of the lungs increases and this causes a decrease in the pressure in the lungs.
5. When the pressure in the lungs is less than atmospheric pressure, a partial vacuum is created and air is sucked into the lungs.
6. Normal expiration is a passive process in which the muscles of the chest and lungs recoil and the volume of the lungs decreases.
7. When the volume of the lungs decreases, the pressure inside the lungs increases and, when it is greater than the atmospheric pressure, air will move out of the lungs to the area of lowest pressure.

8. In active expiration, the abdominal and internal intercostal muscles contract to force the diaphragm upward. This results in a reduction of the size of the thoracic cavity and an increase in the pressure within the lungs. This leads to expiration.

External respiration (pulmonary respiration)

1. External respiration is the exchange of gases between the alveoli of the lungs and the blood in the pulmonary capillaries.
2. In external respiration, oxygen diffuses from the alveolar air into the blood and carbon dioxide diffuses from the blood into the alveolar air.
3. Oxygen is transported by hemoglobin in the blood.
4. Carbon dioxide is transported as bicarbonate ions in the blood plasma.

> **Remember:**
> External respiration = blood gains oxygen and loses carbon dioxide

Internal respiration (tissue respiration)

1. Internal respiration is the exchange of gases between the blood and tissue cells.
2. In internal respiration, oxygen diffuses from the blood into the cells and carbon dioxide diffuses from the cells into the blood.

> **Remember:**
> Internal respiration = blood loses oxygen and gains carbon dioxide

Composition of inspired and expired air

1. Inspired air contains:
   - 21% oxygen
   - 0.04% carbon dioxide
   - 78% nitrogen
   - 0.96% inert gases
   - A variable amount of water vapor.
2. Expired air contains:
   - 16 to 17% oxygen
   - 4 to 4.5% carbon dioxide
   - 78% nitrogen
   - 0.96% inert gases
   - A variable amount of water vapor.

Review

1. Identify the functions of the respiratory system.
2. Identify the two zones into which the respiratory system can be divided.
3. Following the passage of air from the atmosphere into the alveoli, put the following into their correct order:
   - Laryngopharynx
   - Bronchioles
   - Atmosphere
   - Trachea
   - Nasopharynx
   - Bronchi
   - Alveoli
   - Nose
   - Oropharynx
   - Larynx.

4. Describe where and how sound is produced.
5. Explain the function of the epiglottis.
6. Identify the differences between the two lungs.
7. Describe the blood supply to the lungs.
8. Identify the differences between pulmonary ventilation, external respiration, internal respiration, and cellular respiration.
9. Explain how inspiration and expiration occur.
10. Describe the following disorders:
    - Hyperventilation
    - Cystic fibrosis
    - Rhinitis.

Multiple-Choice Questions

1. Which of the following statements is correct?
   a. Tuberculosis is a non-contagious, infectious disease caused by an airborne fungus
   b. Tuberculosis is a contagious, infectious disease caused by an airborne bacterium
   c. Tuberculosis is a non-contagious, infectious disease caused by an airborne bacterium
   d. Tuberculosis is a contagious, infectious disease caused by an airborne fungus

2. Another name for the nostrils is the:
   a. Conchae
   b. Epiglottis
   c. Adenoids
   d. External nares

3. Which portion of the pharynx contains openings from the Eustachian tubes?
   a. Nasopharynx
   b. Oropharynx
   c. Laryngopharynx
   d. Eustachiopharynx

4. What is the main function of the respiratory membrane?
   a. It protects the lungs
   b. It is the site of gaseous exchange
   c. It lubricates and moistens the lungs
   d. It filters out foreign particles

5. Which of the following statements is correct?
   a. During internal respiration blood loses oxygen and gains carbon dioxide
   b. During internal respiration blood loses carbon dioxide and gains oxygen
   c. During internal respiration blood loses oxygen and gains nitrogen
   d. During internal respiration blood loses nitrogen and gains oxygen

6. Which of the following is a major by-product of cellular respiration?
   a. ATP
   b. Nitrogen
   c. Oxygen
   d. Carbon dioxide

7. If the volume of a closed container is reduced, what will happen to the pressure of the gas within it?
   a. It will increase
   b. It will decrease
   c. It will remain the same
   d. None of the above

8. During inspiration, what does the diaphragm muscle do?
   a. It relaxes
   b. It contracts
   c. It stays the same
   d. None of the above

9. Which of the following diseases are classified as chronic obstructive pulmonary disease (COPD)?
   a. Cystic fibrosis, hyperventilation, pulmonary fibrosis
   b. Laryngitis, sinusitis, rhinitis
   c. Influenza, whooping cough, tuberculosis
   d. Asthma, bronchitis, emphysema

10. How is oxygen transported in the blood?
    a. It travels freely in the blood
    b. It is transported as bicarbonate ions in red blood cells
    c. It attaches to hemoglobin in red blood cells
    d. It attaches to white blood cells

The Cardiovascular System

Introduction

Every cell in the body needs oxygen to survive and there is only one way they can get it—through the blood. In turn, this life-giving substance depends on a small, fist-sized organ to pump it around the body—the heart. This vital organ is very simple in its structure, yet it pumps blood through approximately 60,000 miles of vessels to over 60 billion cells. Together, the blood, the heart, and its vessels form the cardiovascular system, and in this chapter you will discover the important role this system plays in your body.

Student objectives

By the end of this chapter you will be able to:

- Describe the functions of the cardiovascular system
- Describe blood, its components, and functions
- Describe the heart and explain how it functions
- Explain what blood pressure is and how it is maintained
- Describe the different types of blood vessels
- Explain the different types of circulation
- Identify the primary blood vessels of the body
- Describe the common pathologies of the cardiovascular system.

> ### Did you know?
>
> Blood makes up 8% of your total body weight, and an average adult male has 8⅘–10½ pints (5–6 liters) of blood in his body, while an average female has 7–8⅘ pints (4–5 liters).

Blood

Functions of blood

Blood is a liquid connective tissue that is slightly sticky and is heavier, thicker, and more viscous than water. It is a vital substance in the body that functions in transportation, regulation, and protection.

Transportation
Blood transports:

- Oxygen from the lungs to cells
- Carbon dioxide from cells to the lungs
- Nutrients from the gastrointestinal tract to cells
- Heat and waste products away from cells
- Hormones from glands to cells.

Regulation
Blood regulates:

- The pH of the body
- The temperature of the body
- The water content of cells.

Protection
Blood protects cells against foreign microbes and toxins, and also has the ability to clot and so protect the body against excessive blood loss.

Components of blood

In a laboratory, blood can be centrifuged (spun) in a glass tube until it separates into three segments:

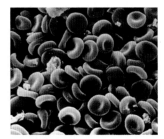

Red blood cells

- Red blood cells sink to the bottom of the tube.
- White blood cells and platelets form a thin layer on top of the red blood cells. This is called the **buffy coat.**
- A straw-colored, watery plasma forms a layer on top.

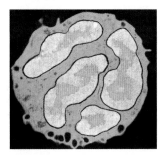

White blood cell

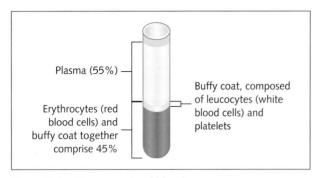

Plasma (55%)

Buffy coat, composed of leucocytes (white blood cells) and platelets

Erythrocytes (red blood cells) and buffy coat together comprise 45%

Figure 9.1 *Components of blood*

This demonstrates that blood is composed of **blood plasma** and cells called **formed elements**.

Blood plasma

A watery, straw-colored liquid that contains dissolved substances comprises 55% of blood. This liquid is called blood plasma, and 91.5% of it is water while the other 8.5% is dissolved substances (solutes). The chart below details the components of blood plasma.

COMPONENTS OF BLOOD PLASMA

Component	Description	Function
Solvent		
Water		• Functions as a **solvent** and suspending medium for carrying other substances • Also absorbs, transports, and releases heat
Solutes		
Proteins	Proteins include albumins, globulins, and fibrinogen	• **Albumins** contribute to the osmotic pressure of the blood and transport fatty acids, some lipid-soluble hormones, and certain drugs • **Globulins** transport lipids and function in defense (antibodies are a type of globulin called gamma globulins, or immunoglobulins) • **Fibrinogen** functions in blood clotting
Electrolytes (ions)	Electrolytes include sodium, potassium, calcium, magnesium, chloride, and bicarbonate	• Function in maintaining osmotic pressure, pH buffering, and regulation of membrane permeability • Also serve as essential minerals
Nutrients	Nutrients from the gastrointestinal tract include amino acids, glucose, fatty acids, and glycerol	Serve as nutrients for the cells
Regulatory substances	Enzymes and hormones	• **Enzymes** catalyze chemical reactions • **Hormones** regulate cellular activity
Gases	Oxygen, carbon dioxide, and nitrogen	• **Oxygen:** Most oxygen is carried in red blood cells, but a minute amount is also transported in the blood plasma • **Carbon dioxide:** Most carbon dioxide is transported in the blood plasma and a small amount is carried by red blood cells • **Nitrogen:** The functions of nitrogen in the blood are not yet known
Wastes	Waste products of metabolism include urea, uric acid, and other substances	Carried to the organs of excretion

Formed elements: erythrocytes, leucocytes

Cells and cell fragments make up 45% of blood. Together these are referred to as formed elements. Red blood cells (erythrocytes) comprise 99% of formed elements, and only 1% are white blood cells and platelets. The chart below details the components of formed elements.

Infobox

· ·

Red blood cells survive in the body for only 120 days. They are produced in the red bone marrow of long bones and are released into circulation at the rate of approximately two million red blood cells per second.

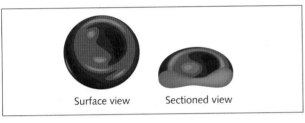

Surface view   Sectioned view

Figure 9.2   *Red blood cell*

A closer look at red blood cells

To ensure there is maximum space within the cells for oxygen transportation, red blood cells do not contain a nucleus and have few organelles. Thus, once in circulation, they cannot reproduce or carry out extensive metabolic reactions. Oxygen is carried by a red pigment protein molecule called **hemoglobin**, and each red blood cell contains approximately 280 million hemoglobin molecules.

Red blood cells are also specially shaped to perform their vital job of transporting oxygen. They are shaped like biconcave discs, and this shape provides a large surface area for the diffusion of gases into and out of the cell. It also gives red blood cells their flexibility and ability to squeeze through even the smallest blood vessels.

Because red blood cells are constantly squeezing through tiny capillaries, their plasma membrane suffers from a great deal of wear and tear and so they do not have a long life span. They are broken down in the spleen and liver, where their breakdown products are then recycled.

Infobox

· ·

Anatomy and physiology in perspective

When a blood vessel is injured there needs to be a quick, localized response that can stop the bleeding before there is excessive blood loss. This process is called **hemostasis** and it occurs in three phases:

1. **Vascular spasm:** If damaged, the smooth muscles in the wall of a blood vessel immediately contract to narrow the vessel and thus reduce blood flow through it. This contraction is thought to be caused by reflexes initiated by pain receptors in the vessels as well as by serotonin, which is released by platelets once they adhere to the damaged site.
2. **Platelet plug formation:** When a blood vessel is damaged, collagen fibers that usually lie under the endothelial cells are exposed and platelets are able to adhere to them. The platelets clump together and release chemicals that attract more platelets to the site. Soon, a mass of platelets called a **platelet plug** or white thrombus forms and seals the injury.
3. **Coagulation (blood clotting):** In addition, blood begins to clot or thicken and form a gel at the site of injury. Blood clotting is a complex process that is promoted by the release of chemicals from platelets. This process results in a mesh of fibrin protein fibers in which blood cells are trapped.

FORMED ELEMENTS		
Component	**Description**	**Function**
Erythrocytes (red blood cells)		
Erythrocytes, or red blood cells, contain the protein hemoglobin, which transports oxygen in the blood		
Erythrocytes	Biconcave discs with no nucleus and few organelles; full of hemoglobin	Transport oxygen

FORMED ELEMENTS

Component	Description	Function
Leucocytes (white blood cells)		
Leucocytes, or white blood cells, function primarily in protecting the body against foreign microbes and in immune responses. They do not contain hemoglobin and therefore do not have the red color that hemoglobin gives red blood cells. Thus, white blood cells are a pale, "whitish" color		
Most white blood cells live for a few hours to a few days, and they are less numerous than red blood cells (for every white blood cell in the body there are approximately 700 red blood cells). White blood cells can be categorized into granulocytes and agranulocytes		
Granulocytes		
Granulocytes have multilobed nuclei and contain granules in their cytoplasm. Their names represent the colors of the dyes that they take up when stained in a laboratory		
Neutrophils	Cytoplasm has very fine, pale pink granules *(neutro = neutral; takes up both red acid and alkaline methylene blue dyes)*	• Engulf and digest foreign particles and remove waste through the process of **phagocytosis**; thus, they are referred to as **phagocytes** • Phagocytes increase rapidly during infection and are attracted in large numbers to areas of infection
Eosinophils	Cytoplasm has large, red-orange granules *(eosino = red acid dye)*	• Destroy certain parasitic worms, phagocytize antigen-antibody complexes, and combat the effects of some inflammatory chemicals • Eosinophils increase during allergies and infections by parasitic worms
Basophils	Cytoplasm has large, blue-purple granules *(baso = alkaline methylene blue dye)*	• The granules in basophils contain **histamine**, which causes the dilation of blood vessels • Basophils release histamine at sites of inflammation and are closely associated with allergic reactions
Agranulocytes		
Agranulocytes have a large nucleus and do not contain cytoplasmic granules		
Lymphocytes	Includes T cells, B cells, and natural killer cells	Lymphocytes play an important role in the immune response and are present in lymphatic tissue, such as lymph nodes and the spleen (immunity is discussed in more detail in chapter 10)
Monocytes	The largest white blood cells	• Some monocytes circulate in the blood and are phagocytes • Other monocytes migrate into the tissues and become **macrophages**, which are large scavenging cells that clean up areas of infection • Monocytes increase in number during chronic infections
Thrombocytes (platelets)	Granular, disc-shaped cell fragments containing no nucleus	• Function in **hemostasis**, which is the process by which bleeding is stopped • Thrombocytes form a platelet plug and release chemicals that promote blood clotting

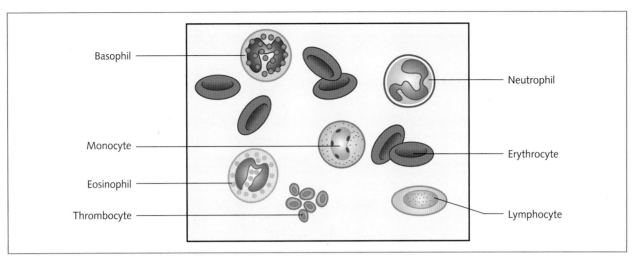

Figure 9.3 *Blood cells*

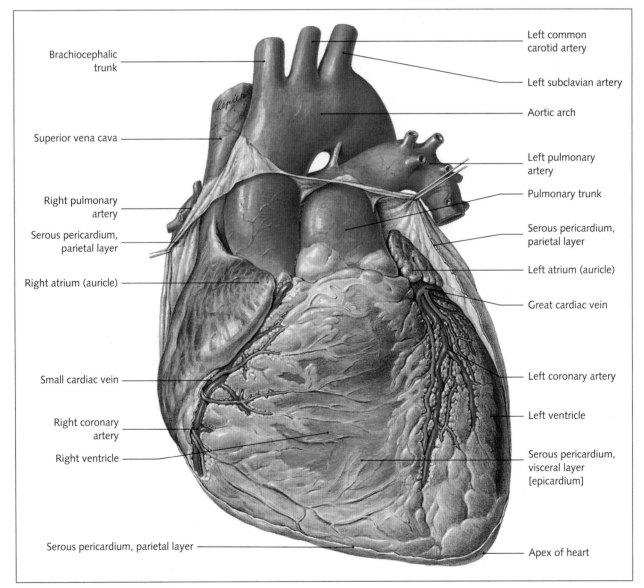

Figure 9.4 *Coronary blood vessels*

Heart

Anatomy of the heart

The heart has the sole but important function of pumping blood around the entire body. Yet, despite its importance, it is actually an uncomplicated structure. The heart is a hollow, muscular organ divided into two halves:

- The right side of the heart receives **deoxygenated** blood from the body and pumps it to the lungs for oxygenation.
- The left side of the heart receives **oxygenated** blood from the lungs and pumps it to the rest of the body.

Each of these halves both receives and delivers blood, and so each has:

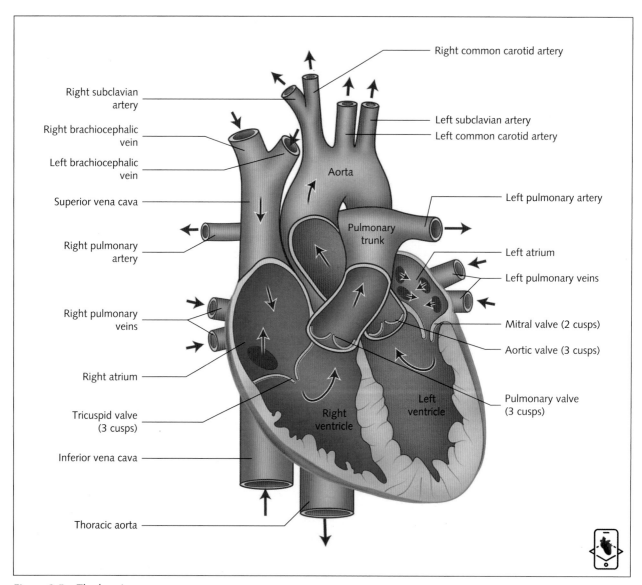

Figure 9.5 *The heart*

- A receiving chamber called an **atrium**, or **auricle**
- A delivering chamber called a **ventricle**.

Separating these chambers are valves. These valves are specially designed to prevent blood from flowing backward.

Location of the heart

The heart lies in the **mediastinum**, which is the partition between the lungs in the thoracic cavity.

- Approximately two-thirds of the heart lies to the left of the median line.
- Its pointed apex rests on the diaphragm at the level of the fifth intercostal space and points toward the left hip.
- Its broader, superior aspect is called the **base**, and it lies beneath the second rib and points toward the right shoulder.

Pericardium: The covering of the heart

Surrounding and protecting the heart is a triple-layered sac called the pericardium. Similar to the pleural membrane of the lungs, the pericardium is composed of:

- The outer **fibrous pericardium,** which is made of tough, inelastic connective tissue that prevents overstretching of the heart and anchors it in the mediastinum
- The inner **serous pericardium,** which is a thin membrane that forms a double layer around the heart; it is made up of:
  - The outer **parietal layer,** which is fused to the fibrous pericardium
  - The inner **visceral layer (epicardium),** which adheres to the heart

- The space between the two layers is called the **pericardial cavity;** it contains a lubricating fluid called **pericardial fluid** that is secreted by the membranes and that reduces friction between them as the heart moves.

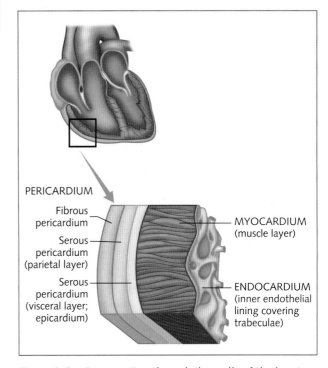

Figure 9.6 *Cross-section through the walls of the heart*

Epicardium, myocardium, and endocardium: The walls of the heart

The power of the heart is quite incredible: it contracts about one hundred thousand times and pumps almost 2,000 gallons (7,500 liters) of blood every single day for its entire lifetime. Can you imagine how hard it must work? In order to beat tirelessly day in, day out, the heart is composed of three layers of tissue:

- **Outer epicardium:** This is also called the visceral layer of the serous pericardium.
- **Middle myocardium:** This is the layer that actually contracts to pump blood. It is a thick layer composed of cardiac muscle tissue, which is involuntary, striated, and arranged in spiral-shaped bundles of branching cells.
- **Inner endocardium:** This is the thin, smooth lining of the inside of the heart. It is composed of flattened epithelial cells and is consistent with the endothelial lining of the blood vessels.

Atria and ventricles: The chambers of the heart

The heart is divided into four compartments, or chambers, lined with endocardium:

- **Superior left and right atria:** The atria (singular = atrium) are the receiving chambers and they receive blood from the veins. They are separated by the **interatrial septum**. The walls of both of these chambers are thin because they only need to deliver blood into the ventricles beneath them.
- **Inferior left and right ventricles:** The ventricles are the delivery chambers and they pump blood into the arteries. They are separated by the **interventricular septum**. The walls of both of these chambers are thick because they need to pump blood out of the heart. The walls of the left ventricle are two to four times thicker than those of the right, because the left ventricle pumps blood throughout the entire body while the right one only pumps it to the lungs.

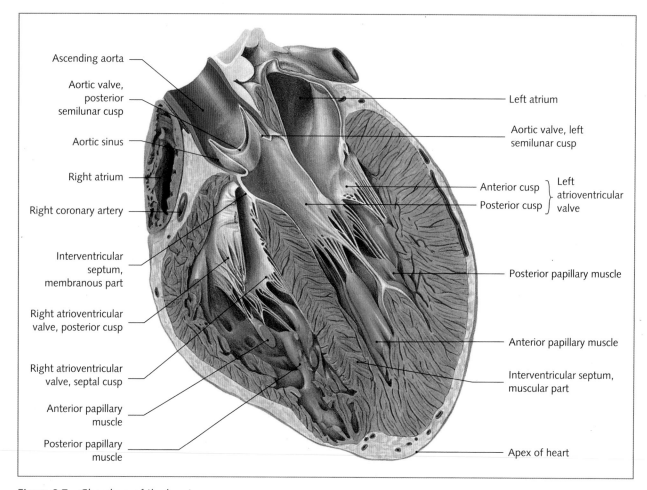

Figure 9.7 *Chambers of the heart*

Atrioventricular and semilunar valves: The valves of the heart

Blood has to flow through the heart in one direction only: from the atria into the ventricles and then into the arteries. It must not flow backward, and to prevent this from happening the heart has four valves. These are composed of dense connective tissue covered by endocardium.

- **Atrioventricular valves (AV valves):** These lie between the atria and the ventricles and prevent blood from flowing back into the atria when the ventricles contract. The valves consist of cusps, or flaps, that are anchored to the inner surface of the ventricles by tendon-like cords called **chordae tendineae.**
  - When the heart is relaxed and the chambers are being filled with blood, the valve flaps hang open in the ventricles
  - When the ventricles contract and the pressure inside the chambers rises, the valves are forced upward and close. The chordae tendineae prevent them from opening upward into the atria, and thus prevent backflow of blood into the atria
  - The right AV valve is called the **tricuspid valve** as it has three cusps
  - The left AV valve is called the **mitral (bicuspid) valve** as it has two cusps

- **Semilunar valves:** These lie between the ventricles and the arteries and prevent blood from flowing back into the ventricles when they relax.
  - The semilunar valves have three cusps that fit together to form a seal when the valves are closed. When the ventricles contract and push blood into the arteries the cusps are forced open and flattened against the walls of the arteries. When the ventricles relax, blood starts to flow backward and fills the cusps so that they close and form a seal that prevents arterial blood from re-entering the heart
  - The semilunar valve between the right ventricle and the pulmonary trunk is called the **pulmonary valve**
  - The semilunar valve between the left ventricle and the aorta is called the **aortic valve**

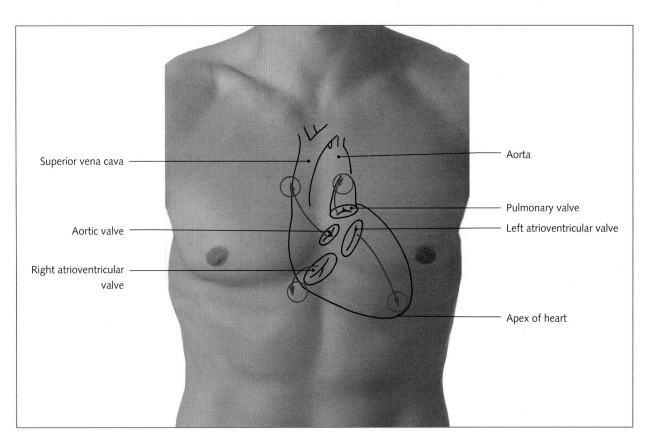

Figure 9.8 *Contour of the heart and its valves*

Pulmonary and systemic circulation: The flow of blood through the heart

The heart is a double pump that pumps blood into two different circulations:

- **Pulmonary circulation:** The **right side** of the heart receives deoxygenated blood from the body and pumps it to the lungs where it is oxygenated. This is referred to as pulmonary circulation.
- **Systemic circulation:** The **left side** of the heart receives oxygenated blood from the lungs and pumps it to the rest of the body. This is referred to as systemic circulation.

We will take an in-depth look at blood vessels shortly, but to begin with it helps to have a basic understanding of the principal vessels of the heart.

These are outlined in the table below. You will see that the coronary sinus and artery are also mentioned. These will be discussed in the following section on coronary circulation.

Study tip

Blood flows through a number of different routes in the body and this flow of blood is referred to as "circulation." Here we have looked at pulmonary and systemic circulation, but these are not the only routes of blood in the body. Later in this chapter we will look at two other circulations: coronary and hepatic portal.

PRINCIPAL BLOOD VESSELS OF THE HEART			
Vessel	**Blood**	**From**	**To**
Arteries Arteries carry blood **away** from the heart and generally carry **oxygenated** blood			
Aorta	Oxygenated	Heart	Most of the body
Coronary artery	Oxygenated	Heart	Heart tissue
Pulmonary artery	Deoxygenated	Heart	Lungs
Note: The pulmonary artery is the only artery in the body that transports deoxygenated blood			
Veins Veins carry blood **toward** the heart and generally carry **deoxygenated** blood			
Superior vena cava	Deoxygenated	Most of the body superior to the diaphragm, except the alveoli and heart	Heart
Inferior vena cava	Deoxygenated	Body inferior to the diaphragm	Heart
Coronary sinus	Deoxygenated	Heart tissue	Heart
Pulmonary vein	Oxygenated	Lungs	Heart
Note: The pulmonary vein is the only vein in the body that transports oxygenated blood			

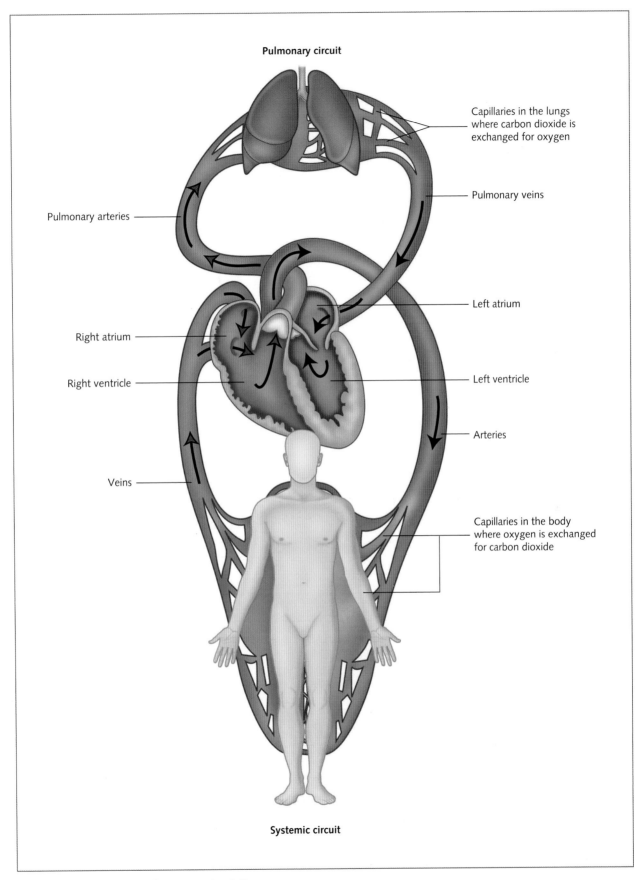

Figure 9.9 *Pulmonary and systemic circulation*

Blood flow through the heart

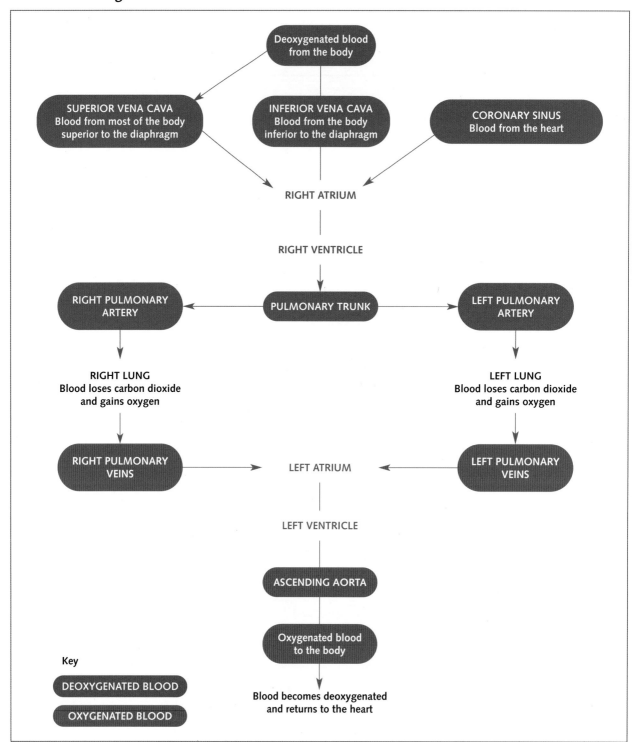

Coronary circulation: The blood supply to the heart

The heart is composed mainly of muscle and, like all muscles, it needs a constant supply of oxygen and nutrients and the constant removal of its waste products in order to function. Thus, it also needs its own blood supply, and this supply is called the **coronary circulation** (**cardiac circulation**). The blood supply to the heart is as shown in the diagram that follows.

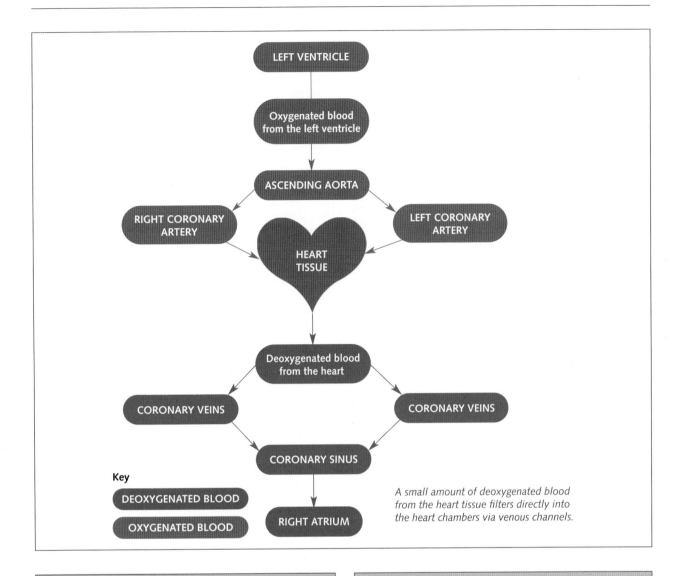

A small amount of deoxygenated blood from the heart tissue filters directly into the heart chambers via venous channels.

Did you know?

The word "coronary" comes from the word *corona*, which means "crown," and the coronary blood vessels encircle the heart just as a crown encircles the head.

Did you know?

Despite its small size and weight, the heart receives 5% of the total blood it pumps. This reflects the amount of oxygen and energy it needs to perform its momentous task.

Physiology of the heart

Regulation of the heart rate

Cardiac muscle cells are unique in that they contract independently of nervous stimulation and thus have what is called a **myogenic rhythm**. However, although the cells contract regularly and continuously, the rhythm of their contraction needs to be controlled to ensure the heart functions as a coordinated whole.

Did you know?

Even though it has no nerve supply once removed from the body, a heart continues to beat for a few minutes until it has depleted any available oxygen.

The rhythm of the heart's contractions is controlled by:

- Specialized cells called **autorhythmic cells**. These cells form the **pacemaker** of the heart, which is called the **intrinsic conduction system, or nodal system**.
- The autonomic nervous system and certain hormones also help control the rate at which the heart beats.

Intrinsic conduction system (nodal system)

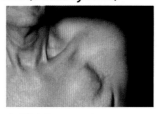

In the right atrial wall of the heart is a mass of autorhythmic cells that initiates impulses and so starts each heartbeat. This is the **sinoatrial node (SA node)** and it is the heart's pacemaker.

Artificial pacemaker

The impulses are then conducted through the myocardium (heart muscle) from the right atrial wall down to the apex of the heart, and then upward into the myocardium of the ventricles. This movement of the impulse results in a "wringing" action, which causes the blood to be ejected upward into the arteries.

> ## Did you know?
> ....
> Other areas of the heart can develop abnormal self-excitability and become pacemakers. These are called **ectopic pacemakers** and can be triggered by substances such as caffeine and nicotine.

> ## Infobox
> ....
> ### Anatomy and physiology in perspective
> If the SA node becomes diseased or damaged, other node fibers can become the pacemaker. However, the rhythm they produce may be too slow for efficient functioning of the heart. When this occurs, a device that sends out small electrical currents can be inserted into the heart. This is called an **artificial pacemaker.**

Impulses are conducted through the heart muscle as follows:

Pacemaker

SINOATRIAL NODE
(SA node)
Function: Initiates impulses and conducts them throughout both atria.
Location: Right atrial wall.

ATRIOVENTRICULAR NODE
(AV node)
Function: Receives impulses from SA node and passes them to AV bundle of His. Impulses are slightly delayed here to give the atria time to finish contracting.
Location: Atrial septum.

ATRIOVENTRICULAR BUNDLE OF HIS
(AV bundle of His)
Function: Is a bundle of fibers that acts as the electrical connection between the atria and ventricles. Receives impulses from AV node and passes them to right and left bundle branches.
Location: Interventricular septum.

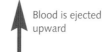
Blood is ejected upward

PURKINJE FIBERS
(Conduction myofibers)
Function: Receive impulses from the bundle branches and conduct them to the ventricular myocardium. Conduct impulses to the apex of the heart first and then upward to the rest of the heart so that the blood is ejected upward into the arteries.
Location: Ventricular myocardium.

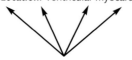

RIGHT AND LEFT BUNDLE BRANCHES
Function: Conduct impulses toward the apex of the heart. Receive impulses from AV bundle of His and conduct them to Purkinje fibers.
Location: Interventricular septum toward the apex of the heart.

Apex of heart

Autonomic and chemical regulation of the heart rate

The number of times the heart beats in one minute is called the **heart rate**, and resting heart rate is normally 60–100 beats per minute (bpm). Although the heart's pacemaker establishes the fundamental rhythm of the heartbeat, it can be modified by the nervous and endocrine systems:

- **Autonomic regulation:** In the brain's medulla oblongata is the cardiovascular center, which receives information from sensory receptors such as proprioceptors, monitoring the positions of limbs and muscles; chemoreceptors, monitoring chemical changes in the blood; and baroreceptors, monitoring blood-pressure changes in the arteries and veins. Information from higher brain centers such as the cerebral cortex and limbic system also send signals to the cardiovascular system. Once all this information has been interpreted the autonomic nervous system responds either sympathetically or parasympathetically to adjust the heart beat:
  - **Sympathetic stimulation:** Cardiac accelerator nerves extend into the SA node, AV node, and most of the myocardium. These nerves stimulate the release of norepinephrine, which, acting as a neurotransmitter, increases the heart rate
  - **Parasympathetic stimulation:** Fibers of the right and left vagus (X) nerves innervate the SA node, AV node, and atrial myocardium. These nerves stimulate the release of the neurotransmitter acetylcholine, which decreases the heart rate
- **Chemical regulation:** Different chemicals can also affect the heart rate:
  - **Hormones** such as epinephrine and norepinephrine, released by the adrenal medulla, increase the heart rate. Their release is stimulated by exercise, stress, and excitement. Thyroid hormones also increase the heart rate
  - **Ions** are electrically charged molecules that play an integral role in the production of impulses in both nerve and muscle fibers. If there is an imbalance in their concentrations the heart rate will be affected

- Certain drugs and dissolved gases can also alter the heart rate

Infobox

Anatomy and physiology in perspective

Other factors also influence our heart rates:

- **Age:** Newborn babies have a high heart rate of approximately 120 bpm. As we age our heart rate slows to approximately 70–75 bpm in adulthood and then begins to increase again in old age.
- **Exercise:** Physical exercise can increase the heart rate to as much as 150–200 bpm.
- **Fitness:** Trained athletes can have a resting heart rate as low as 40–60 bpm.
- **Temperature:** Increases in body temperature increase the heart rate, and decreases in body temperature decrease the heart rate.
- **Emotions:** Excitement, fear, and anxiety all increase the heart rate.

Did you know?

When your body is at rest, your heart can circulate your entire blood content throughout your body within one minute. If you are exercising, it can do this in as little as ten seconds.

Cardiac cycle

Now that you know how often the heart beats and what controls its beating, it is time to look at all the events associated with a heartbeat. This is called the **cardiac cycle**, and one cycle, or heartbeat, automatically follows another throughout life.

A cardiac cycle lasts approximately 0.8 seconds and involves the contraction and relaxation of both the atria and of both the ventricles. While the two atria contract, the ventricles relax, and while the two ventricles contract, the atria relax. As they alternately contract and relax pressure changes occur and blood flows from areas of higher pressure to areas of lower pressure. Two specific terms are associated with a cardiac cycle: **systole** means contraction, and **diastole** means relaxation.

- **Atrial systole:** The SA node stimulates the contraction of the atria, and as the right and left atria contract simultaneously, they empty all their contents into the ventricles.
- **Ventricular systole:** Ventricular contraction is then triggered by the AV node, and as the ventricles contract blood is pushed up against the AV valves, forcing them shut.
    - The AV valves and the semilunar valves are now shut and the pressure within the ventricles rises
    - When this pressure is greater than the pressure in the pulmonary trunk and aorta, the semilunar valves are forced open and blood is ejected from the heart into the vessels
- **Cardiac diastole (relaxation or quiescent period):** At the end of a heartbeat all four chambers are relaxing and thus are in diastole. At this stage the AV valves are closed and the semilunar valves are open.
    - Because the chambers are relaxing, pressure within them drops and this causes blood to flow from the pulmonary trunk and aorta back toward the ventricles. This backflow of blood causes the semilunar valves to close
    - The AV valves and semilunar valves are now closed and as the ventricles continue to relax the space inside them expands and the pressure within them drops
    - When ventricular pressure is below atrial pressure the AV valves open and blood pours into the ventricles

---

Infobox

Anatomy and physiology in perspective

Instead of the "boom, boom, boom" sound we associate with a heartbeat, hearts actually make a "lubb-dup" sound. The long, loud "lubb" is the sound of the AV valves closing, and the short, quick "dup" is created by the semilunar valves snapping shut.

Blood Vessels

Blood is pumped by the heart into vessels that then transport it throughout the body. These vessels form a closed system of tubes that is made up of:

- Vessels that carry blood **away from the heart** toward the tissues are **arteries** and **arterioles**.
- Vessels that branch throughout tissues are **capillaries**.
- Vessels that carry blood away from the tissues **toward the heart** are **veins** and **venules**.

Arteries and arterioles

Blood is ejected from the heart into large, thick-walled vessels called arteries.

Structure of arteries

Arteries consist of a **lumen**, which is a hollow center through which the blood flows, surrounded by a triple-layered wall composed of:

- An outer layer of fibrous tissue called the **tunica adventitia (tunica externa)**
- A middle layer of smooth muscle and elastic tissue called the **tunica media**
- An inner layer of squamous epithelium (endothelium) called the **tunica intima (tunica interna)**.

Types of arteries

Elastic (conducting) arteries: Large arteries whose walls are relatively thin and whose tunica media consists of more elastic fibers than muscle fibers. This enables the arteries to stretch and recoil as they conduct blood from the heart to the medium-sized arteries. The aorta is an example of an elastic artery.

Muscular (distributing) arteries: Medium-sized arteries whose tunica media consists of more smooth muscle fibers and fewer elastic fibers. This large amount of smooth muscle fibers means the walls of muscular arteries are relatively thick and are capable of greater vasoconstriction and vasodilation as they distribute blood to various parts of the body. The brachial artery is an example of a muscular artery.

Arterioles: Tiny arteries that deliver blood to capillaries.

The smooth muscle of arteries is arranged circularly around the lumen so that when it contracts it

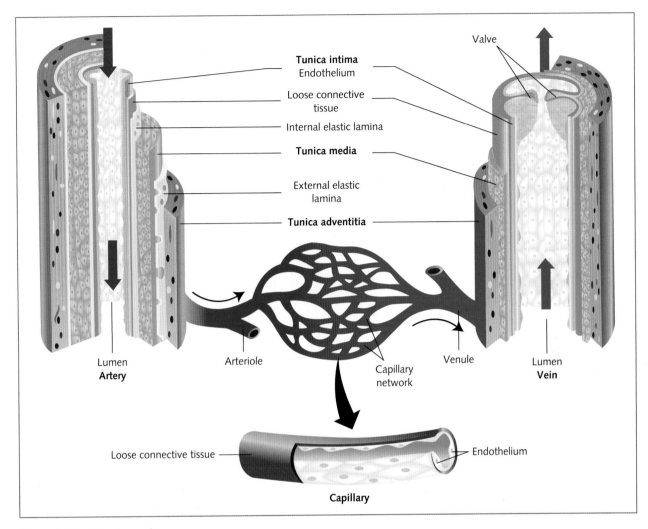

Figure 9.10 *Blood vessels*

narrows the lumen. This narrowing of the lumen is called **vasoconstriction**. When the smooth muscle fibers relax the size of the lumen increases, and this is called **vasodilation**. Vasoconstriction and vasodilation are usually controlled by the autonomic nervous system.

Capillaries

Blood from arteries flows into arterioles and then finally into capillaries, from where nutrients and wastes can be exchanged with tissue cells through interstitial fluid.

The name capillary derives from the Latin word *capillaris*, which means "hairlike," and capillaries are microscopic vessels that network through tissues and connect arterioles and venules in what is referred to as **microcirculation**.

The mechanisms of vasoconstriction and vasodilation enable capillaries to help adjust body temperature:

- **Vasoconstriction:** Narrowing of the vessels results in a reduction in the flow of blood through the capillaries. Thus, heat in the blood is conserved and the body is kept warm.
- **Vasodilation:** Widening of the vessels results in an increase of blood to the surface of the skin. From here, heat in the blood is lost through radiation and the body is cooled.

Structure of capillaries
Capillary walls are made up of only a single layer of endothelium and a basement membrane. This extremely thin layer enables substances such as nutrients, oxygen, and wastes to pass easily between the interstitial fluid surrounding cells and the blood.

Veins and venules

Blood from capillaries drains into venules, which are tiny veins, and then into veins. Veins return blood to the heart.

Structure of veins

The structure of veins is similar to that of arteries in that they consist of a triple-layered wall surrounding a lumen. This wall consists of the tunica adventitia (externa), tunica media, and tunica intima (interna). However:

- The walls of veins are much thinner than those of arteries because there is less muscle and elastic tissue in the tunica media.

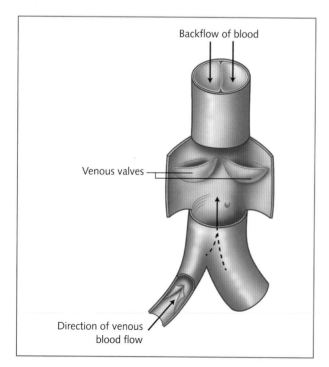

Backflow of blood

Venous valves

Direction of venous blood flow

Figure 9.11 *Venous valves*

- The lumen of a vein is usually larger than that of an artery.
- Some veins, such as those in the limbs, have valves to prevent the backflow of blood as it flows upward toward the heart. These valves are composed of thin folds of tunica intima and form flap-like cusps that project into the lumen of the vein and point toward the heart. If blood moves back toward the feet it causes the cusps to close and so prevent backflow.

Movement of blood through veins

The flow of blood through vessels is dependent on a pressure gradient: blood flows from an area of high pressure into an area of low pressure. Blood passes from the heart into the arteries at a very high pressure and it flows continually along a pressure gradient, always moving into areas of lower pressure.

However, in the larger veins where there is minimal pressure, the pressure gradient is not enough to ensure the flow of blood. Thus, blood is moved through the veins by the milking action of skeletal muscles and the movement of the diaphragm during inspiration, which causes pressure changes in the thoracic cavity. The blood is also prevented from flowing backward by valves.

DIFFERENCES BETWEEN ARTERIES AND VEINS		
Features	Arteries	Veins
Structure	• Thick walls • No valves • Smaller lumen	• Thin walls • Valves • Larger lumen
Function	Carry blood away from the heart	Carry blood toward the heart
Blood pressure	Higher	Lower

Did you know?

Mean arterial blood pressure (MABP) is a measurement of the average blood pressure of a vessel. At the arteriolar end of a capillary it is approximately 35 mm Hg, at the venous end it has dropped to 16 mm Hg, and by the time the blood enters the right ventricle it is 0 mm Hg.

Blood Pressure

The force exerted by blood on the walls of a blood vessel is referred to as blood pressure. It is the force that keeps blood circulating and it is generated by the contractions of the left ventricle.

Blood pressure is highest in the aorta, as this is the artery that receives blood directly from the left ventricle. The pressure then progressively falls as blood moves further and further away from the left ventricle. Thus, pressure is lowest in the veins, and lowest of all in the inferior vena cava.

Measuring blood pressure

Blood pressure is measured in millimeters of mercury (mm Hg), and is measured near the large systemic arteries. In a normal, young adult, blood pressure is 120/80 mm Hg while at rest. The first figure, 120 mm Hg, is the systolic pressure and shows the pressure of the blood during systole, or contraction, of the left ventricle. The second figure, 80 mm Hg, is the diastolic pressure and shows the pressure of the blood during diastole, or relaxation, of the left ventricle.

When measuring blood pressure it is important to be aware that blood pressure varies slightly according to:

- **Time of day:** Blood pressure drops during night-time sleep.
- **Posture:** Blood pressure is lower when lying down.
- **Age:** Blood pressure tends to increase with age.

Factors affecting blood pressure

Blood pressure is increased or decreased by the following factors:

- **Cardiac output:** Cardiac output is the amount of blood pumped out of the heart by the left ventricle in one minute. In a normal adult it is approximately 10½ pints (5 liters). This means that approximately 10½ pints (5 liters) of blood passes through the entire body in one minute. Cardiac output is affected by the heart rate.
  - The heart rate varies with the demands of the body. For example, exercise increases the heart rate. Thus, exercise increases cardiac output and so increases blood pressure. On the other hand, blood loss decreases cardiac output and so decreases blood pressure
  - The heart rate is also affected by the autonomic nervous system, hormones and ions. Refer to the section "Autonomic and chemical regulation of the heart rate," above, for more details
- **Resistance:** The opposition to the flow of blood through the vessels. An increased resistance increases the blood pressure. Resistance is affected by:
  - **Changes in the tunica media of the arterioles:** The tunica media of arterioles is mainly composed of smooth muscle. If this muscle is replaced by inelastic fibrous tissue then this will cause blood pressure to increase. This occurs with aging
  - **Blood viscosity:** The viscosity, or thickness, of blood increases with conditions such as dehydration and decreases with conditions such as anemia or hemorrhaging. An increase in viscosity causes an increase in resistance and thus blood pressure, while a decrease in viscosity causes a decrease in resistance and thus blood pressure

– **Blood vessel length:** Longer blood vessels increase the resistance and thus increase blood pressure. Longer blood vessels are present in people who are obese as additional vessels are necessary to supply the additional adipose tissue

– **Blood vessel radius:** A decrease in the radius of a blood vessel increases resistance and thus increases blood pressure. Arterioles change their diameters by vasoconstricting or vasodilating. This enables them to control the amount of blood flowing to a particular organ. For example, an active organ needs more oxygen and nutrients than a resting one. Blood pressure is increased when arterioles vasoconstrict and decreased when they vasodilate. This change in vessel radius is referred to as **systemic vascular resistance (SVR)** or **total peripheral resistance**

In the classroom

During stressful situations, blood pressure quickly rises in order to prepare the body for "fight or flight." These effects on blood pressure are short-lived, and once the situation has cleared the body quickly returns to homeostasis. Why then do doctors say that stress is a major risk factor or contributor to hypertension? In order to answer this question, have a group discussion around the following:

• What are the physiological (and pathological) effects of frequent, repetitive increases in blood pressure? What changes occur to the blood vessels themselves?

• How does stress affect other risk factors for hypertension, such as cigarette smoking, alcohol consumption, poor diet, and a lack of exercise?

Primary Blood Vessels of Systemic Circulation

Blood vessels are organized into routes that transport blood throughout the body. The word *systemic* refers to the body as a whole, and systemic circulation is the route blood follows from the heart to the tissues and organs of the body and back to the heart. This route is as follows:

• Oxygenated blood from the left ventricle of the heart is ejected into the aorta, which then

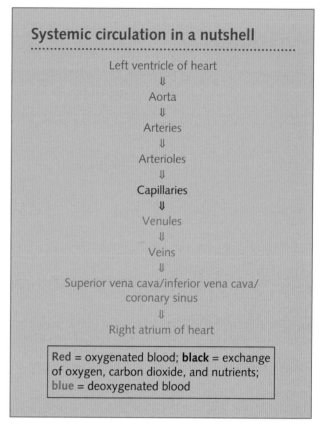

Systemic circulation in a nutshell

Left ventricle of heart
⇓
Aorta
⇓
Arteries
⇓
Arterioles
⇓
Capillaries
⇓
Venules
⇓
Veins
⇓
Superior vena cava/inferior vena cava/ coronary sinus
⇓
Right atrium of heart

Red = oxygenated blood; **black** = exchange of oxygen, carbon dioxide, and nutrients; blue = deoxygenated blood

Did you know?

The diameter of the aorta is approximately the same as that of your thumb.

branches into arteries, arterioles, and finally capillaries.

– Blood traveling through the aorta has a high pressure because it has been ejected with force from the heart. As it travels through the systemic circulation it progressively loses this pressure and by the time it returns to the right atrium of the heart it has almost no pressure at all

– Blood traveling through the aorta is a bright red color because it is oxygenated. As it loses its oxygen and gains carbon dioxide it also loses its bright color, and blood traveling through the veins back to the right atrium is a dark red color

• At the capillaries, nutrients and wastes are exchanged with tissue cells through interstitial fluid. The capillaries connect arterioles to venules.

• Deoxygenated blood then drains into venules, veins, and finally into the superior vena cava, inferior vena cava, or coronary sinus, which return blood to the right atrium.

Aorta

The aorta is the largest blood vessel in the body and it receives oxygenated blood from the left ventricle. Different regions of the aorta are named according to their location or shape, as follows:

- **Ascending aorta:** The aorta extends upward from the left ventricle before arching downward. This upward extension is the ascending aorta.
- **Aortic arch:** Where the aorta arches downward is called the aortic arch.
- **Descending aorta:** The aorta then descends downward behind the heart and through the trunk.
- **Thoracic aorta:** The thoracic aorta follows the spine through the thoracic cavity.
- **Abdominal aorta:** The aorta then descends behind the diaphragm into the abdominopelvic cavity, where it is called the abdominal aorta.
- The aorta finally divides into the **right** and **left common iliac arteries**, which transport blood to the lower limbs.

Superior vena cava, inferior vena cava, and coronary sinus

The heart ejects blood into only one vessel for systemic circulation: the aorta. However, blood from the systemic circulation returns to the heart via three vessels:

- **Superior vena cava:** This begins behind the right first costal cartilage at the union of the right and left brachiocephalic veins, and empties its blood into the superior part of the right atrium. It receives blood from veins superior to the diaphragm. This includes the head, neck, upper limbs, and thoracic wall.
- **Inferior vena cava:** This is the largest vein in the body and begins at the union of the common iliac veins, above the fifth lumbar vertebra. It ascends through the abdomen and thorax and empties its blood into the inferior part of the right atrium. It receives blood from veins inferior to the diaphragm. This includes the abdominal viscera, most of the abdominal walls, and the lower limbs.
- **Coronary sinus:** This begins in the coronary sulcus, a groove that separates the atria and ventricles, and empties its blood into the right atrium. It receives blood from the cardiac veins, which drain the myocardium of the heart.

Now that you have a basic understanding of the main vessels of the heart, we will look at the primary blood vessels that connect the different regions of the body to the heart.

Study tip

When learning the names of blood vessels, remember that they often tell us which regions or organs the vessels serve, or let us know which bones they follow. For example, the brachial artery is found in the arm.

Guide to flowcharts of the blood vessels of the body

Some of the primary blood vessels of the body have been described in flow charts on the following pages. To help you understand these charts please note the following features of the charts:

Color: The color of the boxes and arrows represents the type of blood transported. Arteries carrying **oxygenated** blood are colored red. Veins carrying **deoxygenated** blood are colored blue.

Colored boxes: The primary vessels associated with an area are in colored boxes. These are the vessels you will need to learn for that particular area. The other vessels are simply to help you picture the flow of the blood.

Direction of arrows: The direction of the arrows represents the direction of blood flow. In general, blood flowing in arteries flows downward from the heart to the rest of the body and blood flowing in veins moves upward from the rest of the body to the heart.

Right/left side representation: Most blood vessels of the body are the same on both sides of the body. Thus, for ease of learning, the left and right sides are not noted. However, if there are differences between the left and right sides of the body, then both sides are represented.

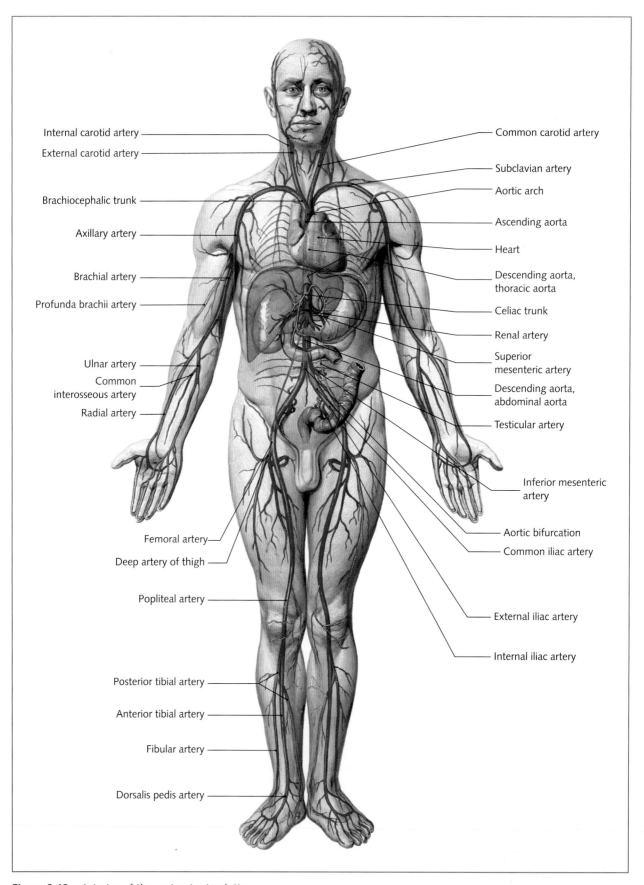

Internal carotid artery

External carotid artery

Brachiocephalic trunk

Axillary artery

Brachial artery

Profunda brachii artery

Ulnar artery

Common interosseous artery

Radial artery

Femoral artery

Deep artery of thigh

Popliteal artery

Posterior tibial artery

Anterior tibial artery

Fibular artery

Dorsalis pedis artery

Common carotid artery

Subclavian artery

Aortic arch

Ascending aorta

Heart

Descending aorta, thoracic aorta

Celiac trunk

Renal artery

Superior mesenteric artery

Descending aorta, abdominal aorta

Testicular artery

Inferior mesenteric artery

Aortic bifurcation

Common iliac artery

External iliac artery

Internal iliac artery

Figure 9.12 *Arteries of the systemic circulation*

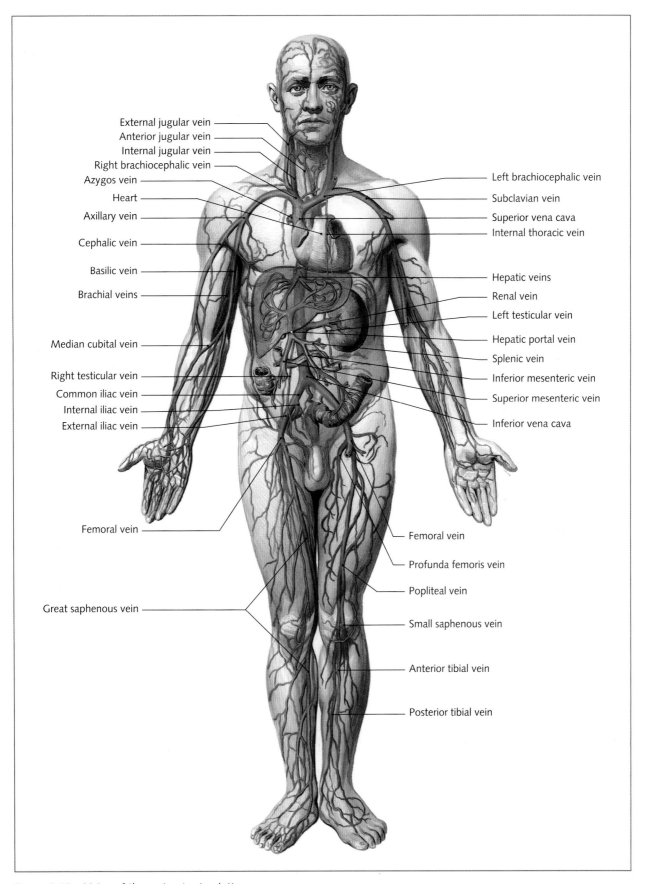

Figure 9.13 *Veins of the systemic circulation*

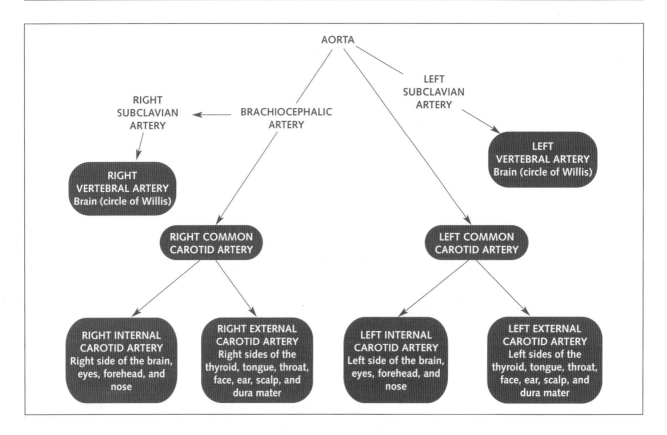

Primary blood vessels of the head, face, and neck

Arteries

The paired arteries supplying the head, face, and neck are the **common carotid arteries** and the **vertebral arteries**.

The right common carotid artery arises from the brachiocephalic artery, while the left one arises directly from the aorta. The common carotid arteries divide into the **internal** and **external carotid arteries**. The vertebral arteries arise from the subclavian arteries, which feed off the aorta.

Veins

Most blood draining from the head passes into three pairs of veins: the **internal jugular veins**, the **external jugular veins** and the **vertebral veins**.

The internal jugular veins unite with the subclavian veins to form the brachiocephalic veins.

The external jugular veins and the vertebral veins feed into the subclavian veins.

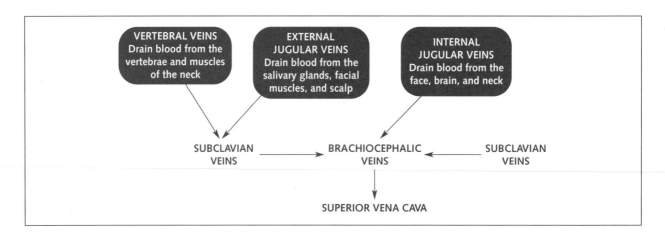

Did you know?

The base of the brain is surrounded by a complete circle of blood vessels called the **circle of Willis (cerebral arterial circle)**. The two internal carotid arteries and the two vertebral arteries contribute to the formation of this circle, and this multiple supply of arterial blood ensures that there are alternate routes to the brain should one of the arteries become damaged. In addition, the circle of Willis helps equalize blood pressure to the brain.

Primary blood vessels of the upper limbs

Arteries

The right and left subclavian arteries transport blood to the upper limbs. These arteries become the **axillary**, then **brachial, radial, ulnar, palmar,** and finally **digital arteries,** and are named after the regions through which they pass. Be aware that on the right side of the body blood flows from the aorta into the brachiocephalic artery and then into the right subclavian artery, while on the left side of the body it flows from the aorta directly into the left subclavian artery.

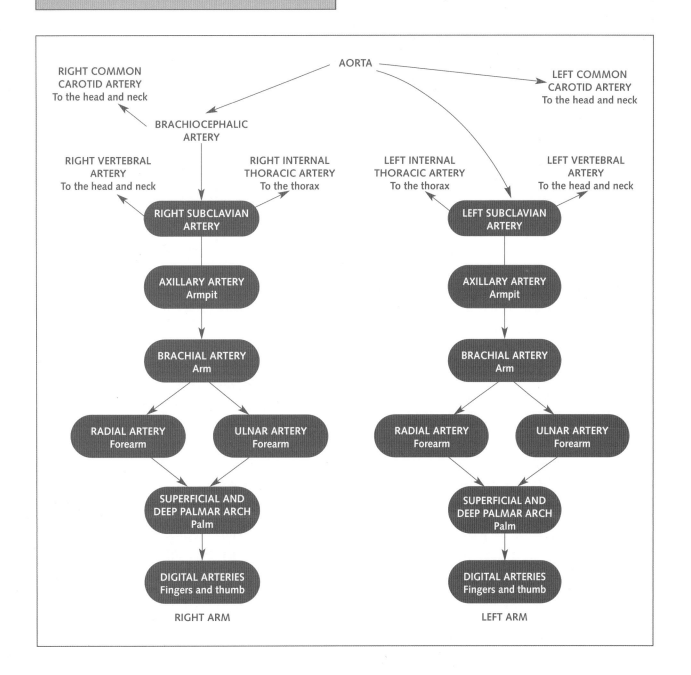

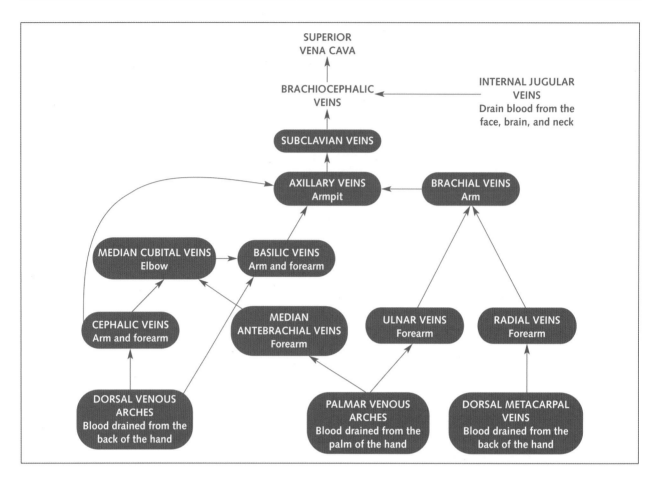

Veins

Veins of the upper limb are divided into two groups: superficial veins and deep veins. The superficial veins are the **cephalic, median cubital, basilic** and **median antebrachial veins.**

- The cephalic vein drains the lateral (radial) aspect of the arm, beginning at the back of the hand and emptying into the axillary vein.
- At the elbow the cephalic gives off a branch called the median cubital vein, which slants upward to join the basilic vein.
- The basilic vein begins at the back of the hand and drains the medial (ulnar) aspect of the arm, emptying into the axillary vein.
- The median antebrachial veins begin at the palm of the hand, ascend on the medial (ulnar) aspect of the forearm, and end in the median cubital veins at the elbow.
- The deep veins follow the course of the arteries and have the same names: **dorsal metacarpal, palmar venous arch, ulnar, radial, brachial, axillary** and **subclavian veins.**

Primary blood vessels of the thorax

Arteries

The **thoracic aorta** gives off paired branches of arteries that supply the thorax. These are divided into two groups and are named after the regions or organs they supply. They include the:

- Arteries that feed the viscera and are collectively called the **visceral branches:**
  - **Pericardial arteries** supply the pericardium
  - **Bronchial arteries** supply the lungs
  - **Esophageal arteries** supply the esophagus
  - **Mediastinal arteries** supply the mediastinum
- Arteries that feed the body-wall structures and are collectively called the **parietal branches:**

Did you know?

Blood is usually drawn from the median cubital vein for blood tests.

- – **Posterior intercostal** and **subcostal arteries** supply the muscles and skin of the thorax, the mammary glands, and the vertebral canal
- – **Superior phrenic arteries** supply the diaphragm

Note: A flow chart of the thoracic arteries has not been included here. This is because most syllabi require that you learn only the thoracic aorta. The other arteries named here have been included for reference only.

Veins

The thorax is drained by a network of veins on either side of the vertebral column called the **azygos system**. This includes the **azygos, hemiazygos,** and **accessory hemiazygos veins,** which receive blood from smaller veins carrying return blood from the parietal and visceral branches of the thoracic aorta. The names of these veins correspond to those of the arteries. The azygos system ultimately feeds into the superior vena cava or the brachiocephalic veins. Both these veins are considered the principal veins of the thoracic region.

- **Superior vena cava:** This is a large vein that receives blood from veins draining the head, neck, upper limbs, and thoracic wall.
- **Brachiocephalic veins:** The left and right brachiocephalic veins are formed by the union of the subclavian and internal jugular veins, and they themselves unite to form the superior vena cava. The brachiocephalic veins drain blood from the head, neck, upper limbs, mammary glands, and superior thorax.

Note: A flow chart of the thoracic veins has not been included here. This is because most syllabi require that you learn only the superior vena cava and brachiocephalic veins. The other veins named here have been included for reference only.

Primary blood vessels of the abdomen

Arteries

The **abdominal aorta** gives off paired and unpaired branches of arteries that supply the abdominopelvic region. Similar to the arteries of the thorax, the abdominal arteries are divided into two groups and named after the regions or organs they supply. They include the:

- Arteries that feed the viscera and are collectively called the **visceral branches:**
  - – The **celiac artery** divides into three branches:
    - ○ The **common hepatic artery** branches into smaller arteries supplying the liver, gall bladder, and parts of the stomach, duodenum, and pancreas
    - ○ The **left gastric artery** supplies the stomach, and its esophageal branch supplies the esophagus
    - ○ The **splenic artery** branches into smaller arteries supplying the spleen, pancreas, and stomach
  - – **Superior** and **inferior mesenteric arteries** supply the small and large intestines
  - – **Suprarenal arteries** supply the adrenal glands
  - – **Renal arteries** supply the kidneys
  - – **Gonadal arteries** (testicular or ovarian) supply the gonads
- Arteries that feed the body-wall structures and are collectively called the **parietal branches:**
  - – **Inferior phrenic arteries** supply the diaphragm
  - – **Lumbar arteries** supply the spinal cord and muscles and skin of the lumbar region
  - – **Median sacral arteries** supply the sacrum, coccyx, and rectum

Note: A flow chart of the abdominal arteries has not been included here. This is because most syllabi require that you learn only the abdominal aorta. The other arteries named here have been included for reference only.

Veins

Blood from the abdomen returns to the heart via the **inferior vena cava.**

This large vein receives blood from smaller veins carrying return blood from the parietal and visceral branches of the abdominal aorta. The names of these veins correspond to those of the arteries (**renal, gonadal, suprarenal, inferior phrenic, hepatic,** and **lumbar**).

However, blood from the digestive organs (the gastrointestinal tract, spleen, pancreas, and gall bladder) does not flow directly into the inferior vena cava. It first passes through the liver via the **hepatic portal circulation** (see next section).

After it has passed through the liver it drains into the **hepatic veins** and then into the inferior vena cava.

The right and left **common iliac veins** drain most of the blood from the lower limbs and pelvis and unite to form the inferior vena cava.

Hepatic portal circulation

Blood from tissues usually flows through one capillary bed before it is returned to the heart. However, blood from the digestive organs passes through a second capillary bed at the liver before it is returned to the heart. This is necessary for two reasons:

- Blood from the digestive organs is rich with absorbed nutrients—the liver stores or modifies these nutrients in order to maintain correct nutrient concentrations in the blood.
- Blood from the digestive organs may contain harmful substances—the liver detoxifies the blood to ensure these substances are not transported to the rest of the body.

The liver receives blood from two major vessels:

- The liver receives nutrient-rich, deoxygenated blood directly from the digestive organs through the hepatic portal vein, which drains blood from the:
    - **Superior mesenteric vein,** which receives blood from veins draining the small intestine, portions of the large intestine, stomach, and pancreas
    - **Splenic vein,** which receives blood from veins draining the stomach, pancreas, and portions of the large intestine
    - **Inferior mesenteric vein,** which joins the splenic vein and receives blood from veins draining portions of the large intestine
    - **Right and left gastric veins,** which drain the stomach
    - **Cystic vein,** which drains the gall bladder
- The liver receives oxygenated blood via the **hepatic artery,** which branches off the **celiac artery.**

All blood leaves the liver through the hepatic veins, which drain into the inferior vena cava.

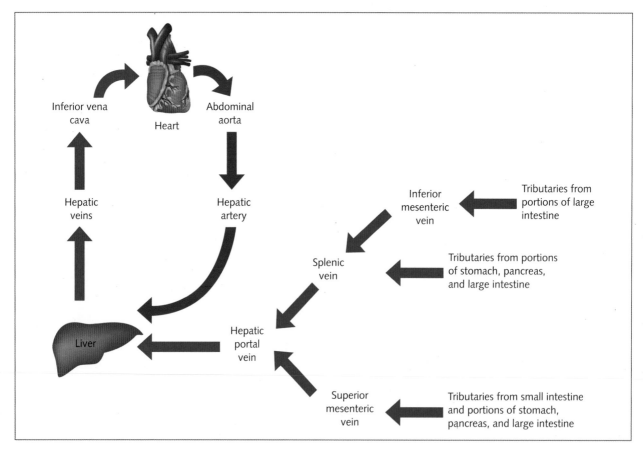

Figure 9.14 *Hepatic portal circulation*

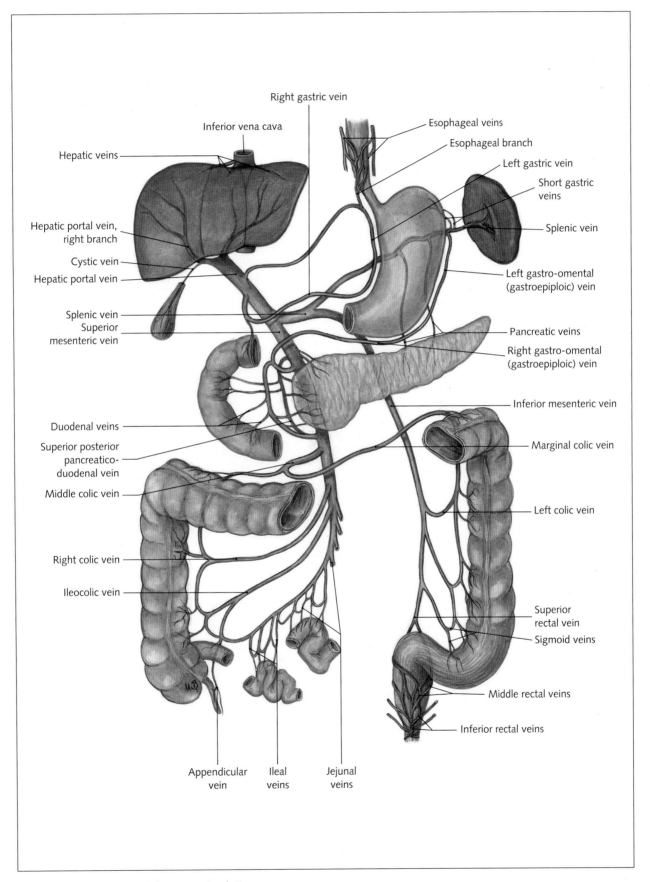

Figure 9.15 *Hepatic portal venous circulation*

Primary blood vessels of the pelvis and lower limbs

Arteries

The abdominal aorta divides into the **right** and **left common iliac arteries**, which in turn divide into the **internal** and **external iliac arteries**:

- The **internal iliac arteries** supply most of the pelvic viscera and wall.
- The **external iliac arteries** enter the thigh and become the **femoral arteries**.
- As the femoral arteries descend through the leg they become the **popliteal arteries**, which divide into the **anterior** and **posterior tibial arteries**.
- The anterior tibial artery continues over the top of the foot as the **dorsalis pedis artery**.
- The posterior tibial artery gives off the **fibular branch** and then becomes the **plantar artery** (medial and lateral plantar), supplying the sole of the foot.
- Together with the **dorsalis pedis**, the plantar artery and its branches form the **plantar arch**, from which the **digital arteries** arise.

Veins

Veins of the lower limb are divided into two groups: superficial veins and deep veins:

- Superficial veins are the **great saphenous** and **small saphenous veins**.
  - The **great saphenous vein** is the longest vein in the body and runs up the inner thigh, beginning at the dorsal venous arch and emptying into the femoral vein in the groin
  - The **small saphenous vein** begins behind the ankle joint and ascends the back of the leg, where it joins the **popliteal vein** behind the knee

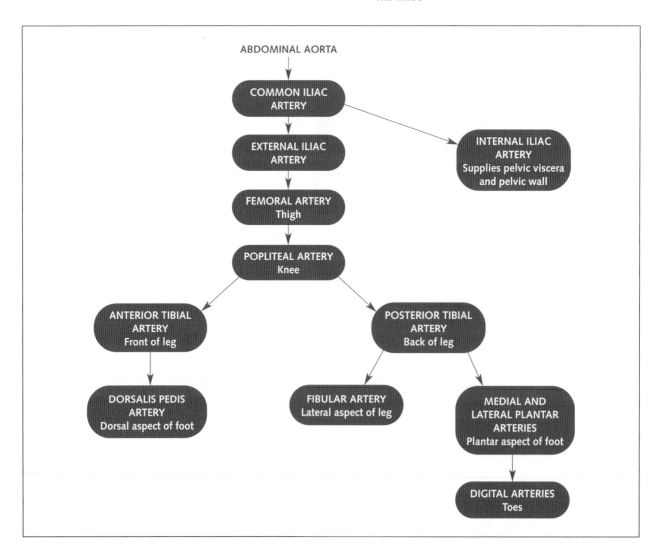

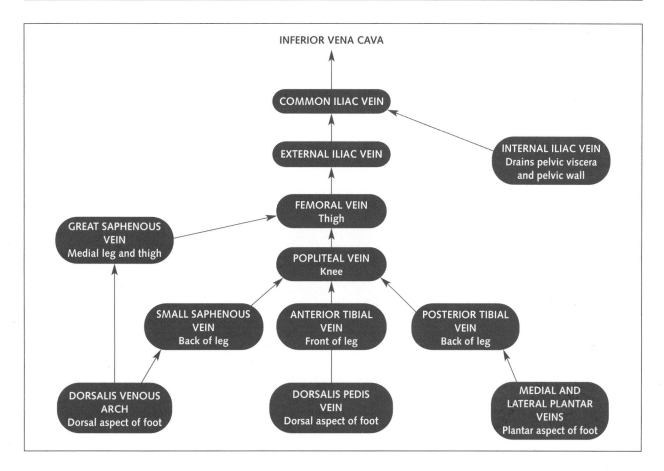

- The deep veins follow the course of the arteries and have the same names: **anterior tibial, posterior tibial, popliteal, femoral, external iliac, internal iliac,** and **common iliac veins.**

Common Pathologies of the Cardiovascular System

To a certain extent, the health of the cardiovascular system is dependent on one's lifestyle. Leading a healthy lifestyle that ensures you do not become obese or develop high blood pressure, avoiding smoking cigarettes, and exercising regularly can help to keep your heart and blood vessels healthy.

Red flags

- **Heart attack:** Someone having a heart attack may experience any of the following sensations (or occasionally none at all):
  - Chest pain or discomfort often described as a squeezing pain or sensation of pressure/fullness; this discomfort can spread to the shoulders, back, neck, face, arms, or upper abdomen
  - Shortness of breath
  - Light-headedness, dizziness, fainting
  - Sweating
  - Nausea
  - Anxiety
- **Sepsis:** This is an extreme inflammatory response to an infection that can be caused by bacteria in the blood (**septicemia**) or by a localized infection such as pneumonia; it can quickly develop into septic shock, which is life-threatening. Signs and symptoms of sepsis include:
  - Rapid breathing
  - Mental confusion
  - Fever
  - Chills
  - Shaking
  - Warm skin
  - Rapid heartbeat
- **Shock:** There are many causes of shock, including trauma, allergic reactions, infection, poisoning, heatstroke, or severe burns. When people go into shock their organs do not receive enough oxygen

Infobox

Anatomy and physiology in perspective

As a health professional you will find many of your clients are on medication for cardiovascular conditions such as hypertension or angina pectoris. It is important to have a basic understanding of these medications so that you know when it is safe, and when it is not safe, for you to treat your client. Listed below are the most commonly used heart medications that some of your patients may be taking. Please note, only a few generic examples have been given and we suggest you find out your country's trade names of these medications so that you can recognize them easily.

Anticoagulants

Anticoagulants help prevent the formation, or enlargement, of blood clots (thrombi) and include *heparin* and *warfarin*. Clients who are taking anticoagulants are at an increased risk of hemorrhage as well as hypersensitivity reactions such as skin rashes, and are **contraindicated** to most complementary therapies.

Antiplatelet drugs

Antiplatelet drugs such as *aspirin* and *clopidogrel* help prevent the formation of blood clots by reducing the adhesion of blood platelets. They are sometimes used in combination with other medications.

Statins (HMG CoA reductase inhibitors)

Statins such as *simvastatin* and *lovastatin* are used to help lower LDL cholesterol by inhibiting the enzyme involved in the synthesis of cholesterol. They can have adverse side effects on the liver and cause muscle weakness (myopathy).

Calcium channel blockers

Calcium channel blockers such as *amlodipine* and *nifedipine* are vasodilators and are used to treat hypertension or angina pectoris.

Beta-adrenergic blocking agents

Beta-adrenergic blocking agents, or "beta-blockers," include *atenolol* and *metoprolol* and are used to decrease heart rate and contractility. They are used as long-term treatment for exertional angina and should never be withdrawn abruptly.

Diuretics and angiotensin-converting enzyme (ACE) inhibitors

Diuretics such as *hydrochlorothiazide* and *furosemide*, as well as ACE inhibitors such as *captopril* and *enalapril*, help to lower blood pressure and are used in the long-term treatment of hypertension. They act on the urinary system and are discussed in more detail in chapter 12.

---

and this can result in permanent organ damage or death. Signs and symptoms vary, but can include:

– Low blood pressure, weakness, and fatigue
– Dizziness or fainting
– Rapid pulse
– Rapid breathing
– Skin that is cool and clammy to touch
– Skin that is pale or ashen in color
– Nausea and vomiting
– Enlarged pupils
– Anxiety, confusion, or other changes in mental behavior

Blood disorders

Blood disorders are sometimes difficult to diagnose as their signs and symptoms can indicate many other types of disorders. Therefore, it is usually necessary to have blood tests done in order to diagnose blood disorders properly.

General signs and symptoms of blood disorders can include fatigue, weakness, shortness of breath, dizziness, excessive bleeding, and easy bruising.

Anemia

Reduction in the oxygen-carrying capacity of the blood and characterized by a reduced number of red blood cells, or a reduction in the amount of hemoglobin, in the blood. It can be caused by a loss of blood, a lack of iron, or the destruction or impaired production of red blood cells. Signs and symptoms of anemia include fatigue, paleness, breathlessness on exertion, lowered resistance to infection, and an intolerance to the cold. There are many different types of anemia, including:

- **Iron-deficiency anemia:** The body needs iron to produce red blood cells, and if it is lost through bleeding or if there is a lack of iron due to an inadequate supply or poor absorption of dietary iron, then anemia can occur. Iron-deficiency anemia is common in menstruating females and also affects infants, pregnant women, and the elderly.
- **Pernicious anemia (vitamin-deficiency anemia):** This results from low levels of vitamin B12 (cyanocobalamin). This can be caused by either low dietary levels of vitamin B12 or from the inability of the stomach to produce intrinsic factor, which is necessary for the absorption of vitamin B12 in the small intestine.
- **Sickle-cell anemia:** This is a genetic disorder that is more common in people who live in malarial areas such as sub-Saharan Africa and tropical Asia. In sickle-cell anemia the hemoglobin molecule is abnormally shaped and bends the red blood cells into sickle, or crescent, shapes. These cells then rupture easily, and this destruction of the red blood cells leads to chronic anemia. Ironically, people with sickle-cell anemia have a high resistance to malaria.
- **Thalassemia:** This is an inherited disorder in which hemoglobin production is impaired. There are different types of thalassemias but most of them cause varying degrees of fatigue and weakness.

Blood-clotting disorders

Hemostasis is the way in which the body stops bleeding, and it comprises a series of processes that involve the constriction of blood vessels and the clotting of the blood. This clotting is balanced by the breakdown of the clots once vessels have healed, thus ensuring that the blood remains fluid. However, sometimes the blood does not clot properly or the clots do not dissolve properly and so disorders occur. Some of these disorders include:

- **Hemophilia:** This is a hereditary disorder in which blood clots very slowly owing to a deficiency of certain clotting factors. The severity of the disorder varies: in mild hemophilia the person may bleed more than expected after injuries or surgery, while in severe hemophilia a slight bump can trigger chronic internal bleeding, which can be fatal.
- **Pulmonary embolism:** This is the blocking of the pulmonary artery by an **embolus** (which can be

a clot). This disorder is discussed in more detail in chapter 8.
- **Thrombophilia:** Condition where the blood clots easily or excessively, and patients are at risk of developing blood clots, usually in veins. Thrombophilia can be hereditary or can develop after birth owing to a variety of factors.
- **Thrombosis:** This is a condition in which a blood clot, or **thrombus**, is produced. If it is large enough, a blood clot can obstruct the flow of blood to an organ:
  - **Coronary thrombosis** is the formation of a blood clot in the coronary artery, and it can lead to the obstruction of the flow of blood to the heart
  - **Deep vein thrombosis (DVT)** is a deep vein clot, called a **phlebothrombosis**, in the legs and is usually characterized by the leg becoming swollen and tender. The clot may become detached and block the pulmonary artery (**pulmonary embolism**). Risk factors of DVT include thrombophilia, prolonged bed rest, pregnancy, and surgery

Dyslipidemia

Dyslipidemia refers to abnormal levels of lipids in the bloodstream, whereas the term **hyperlipidemia** refers to abnormally high levels of lipids. The most common hyperlipidemias are high cholesterol levels (**hypercholesterolemia**) and high triglyceride levels (**hypertriglyceridemia**) and these are major risk factors for cardiovascular disease. Hyperlipidemia has few signs or symptoms and is usually discovered through blood tests. However, individuals who are overweight, do not exercise regularly, and have a family history of the condition are more at risk of developing hyperlipidemia.

Hematoma

Collections of blood outside of a blood vessel that are usually caused by damage to the blood-vessel wall through trauma or injury. They can also be associated with medications such as anticoagulants, or diseases that decrease the blood's clotting abilities. Signs, symptoms, and severity of hematomas depend on their location and size. For example, an intracranial epidural hematoma is the accumulation of blood in the space between the dura and cranial bones and it is considered to be one of the most dangerous and fatal complications of head injury. On the other hand, a subungual hematoma is the collection of blood under the nail and can result from slamming your finger in the door.

Nosebleeds (epistaxis)

Bleeding through the nose is commonly caused by nose picking or injury to the nose. However, it can sometimes develop as a side effect of taking aspirin or anticoagulant drugs, or it can be associated with fever, high blood pressure, or blood disorders. Common nosebleeds are usually easily controlled at home and should subside within ten minutes. If the bleeding is severe and prolonged, medical help should be sought.

Septicemia

Serious bloodstream infection commonly known as **blood poisoning**. If the infectious agent is a bacterium, then septicemia is called **bacteremia**. It occurs when infection elsewhere in the body—for example, the lungs—enters the bloodstream, or after medical or dental procedures involving the insertion of foreign bodies such as catheters.

Heart and blood-vessel disorders

Risk factors in heart disease

Statistics show that your lifestyle influences your risk of suffering from heart disease and that simple changes to your lifestyle can often reduce your chances of developing it. Factors that increase your chance of suffering from a disease are called **risk factors**, and the following are major risk factors in heart disease:

- Obesity
- Lack of regular exercise
- High blood cholesterol level
- High blood pressure
- Cigarette smoking
- Diabetes mellitus
- Family history of heart disease at an early age
- Gender: Men are more at risk of heart disease than women; however, after the age of 70 years the risk is equal in both sexes.

Aneurysm

Abnormal swelling or bulge in the walls of a blood vessel. The swelling weakens the walls, which can rupture, causing internal bleeding, or it can put pressure on surrounding tissues and nerves. The blood vessels of the brain and the aorta are the most commonly affected sites, and causes of aneurysms include trauma, infection, connective-tissue disorders, inflammation, high blood pressure, and fatty plaques.

Angina pectoris

Temporary sensation of a chest pain, which often spreads to the arms or jaw, or of suffocation. It is caused by a lack of oxygen to the heart muscle. This pain is usually induced by exercise or emotional distress and relieved by rest. Angina is usually caused by coronary artery disease in which the coronary arteries have become narrowed so that blood flow to the heart is reduced.

Arrhythmia (abnormal heart rate rhythms)

Abnormal heart rate rhythms are irregular sequences of heartbeats. A normal heart rate is usually 60–100 bpm and anything above or below this rate is considered abnormal (except in very fit, young people who can have a heart rate below 60). Signs and symptoms of abnormal rhythms vary from not being felt at all to palpitations (an awareness of the heartbeat) to weakness, light headedness, dizziness, and fainting. The most common cause of abnormal heart rates is heart disease, although they can also be caused by certain drugs or congenital birth defects.

- **Bradycardia** is an abnormally slow heart rate, usually taken as below 50 bpm. Bradycardia can be triggered by pain, hunger, fatigue, diarrhea, or vomiting.
- **Tachycardia** is an abnormally fast heart rate; it can be triggered by exercise, stress, alcohol, cigarette smoking, or stimulant drugs.

Arteriosclerosis

Hardening of the arteries that can be related to many different diseases and is a condition in which arterial walls become thicker and less elastic.

Atherosclerosis

Type of arteriosclerosis in which fatty substances, especially cholesterol and triglycerides, deposit on the inner walls of arteries and develop into atherosclerotic plaques, which obstruct the flow of blood through the arteries and cause the arteries to harden. Atherosclerosis is symptom-free until the artery has narrowed by more than 70%. Then signs and symptoms will vary according to where the narrowing or blockage occurs in the body. For example, blockage of coronary arteries can cause angina pectoralis or a heart attack, while blockage of the carotid arteries to the brain can result in a stroke. Risk factors for atherosclerosis include cigarette smoking, high cholesterol levels, high blood pressure, diabetes mellitus, obesity, a lack of exercise, and high blood levels of an amino acid called homocysteine.

Cardiac failure
Condition where the heart cannot pump enough blood to meet the demands of the body. Although it is often the end result of many conditions that affect the heart, cardiac failure can also occur suddenly under conditions of high cardiac demand. Signs and symptoms may include tachycardia, edema, fatigue, and breathlessness. Common conditions that are linked to cardiac failure include coronary artery disease, hypertension, and diabetes mellitus.

Coronary artery disease
Condition where the main arteries to the heart become narrowed and blood flow to the heart is reduced. Causes of coronary artery disease are atherosclerosis, coronary artery spasm, or a coronary thrombosis.

Gangrene
Death and decay of tissue due to a lack of blood supply. It can be caused by many conditions, including diseases such as diabetes mellitus, injury, frostbite, or severe burns.

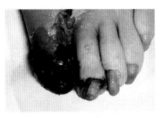

Gangrene

Hemorrhoids (piles)
Enlarged, dilated, and often twisted veins located in the rectum and anus. They can be caused by repeated straining during defecation (usually due to constipation), frequent heavy lifting, or additional pressure resulting from pregnancy. The main sign of hemorrhoids is small amounts of bleeding after a bowel movement.

Hypertension
Abnormally high blood pressure. Normal blood pressure is 120/80 mm Hg and hypertension is defined as a systolic pressure higher than 140 mm Hg, or a diastolic pressure higher than 90 mm Hg, or both (these pressures are taken in a resting adult). Hypertension can be caused by a number of factors, but risk factors include being older than 75 years of age, obesity, poor diet, lack of exercise, stress, metabolic defects, and genetics. Hypersecretion of aldosterone by the adrenal cortex and kidney disease can also cause hypertension.

Hypotension
Blood pressure that is low enough to cause signs and symptoms such as dizziness and fainting. Although low blood pressure is generally healthy, it can cause an insufficient supply of blood to the brain, resulting in fainting and dizziness, or an insufficient supply of blood to the heart, resulting in shortness of breath or chest pain. Hypotension can be caused by a number of factors, including heart disease, infections, and excess fluid or blood loss.

Intermittent claudication
Pain in the lower limbs that is brought on by exercise, e.g., while walking. It improves with rest. Intermittent claudication is associated with atherosclerosis.

Myocardial infarction (heart attack)
Death of an area of heart muscle due to an interruption in the supply of blood to the heart. It is most commonly caused by a blood clot in a coronary artery that has already been partially narrowed by atherosclerotic plaques. The main symptom of a heart attack is severe pain in the middle of the chest, back, jaw, or left arm. This pain is not alleviated by rest. Occasionally, no pain is felt at all. Other signs and symptoms include sweating, nausea, shortness of breath, faintness, and a heavily pounding heart.

Palpitations and panic attacks
A palpitation is an awareness of the heart beating. One is not normally aware of the sensation of the heart beating but occasionally it can be felt—for example, during strenuous exercise or an extremely emotional experience. Panic attacks are episodes occurring in anxiety disorders. Symptoms of panic attacks vary and can include palpitations, chest pain, dizziness, chills, nausea, and feelings of unreality.

Phlebitis

Inflammation of the walls of a vein and characterized by localized pain, tenderness, redness, and heat. Phlebitis often occurs in the legs as a complication of varicose veins and it can lead to the development of a thrombosis.

Raynaud's disease

Condition in which the arterioles of the fingers and toes constrict abnormally when exposed to cold. It can also be triggered by strong emotions. Signs and symptoms

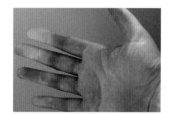

Raynaud's disease

include numbness, tingling, or pins-and-needles sensations in the fingers and toes, and the ends of the fingers or toes become pale and bluish. Rewarming the affected areas restores normal color and sensation. The cause of Raynaud's disease is not always known, but it can accompany disorders such as rheumatoid arthritis or atherosclerosis.

Septal defect (hole in the heart)

Congenital conditions in which babies are born with a hole in the wall (septum) that separates the left and right sides of the heart. Atrial septal defects (ASDs) are located between the atria, while ventricular septal defects (VSDs) are located between the ventricles. Septal defects enable blood to pass through the heart in the wrong direction and this can cause cyanosis. Small septal defects often heal as the child grows, while larger ones need to be treated.

Varicose veins (varices)

Abnormally enlarged veins that are most common in the veins of the legs but can occur in other areas of the body. They can be inherited, occur during pregnancy, or be caused

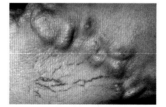

Varicose veins (varices)

by an obstruction to the flow of blood. Affected veins lengthen and widen and the valve cusps within them separate. This results in the backflow of blood, which in turn causes the veins to become even larger and more distended. Varicose veins can result in pain, itchiness, phlebitis, and varicose ulcers.

NEW WORDS	
Autorhythmic cells	Muscle or nerve cells that generate an impulse without an external stimulus; i.e., they are self-excitable
Diastole	Relaxation of the heart muscle during the cardiac cycle
Hemostasis	The stopping of bleeding
Macrophage	Large scavenger cell
Phagocytosis	The engulfment and digestion of foreign particles by phagocytes
Solvent	A medium (usually a liquid) in which substances (solutes) can be dissolved
Systole	Contraction of the heart muscle during the cardiac cycle
Vasoconstriction	The constriction of blood vessels
Vasodilation	The dilation of blood vessels

Study Outline

Blood

Functions of the blood

Blood functions in transportation, regulation, and protection.

Components of blood

1. Blood is composed of blood plasma and formed elements.
2. Blood plasma is composed of water, which acts as a solvent, and solutes that include proteins, electrolytes, nutrients, regulatory substances, gases, and wastes.
3. Formed elements include erythrocytes (red blood cells), leucocytes (white blood cells), and thrombocytes (platelets).

4. Erythrocytes transport oxygen.
5. Leucocytes protect the body against foreign microbes and function in the immune response.
6. Thrombocytes function in stopping the bleeding process (hemostasis).

> Even Red Ladies Will Throw Plates
> Erythrocytes, Red blood cells, Leucocytes, White blood cells, Thrombocytes, Platelets

Heart

The heart pumps blood around the body.

Anatomy of the heart

1. The heart is located in the mediastinum between the lungs in the thoracic cavity.
2. The heart is covered and protected by a triple-layered sac called the pericardium. The pericardium is composed of the outer fibrous pericardium and the inner serous pericardium, which forms a double layer (the outer parietal layer and the inner visceral layer).
3. The walls of the heart are composed of three layers: the outer epicardium, the middle myocardium, and the inner endocardium.
4. The heart is divided into two halves: the left and right sides.
5. Each side of the heart is composed of two chambers: an atrium for receiving blood into the heart and a ventricle for pumping blood out of the heart.
6. Blood is prevented from flowing backward by heart valves: atrioventricular valves (AV) separate the atria and ventricles, while semilunar valves separate the ventricles and arteries.
7. The right AV valve is the tricuspid valve. The left AV valve is the mitral (bicuspid) valve.
8. The right semilunar valve is the pulmonary semilunar valve. The left semilunar valve is the aortic semilunar valve.

Pulmonary and systemic circulation

1. Each side of the heart pumps blood into a different circulation: the pulmonary and systemic circulations.
2. Pulmonary circulation: The right side of the heart receives deoxygenated blood from the body and pumps it to the lungs for oxygen.
3. Systemic circulation: The left side of the heart receives oxygenated blood from the lungs and pumps it to the rest of the body.
4. The principal arteries of the heart are the aorta, coronary artery, and pulmonary artery.
5. The principal veins of the heart are the superior vena cava, inferior vena cava, coronary sinus, and pulmonary vein.

Coronary circulation

The coronary circulation is the blood supply of the heart tissue.

Physiology of the heart

Regulation of the heart rate

1. Cardiac muscle cells have a myogenic rhythm and contract independently of nervous stimulation.
2. The rhythm of the heart is mainly controlled by the intrinsic conduction system (nodal system).
3. The sinoatrial node (SA node) is the heart's pacemaker. It initiates impulses that are then conducted through the atrioventricular node (AV node), to the atrioventricular bundle of His (AV bundle of His), to the right and left bundle branches, and finally to the Purkinje fibers (conduction myofibers).
4. The heart rate is the number of times the heart beats in one minute. Resting heart rate is normally 60–100 bpm.
5. The heart rate can be modified by the autonomic nervous system: sympathetic stimulation increases the heart rate and parasympathetic stimulation decreases the heart rate.
6. The heart rate can also be modified by chemicals such as hormones, ions, certain drugs, and gases.

Cardiac cycle

1. The cardiac cycle is all the events associated with a heartbeat.
2. Starting from the end of the previous heartbeat, a cardiac cycle involves cardiac diastole (relaxation), in which the chambers begin to fill with blood; atrial systole (contraction), in which the atria contract and empty their contents into the ventricles; ventricular systole, in which the ventricles contract and pump blood into the arteries; and then the cycle returns to cardiac diastole.

Blood vessels

1. Arteries and arterioles carry blood away from the heart toward the tissues.

> Arteries
> **A = Away**

2. Capillaries branch throughout tissues and are the site for the exchange of nutrients, oxygen, and waste between the blood and interstitial fluid.
3. Veins and venules carry blood away from tissues toward the heart.
4. In general (except for the vessels of the pulmonary circulation), arteries and arterioles carry oxygenated blood, while veins and venules carry deoxygenated blood.

Arteries

1. Arteries are composed of a lumen surrounded by the tunica intima (interna), then the tunica media, and finally the outer tunica adventitia (tunica externa).
2. Elastic (conducting) arteries are large arteries that conduct blood from the heart to the medium-sized arteries.
3. Muscular (distributing) arteries are medium-sized arteries that distribute blood to various parts of the body.
4. Arterioles are tiny arteries that deliver blood to capillaries.

Capillaries

1. The walls of capillaries consist of a single layer of endothelium and a basement membrane.
2. Capillaries are extremely thin to allow for the rapid exchange of substances.

Veins

1. The structure of veins is similar to that of arteries, except that their walls are thinner and their lumen is larger.
2. Some veins have valves to prevent backflow of blood.
3. Blood is moved through veins by the milking action of skeletal muscles and the movement of the diaphragm.

Blood pressure

1. Blood pressure is the force exerted by blood on the walls of a vessel.
2. Blood pressure is highest in the aorta and lowest in the inferior vena cava.
3. In a normal adult, blood pressure is approximately 120/80 mm Hg. The first figure is the systolic pressure and the second is the diastolic pressure.
4. Blood pressure is affected by cardiac output and resistance.
5. Cardiac output is affected by the heart rate.
6. Resistance is affected by changes in the tunica media of arterioles, blood viscosity, and blood vessel length and radius.

Primary blood vessels of systemic circulation

1. In systemic circulation, oxygenated blood is ejected from the left ventricle into the aorta, which branches into arteries and then into arterioles, which transport oxygenated blood to the capillaries. At the capillaries the blood loses its oxygen and nutrients and gains carbon dioxide and wastes. Deoxygenated blood then drains into venules, which lead into veins, which finally drain into the superior vena cava, inferior vena cava, and coronary sinus. These three vessels all empty deoxygenated blood into the right atrium of the heart.
2. Please refer to the flowcharts in the main text of this chapter for summaries of the vessels of the body.

Review

1. Describe the functions of the blood.
2. Identify the main components of blood.
3. Explain the functions of erythrocytes.
4. Explain the functions of leucocytes.
5. Explain the functions of thrombocytes.
6. Describe the pericardium.
7. Describe the walls of the heart.
8. Identify the chambers of the heart and explain their functions.
9. Name the vein in the body that transports oxygenated blood.

10. Identify which vessels transport blood to the heart tissue.
11. Explain the nodal system.
12. Identify where in the body the sinoatrial node is located.
13. Explain what effect parasympathetic stimulation has on the heart rate.
14. Describe the stages of a cardiac cycle.
15. Identify the differences between arteries, capillaries, and veins.
16. Explain what blood pressure is.
17. Describe the route blood takes through the body, beginning when it leaves the heart and ending when it returns to the heart.
18. Identify the blood vessel that receives oxygenated blood from the left ventricle.
19. Name the three vessels that deposit deoxygenated blood into the heart.
20. Describe the following disorders:
    - Deep vein thrombosis
    - Angina pectoris
    - Sickle-cell anemia
    - Varicose veins.

Multiple-Choice Questions

1. Water functions as:
   a. An electrolyte in the blood
   b. An ion in the blood
   c. A solvent in the blood
   d. A solute in the blood

2. Which of the following is the pacemaker of the heart?
   a. Sinoatrial node
   b. Atrioventricular bundle of His
   c. Purkinje fibers
   d. None of the above

3. Which of the following conducts blood from the heart to medium-sized arteries?
   a. Arterioles
   b. Muscular arteries
   c. Elastic arteries
   d. Capillaries

4. The superior vena cava:
   a. Drains blood from the head, neck, upper limbs, and thoracic wall
   b. Drains blood from the abdominal viscera, most of the abdominal walls, and the lower limbs
   c. Drains blood from the myocardium of the heart
   d. Drains blood from the lower limbs

5. Where in the body is the axillary vein located?
   a. The head
   b. The neck
   c. The armpit
   d. The abdomen

6. Where in the body is the great saphenous vein located?
   a. The abdomen
   b. The groin
   c. The leg
   d. The foot

7. Which of the following statements is correct?
   a. Anemia is a reduction in the oxygen-carrying capacity of the blood
   b. Anemia is characterized by a reduced number of white blood cells
   c. Anemia cannot occur in menstruating females
   d. Anemia is a blood-clotting disorder

8. Which of the following best describes hypotension?
   a. High clotting ability
   b. Low clotting ability
   c. High blood pressure
   d. Low blood pressure

9. Which of the following is not a type of white blood cell?
   a. Neutrophil
   b. Lymphocyte
   c. Erythrocyte
   d. Basophil.

10. Which of the following is considered a normal blood pressure in a healthy, resting adult?
   a. 120/80
   b. 140/100
   c. 160/80
   d. 180/100

10

The Lymphatic and Immune System

Introduction

To understand the importance of a system it sometimes helps to try to imagine your body without it. Imagine what would happen to you if your body could not return excess fluid to the bloodstream. Or if your body had no means of transporting fats and fat-soluble vitamins. Or if you could not defend yourself against invasion from disease. These are sobering thoughts.

Although the lymphatic and immune system often appears to be simple, it is of the utmost importance to the health and maintenance of our bodies. In this chapter you will discover more about this system and how it works closely with the cardiovascular system to maintain your health.

Student objectives

By the end of this chapter you will be able to:

- Describe the functions of the lymphatic and immune system
- Explain the organization of the lymphatic and immune system
- Identify the location of major lymphatic vessels, nodes, and organs
- Describe the organs of the lymphatic and immune system
- Explain non-specific resistance to disease and immunity.

Functions of the Lymphatic and Immune System

At first glance, the lymphatic system does not seem as impressive as some of the other systems of the body. It first appears as a simple system that transports a clear, straw-colored fluid from the interstitial spaces surrounding cells to the blood. However, on closer examination you see that this system does so much

more: it drains interstitial fluid to prevent tissues from becoming waterlogged, transports dietary lipids, and protects the body against invasion.

Before we look at the lymphatic system, it is a good idea to ensure you understand the following vocabulary (some of which you may have encountered already):

Antibody	A specialized protein that is synthesized to destroy a specific antigen
Antigen	Any substance that the body recognizes as foreign
Lymphocyte	A type of white blood cell involved in immunity; B cells and T cells are types of lymphocytes
Macrophage	A scavenger cell that engulfs and destroys microbes
Microbe (microorganism)	An organism that is too small to be seen by the eye; microbes include bacteria, viruses, protozoa, and some fungi
Pathogen	A disease-causing microorganism
Phagocyte	A cell that is able to engulf and digest microbes; phagocytes include macrophages and some types of white blood cells

Drainage of interstitial fluid

Every cell is bathed in a dilute saline solution called interstitial fluid. Every day, approximately 44 pints (21 liters) of blood plasma and its components—such as protein particles, fat molecules, and debris—leak out of blood vessels and into the interstitial fluid. Most of this is reabsorbed back into the bloodstream; however, about 6³⁄₁₀ pints (3 liters) is not reabsorbed. If this fluid is not somehow returned to the bloodstream then the tissues will become waterlogged and blood volume will fall. The lymphatic system plays a vital role in draining this excess fluid and returning it to the bloodstream.

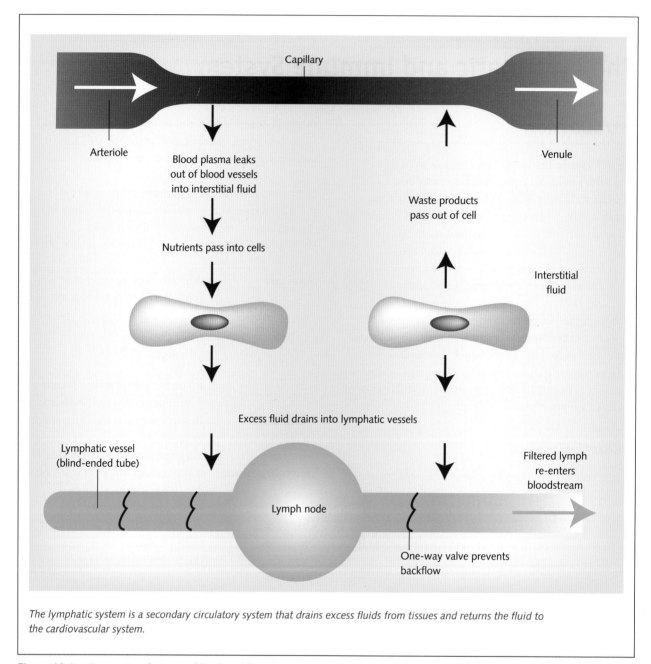

The lymphatic system is a secondary circulatory system that drains excess fluids from tissues and returns the fluid to the cardiovascular system.

Figure 10.1 *Connection between blood and lymph*

Transportation of dietary lipids

Located in the lining of the small intestine are fingerlike projections called **villi**. Inside each of these villi are blood capillaries and specialized lymphatic vessels called **lacteals**. Lacteals absorb lipids and lipid-soluble vitamins (vitamins A, D, E, and K) and transport these substances into larger lymphatic vessels, which finally deposit their contents into the bloodstream. The fluid inside the lacteals is a creamy white color due to its fat content and is called **chyle**.

Protection against invasion: The immune response

In addition to the lymphatic vessels that drain interstitial fluid and transport lipids, the lymphatic system also contains specialized tissues and organs that are involved in protecting the body against invasion. Phagocytic cells and lymphocytes are located in these organs and they function in defending the body through what is known as the immune response.

A closer look at white blood cells

Throughout this chapter you will hear about macrophages, phagocytes, lymphocytes, B cells, and T cells. So let's get a basic understanding of what these are.

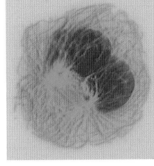

Macrophage

White blood cells (**leucocytes**) are pale, colorless cells that are derived from stem cells in red bone marrow. Although they are called "blood" cells, they circulate in both blood and lymph and they are the body's police, army, and general cleaners.

Every single cell in the body has its own "identification papers": a specific arrangement of protein molecules on the surface of its plasma membrane. If its identification papers are faulty, or if it is recognized as being foreign to the body, it is called an **antigen** and is destroyed as quickly as possible by the body's white blood cells. These white blood cells include **feeding cells** and **lymphocytes**.

Feeding cells

Feeding cells are the general cleaners of the body and they clean up old, dead, or foreign material, including bacteria, dust particles, and even dead cells of the body. Feeding cells are often found in connective tissue, organs such as the spleen and liver, and lymphoid tissue, and they flock in their thousands to sites of injury.

Once a feeding cell comes into contact with an attacker, cytoplasmic projections extend toward the attacker like multiple hands and pull it inward. Then the feeding cell engulfs the attacker, isolates it in an internal cavity and empties enzymes on to it that break the attacker down. Thus, they literally "eat" their prey through a process called **phagocytosis**.

Macrophages, granulocytes, and **monocytes** are all types of feeding cells.

Lymphocytes

Lymphocytes are the trained army personnel of the body. They do not eat their attackers; instead, they kill them with **antibodies** or poison, and in order to do this they first need to be trained, or made "immune competent." After being born in bone marrow, lymphocytes migrate to either lymphoid tissue or the thymus. These are the body's "military training academies," and it is here that lymphocytes specialize and mature.

- **Lymphoid tissue:** Lymphocytes that have migrated to the lymphoid tissue and lymph nodes learn to react to antigens and develop receptors on their surfaces that bind to specific antigens. These lymphocytes are now called **B cells** and every B cell is able to bind to only one specific antigen. B cells circulate in blood or lie in wait in lymph nodes, and when they come across their specific enemy antigen, they bind to it. In the process of binding to the antigen, a signal is transmitted to the nucleus of the B cell, which then divides the cell into many new clones called **plasma cells**. It is these plasma cells that then manufacture antibodies, which bind to the antigen and stop it from penetrating body cells and causing disease.
  - **Complement system:** Special molecules in the blood act as "dynamite" to help antibodies destroy their enemies. These molecules are called **complement factors** and when an antibody binds to an antigen the complement factors flock to the site of battle. Once all the complement factors have arrived, they perforate the membrane of the enemy cell
- **Thymus:** Those lymphocytes that have migrated to the thymus become trained in killing foreign cells and are called **T cells**. Unlike B cells, T cells do not produce antibodies that attack their enemy. Instead, they attack the enemy directly. T cells include:
  - **Helper cells:** Helper cells help B cells and feeding cells
  - **Killer cells:** Killer cells kill the body's own cells that have been invaded by antigens, and also kill tumor cells in the body
  - **Suppressor cells:** Suppressor cells suppress the aggression of some lymphocytes

Now that you have a basic understanding of the battleground within your body, it is time to get back to the lymphatic system.

Organization of the Lymphatic and Immune System

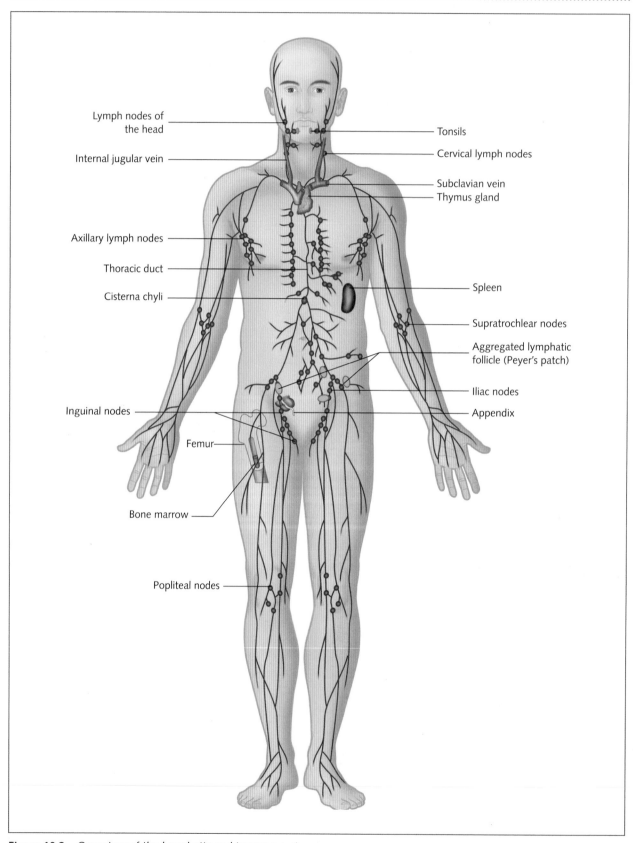

Figure 10.2 *Overview of the lymphatic and immune system*

The lymphatic system consists of:

- Lymph
- Lymphatic capillaries
- Lymphatic vessels, trunks, and ducts
- Lymph nodes (glands)
- Lymphatic organs
- Lymphatic nodules (mucosa-associated lymphoid tissue).

Lymph

The word *lymph* means "clear water" and, as mentioned earlier, lymph is a clear, straw-colored fluid derived from interstitial fluid. It is similar in composition to blood plasma and contains:

- **Protein molecules** that are too large to return to the blood circulation via the capillaries
- **Lipid molecules** that have been absorbed through lacteals located in the lining of the small intestine
- **Foreign particles** such as bacteria that can cause disease
- **Cell debris** from damaged tissues

- **Lymphocytes**, which are a type of white blood cell that functions in the immune response.

Lymph is only found in lymphatic vessels.

Lymphatic capillaries

Lymphatic capillaries are tiny, closed-ended vessels similar to blood capillaries. However, they have a larger diameter than blood capillaries and a unique structure that permits fluid to flow into them but not out of them. Lymphatic capillaries are found throughout the body except in avascular tissue, the central nervous system, splenic pulp (to be discussed shortly), and bone marrow. Interstitial fluid is absorbed into lymphatic capillaries. Once inside the capillaries the fluid is called lymph and it is transported by the tiny lymphatic capillaries into larger vessels called lymphatic vessels.

Lymphatic vessels

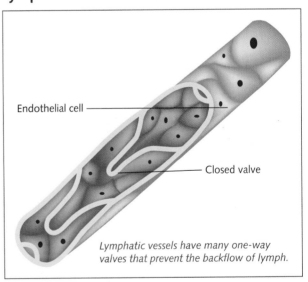

Lymphatic vessels have many one-way valves that prevent the backflow of lymph.

Figure 10.4 *A lymphatic vessel*

Lymphatic vessels and trunks

Lymphatic vessels carry lymph from the capillaries through a number of lymph nodes and into large vessels called lymphatic trunks. These trunks are named after the areas they serve and are the:

- Lumbar trunk
- Intestinal trunk
- Right and left bronchomediastinal trunks
- Right and left subclavian trunks
- Right and left jugular trunks.

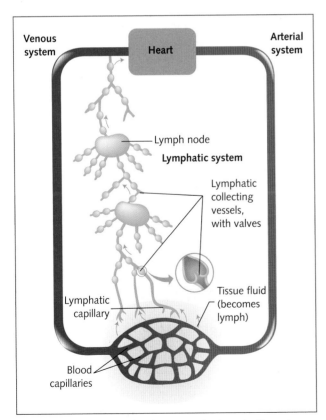

Figure 10.3 *Relationship between the lymphatic and cardiovascular systems*

Lymphatic ducts

The lymphatic trunks carry lymph into two main channels: the **thoracic duct** (**left lymphatic duct**) and the **right lymphatic duct**. These eventually empty their contents into the left and right subclavian veins, respectively.

- **Thoracic duct:** The thoracic duct, or left lymphatic duct, is the main collecting duct of the lymphatic system. It originates near the second lumbar vertebra at a dilation called the **cisterna chyli**, and receives lymph from:
  - The left side of the head, neck and chest
  - The left arm
  - The entire body below the ribs
- **Right lymphatic duct:** The right lymphatic duct receives lymph from only the upper right side of the body.

Movement of lymph through the lymphatic vessels

Unlike blood, which is pumped around the body by the heart, lymph has no pump to move it through its vessels. Instead, certain mechanisms combine to ensure the flow of lymph:

- **Smooth muscle** found in the walls of lymphatic vessels contracts rhythmically to move lymph
- **Skeletal muscles** contract to create a milking action
- **Breathing movements** cause pressure changes in the thoracic cavity
- **One-way valves** prevent the backflow of lymph in the vessels.

> ### Study tip
> ....
>
> Compare the movement of lymph through lymphatic vessels to the movement of venous blood through veins. You will see that they are moved by similar mechanisms.

> ### Did you know?
> ....
>
> Snake venom is transported through the lymphatic system of the body. That is why it is recommended to keep the affected limb as still as possible and apply a pressure bandage in order to slow the movement of lymph.

Lymph nodes (glands)

As lymph travels through the vessels toward the lymphatic ducts, it passes through a number of nodes, or glands, before it is returned to the bloodstream. The function of these nodes is to filter the lymph and remove or destroy any potentially harmful substances before the lymph is returned to the blood.

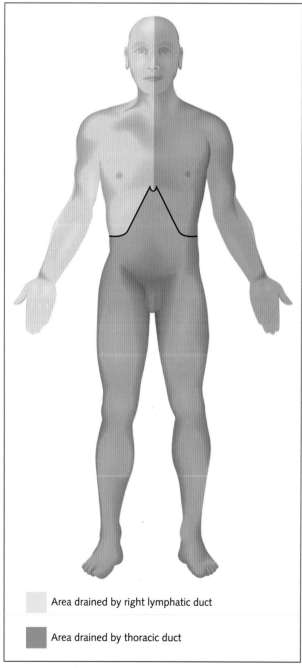

Area drained by right lymphatic duct

Area drained by thoracic duct

Figure 10.5 *Areas drained by the lymphatic ducts*

They also produce lymphocytes that function in the immune response.

Location of lymph nodes

Lymph nodes are scattered along the length of the lymphatic vessels, with higher concentrations of them being strategically placed in sites where there is a greater risk of infection. There are many concentrations of nodes, and a few of the primary ones are listed in the chart following.

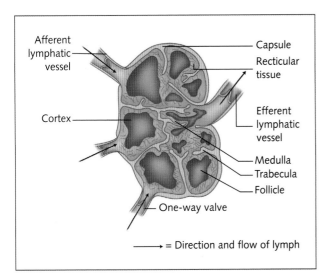

Figure 10.6 *Cross-section of a lymph node*

PRIMARY LYMPH NODES	
Name	**Location**
Lymph nodes of the head and neck	
Superficial parotid nodes (anterior auricular)	In front of ears
Mastoid nodes (posterior auricular)	Behind ears
Submandibular nodes	Beneath mandible
Submental nodes	Beneath chin
Occipital nodes	Base of skull
Deep cervical nodes	Deep within neck
Superficial cervical nodes (includes medial and lateral nodes)	Side of neck
Lymph nodes of the body	
Axillary nodes	Armpit
Supratrochlear nodes	Elbow crease

PRIMARY LYMPH NODES	
Name	**Location**
Ileocolic nodes	Abdomen (near the diaphragm)
Iliac nodes	Abdomen
Inguinal nodes	Groin
Popliteal nodes	Knee

Structure of lymph nodes

Lymph nodes are oval-shaped and vary in size from $\frac{1}{32}$ to 1 in (1 to 25 mm). They are specially structured to allow lymph to flow slowly through them and be filtered of potentially harmful particles and substances.

- Lymph nodes are enclosed in a capsule of dense connective tissue from which strands extend into the node. These strands are called **trabeculae** and they divide the node into compartments. The trabeculae combine together with a network of reticular fibers and fibroblasts to form a framework that supports the continually changing lymphatic tissue within it.
- The lymphatic tissue that makes up lymph nodes consists of:
  - An outer **cortex** of lymphocytes that are arranged into structures called **follicles** The outer rim of these follicles is composed of T cells and macrophages, while in the central areas B cells produce antibody-secreting plasma cells
  - An inner **medulla** of lymphocytes, macrophages, and plasma cells

Lymph can flow in only one direction: from the capillaries toward the ducts. This means that it also only flows through lymph nodes in one direction. The vessels that bring lymph into the nodes are called **afferent vessels** and the vessels that take lymph away from the nodes are called **efferent vessels**.

Lymph flows very slowly through the nodes and as it flows any foreign particles or substances in it are trapped by the reticular fibers of the nodes. Macrophages, antibodies, and lymphocytes then all work to protect the body against these foreign substances. How they do this will be discussed shortly, under the heading "Immunity (the immune response)."

Lymphatic organs

Lymphatic tissue, or lymphoid tissue, plays an essential role in protecting the body from invaders and is responsible for the production of lymphocytes and antibodies.

Thymus gland

The thymus gland is located in the mediastinum, behind the sternum and between the lungs. Not all the functions of the thymus gland are yet known; however, it is known that the gland

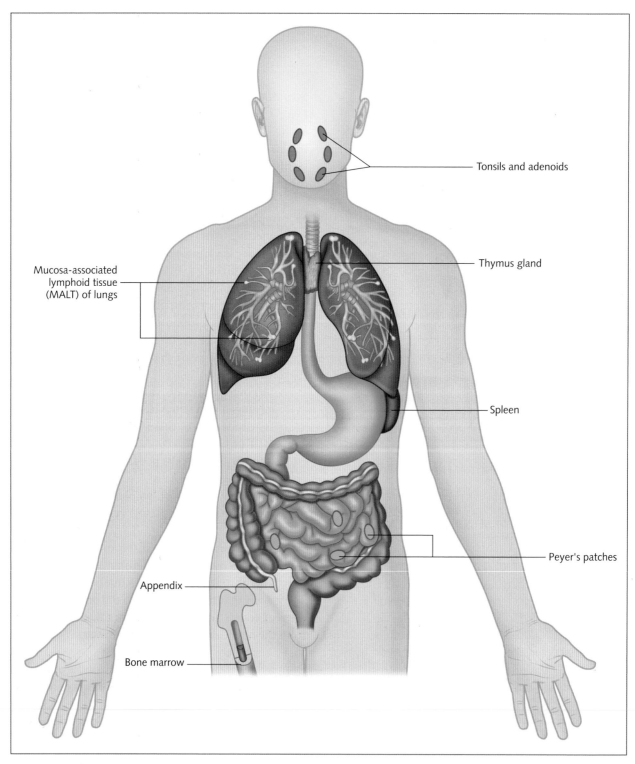

Figure 10.7 *Lymphatic organs and nodules*

produces hormones such as thymosin that help the development and maturation of T cells.

Spleen

The spleen is the largest single mass of lymphatic tissue in the body. It is located in the abdomen, behind and to the left of the stomach. Although it is an organ of the lymphatic system, it is important to remember that the spleen does not filter lymph. Instead, it filters and stores blood. Functions of the spleen include:

- Filtering and cleaning blood
- Destroying old, worn-out red blood cells
- Storing platelets and blood
- Producing lymphocytes.

Similar to lymph nodes, the spleen is enclosed in a dense connective tissue from which trabeculae extend, and, together with reticular fibers and fibroblasts, these trabeculae form the framework of the spleen. The functional part of the spleen consists of two different tissues:

- **White pulp**, which functions in immunity and is the site of antibody-producing plasma cells
- **Red pulp**, which functions in the phagocytosis of bacteria, red blood cells, and platelets.

Lymphatic nodules (mucosa-associated lymphoid tissue)

Lymphatic nodules, or mucosa-associated lymphoid tissue (MALT), are concentrations of lymphatic tissue that are strategically positioned to help protect the body from pathogens that have been inhaled or digested or have entered the body via external openings. Thus, they are scattered throughout the mucous membranes that line systems exposed to the external environment. These include the:

- Gastrointestinal tract
- Respiratory airways
- Urinary tract
- Reproductive tract.

Specific groups of lymphatic nodules include the:

- **Tonsils:** These lie at the back of the mouth and help protect the body against pathogens that may have been inhaled or digested.

- **Peyer's patches:** These are found in the ileum of the small intestine and help protect the body against pathogens that have been digested.
- **Appendix:** This is located at the end of the cecum. Its function is not yet known.

Did you know?

The thymus gland is at its largest in a 10–12-year-old child. Once a child reaches puberty the gland begins to atrophy and thymic tissue is replaced by adipose and areolar tissue.

Did you know?

If damaged, the spleen can be removed and most of its functions can be taken over by other structures, such as the liver and red bone marrow.

Fluid flow through the body in a nutshell

Arteries
Blood plasma

⇓

Blood capillaries
Blood plasma

⇓

Interstitial spaces
Interstitial fluid

⇓

Lymphatic capillaries
Lymph

⇓

Lymphatic vessels
Lymph

⇓

Lymphatic ducts
Lymph

⇓

Subclavian veins
Blood plasma

Resistance to Disease and Immunity

Our bodies are constantly at war, fighting off pathogens trying to invade them from all directions. Bacterial attack, fungal attack, viral attack, chemical attack … and so the list continues. The body employs two approaches to defend itself against this multitude of invaders:

- Firstly, the body has a number of defense mechanisms that immediately provide general protection against a variety of invaders. This approach is known as **non-specific resistance to disease.**
- Secondly, the body employs specialized lymphocytes that recognize and combat specific pathogens. This is called the **immune response,** or **immunity.**

Non-specific resistance to disease

The body has a number of different defense mechanisms that are in place to firstly ward off invading microbes and secondly help the body deal with any microbes that actually enter into the system. These mechanisms include:

- Mechanical and chemical barriers
- Natural killer cells and phagocytes
- Inflammation
- Fever.

Mechanical and chemical barriers

The body's first line of resistance to invaders is its mechanical and chemical barriers.

Mechanical barriers include:

- **The skin:** The skin's many layers of tough cells provide a strong barrier against invading microbes. The top layer of the skin is also shed regularly and this helps remove any microbes that are on the surface of the skin.
- **Mucous membranes:** These trap microbes and also contain hairs or cilia that move microbes and dust away from vital areas.
- **Lacrimal apparatus:** This produces tears that wash away microbes and dirt.
- **Saliva:** This washes away microbes and dirt from the mouth.

- The processes of **urination, defecation,** and **vomiting:** All of these expel invaders from the body.

Chemical barriers include:

- **Sebum:** This acts as a protective film over the skin and helps inhibit the growth of many bacteria and fungi.
- **Perspiration:** This helps wash microbes off the surface of the skin and contains an antibacterial substance called **lysozyme** (discussed shortly).
- **Gastric juice:** This contains hydrochloric acid, which destroys most ingested microbes.
- **Vaginal secretions:** These secretions' acidity discourages bacterial growth.

Also included in chemical barriers are **antimicrobial substances,** which destroy microbes. Examples of these include:

- **Lysozyme:** This is an enzyme found in certain body secretions, such as tears and saliva. It catalyzes the breakdown of the cell walls of certain bacteria.
- **Interferons:** These are substances produced to protect uninfected cells from viral infection.
- **Complement system:** This comprises a group of proteins in blood plasma and on plasma membranes. These proteins are usually inactive, but are activated when antigens and antibodies combine to form an immune complex. When activated, these proteins enhance, or "complement," some immune, allergic, and inflammatory processes.

Natural killer cells and phagocytes

If microbes still manage to enter the body, they then face the body's second line of defense: natural killer cells and phagocytes.

- **Natural killer cells (NK cells):** Natural killer cells are a type of lymphocyte that can kill a variety of microbes as well as some tumor cells. It is not yet known exactly how they recognize or destroy their targets, yet they are found in the spleen, lymph nodes, red bone marrow, and blood.
- **Phagocytes:** The name "phagocyte" literally means "eating cell," and phagocytes are a type

of lymphocyte that ingests microbes and foreign matter. There are two main types of phagocyte:

- **Neutrophils:** These white blood cells were discussed in chapter 9
- **Macrophages:** Macrophages are scavenging cells that develop from monocytes (a type of white blood cell). Wandering macrophages are mobile, while fixed macrophages are found in the skin, liver, lungs, nervous system, spleen, lymph nodes, and red bone marrow

Inflammation

Despite its formidable defense system, the body can still be injured. If tissue cells are damaged through cuts, burns, or microbial invasion, the body responds through a process called **inflammation**. This is the body's response to injury and is a defensive reaction whose purpose is to help prevent the spread of further damage, to prepare the site for repair, and to help clear the area of microbes and toxins.

Inflammation has four key signs and symptoms:

- Swelling
- Heat
- Redness
- Pain.

Occasionally, loss of function of the affected area can be a fifth sign. Inflammation is a long process, which occurs as follows:

- **Vasodilation and increased permeability of blood vessels:** Immediately after the tissue has been damaged, blood vessels vasodilate and become more permeable. This is partly caused by the release of **histamine**, a chemical present in most tissues. Vasodilation results in more blood flowing to the damaged area and more defensive materials—such as antibodies, phagocytes, and clot-forming chemicals—leaving the blood and entering the injured site. This flow of blood to the area causes the swelling, heat, and redness of inflammation. The pain that usually accompanies inflammation is caused by either injury or irritation to nerve fibers. It can also result from increased pressure caused by the swelling.
- **Phagocyte migration and tissue repair:** About an hour after the inflammatory process has begun, large numbers of phagocytes leave the bloodstream and enter the injured site. Neutrophils are the first

type of phagocyte to appear. They engulf microbes and foreign materials but soon exhaust themselves and rapidly die off. They are then followed by wandering macrophages, which engulf the damaged tissue, invading microbes, and worn-out neutrophils. As the tissue repairs, pus forms. This is a collection of dead cells and fluid. Pus formation continues until the infection has subsided.

Fever

A fever is an abnormally high temperature and it is the body's way of dealing with infection. Toxins released by microbes can increase the body's temperature, and this increase in temperature intensifies the effects of the body's own antimicrobial substances, inhibits microbial growth, and increases the speed of tissue repair.

Infobox

Anatomy and physiology in perspective

Have you ever wondered how pain and fever medications such as aspirin, diclofenac, or ibuprofen work? These drugs are classified as non-steroidal anti-inflammatory drugs (NSAIDs), and prevent the formation of two important molecules: prostaglandins and thromboxane. Almost every tissue in the body responds to prostaglandins, which are lipids that play a role in the formation of pain, fever, and inflammation in the body, while thromboxane is necessary for blood clotting and vasoconstriction. If the formation of both of these is inhibited then you can understand how NSAIDs help reduce pain, inflammation, and fever.

Immunity (the immune response)

There are two key differences between immunity and non-specific resistance to disease. Firstly, immunity involves a very specific and focused recognition and response to foreign molecules. Secondly, immunity involves memory.

Recognition of and response to foreign molecules

Immunocompetent cells

Any substance that the body recognizes as foreign and that provokes a response from the immune system is called an antigen.

The body's lymphocytes that are responsible for responding to antigens are referred to as immunocompetent cells, and there are two types:

- **B cells:** These develop and mature in red bone marrow throughout life. They develop into plasma cells and are able to synthesize and secrete antibodies.
- **T cells:** These develop in red bone marrow and then migrate to the thymus gland, where they mature. Two types of T cells exist: **CD4+ cells** and **CD8+ cells.** Before T cells are released into the system, they acquire distinctive surface proteins that are capable of recognizing specific antigens and are called **antigen receptors.**

B cells and T cells respond differently to pathogens. B cells secrete antibodies, while T cells develop antigen receptors. We will now look at how these cells function in the immune response.

Types of immune responses

There are two types of immune responses and pathogens can provoke either one type of response, or both types at the same time.

Cell-mediated (cellular) immune responses (CMI responses): In cell-mediated immune responses, cells attack antigens directly. CD8+ T cells reproduce into "killer cells," which leave lymphatic tissues to seek out and destroy antigens. This is the most common response to intracellular pathogens such as fungi, parasites, and viruses, as well as some cancer cells and tissue or organ transplants.

Remember:
In **cell**-mediated responses, **cells** attack cells.

Antibody-mediated (humoral) immune responses (AMI responses): In antibody-mediated immune responses, antibodies bind to antigens and inactivate them. B cells develop into plasma cells, which secrete antibodies. Antibodies then leave the lymphatic tissue to circulate in the blood and lymph and bind to the particular antigen for which they were made. Once bound to this antigen they destroy it. This response is more common against antigens that are dissolved in body fluids and pathogens such as bacteria that have multiplied in body fluids.

Remember:
In **antibody**-mediated responses, **antibodies** attack cells.

If CD8+ T cells develop into killer cells and B cells develop into antibody-secreting plasma cells, then you may be wondering what CD4+ T cells do. They become "helper" T cells that aid both CMI and AMI responses.

Immunological memory (acquired immunity)

Immunity involves immunological memory. This is the body's ability to remember and recognize antigens that have previously triggered an immune response. Some antibodies and lymphocytes can live for many years, even decades, and are the memory cells of the immune system. The immune system's initial response to antigens, called the **primary response**, is slow, and it can take several days before antibodies are detected in blood serum.

These antibodies also gradually decline unless there is another encounter with the same antigen. If the same antigen is encountered again, a **secondary response** occurs. This is a quicker, more intense response in which the body recognizes and remembers the antigen and so quickly produces more antibodies. Secondary responses can be so quick and successful that you may not even be aware of them.

Immunity can be acquired naturally or artificially, as well as actively or passively, as detailed in the chart following.

TYPES OF IMMUNITY	
Type of immunity	**How is it acquired?**
Naturally acquired immunity	
Naturally acquired active immunity	The body is stimulated to produce its own antibodies through actively having the disease
Naturally acquired passive immunity	This is the transference of antibodies from mother to fetus across the placenta or from mother to baby through breastfeeding
Artificially acquired immunity	
Artificially acquired active immunity	Antigens are introduced to the body in the form of vaccinations that induce an active immune response but do not make the recipient ill
Artificially acquired passive immunity	Ready-made antibodies are injected into the recipient

Infobox

Anatomy and physiology in perspective

Vaccinations (immunizations) are based on the principle of immunological memory. Vaccinations are pretreated to be immunogenic but not pathogenic. This means that they can activate a primary response in a person, while not causing the person to become significantly ill. Thus, when the person next encounters the antigen, there is immediately a secondary response to it.

Common Pathologies of the Lymphatic and Immune System

Red flags

- **Chronic fever** of unknown origin
- **Recurring fever** accompanied by night sweats and weight loss
- **Anaphylaxis** is a severe allergic reaction that requires immediate attention; below is a list of possible signs and symptoms, but please note a person will not necessarily have all of them at the same time:
  - Wheezing, difficult or noisy breathing
  - Swelling and/or tightness of the throat
  - Swelling of the tongue and difficulty talking or swallowing
  - Anxiety
  - Dizziness, faintness, or collapse due to low blood pressure
  - Sweating or flushing
  - Diarrhea or abdominal pain
  - Loss of consciousness

Allergy (hypersensitivity)

Overreaction to a substance that is normally harmless to most people. Any substance that invokes an allergic reaction is called an **allergen**, and foods such as milk, peanuts, shellfish, and eggs are common allergens, as are some antibiotics, vitamins,

Infobox

Anatomy and physiology in perspective

Histamine is a chemical messenger that plays a major role in allergies. Its many functions include:

- Contraction of smooth muscle fibers in the lungs and gastrointestinal tract causing bronchoconstriction and intestinal cramping
- Vasodilation, increased permeability, and increased protein leakage of blood vessels, resulting in low blood pressure, swelling, itching, and redness (inflammation).

Antihistamines are a class of drugs that block histamine receptors throughout the body and so control an allergic response. In addition to blocking histamine receptors, these drugs also block other receptors and can cross the blood–brain barrier. This is why many antihistamines have a sedative effect.

drugs, venoms, cosmetics, plant chemicals, pollens, dust, and molds.

Allergic reactions can only occur if a person has been previously exposed to the allergen and so developed antibodies to it. Symptoms of allergic reactions can range from a running nose and streaming eyes to anaphylactic shock, in which there is swelling, heart and lung failure, and possibly death.

Lymphadenitis

Inflammation or enlargement of one or more lymph nodes and usually caused by an infection. Infected lymph nodes swell and are tender and painful.

Lymphedema

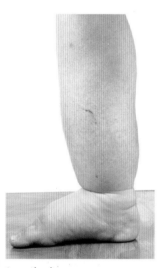

Accumulation of lymph in the tissues. It results in swelling and most often affects the legs. Lymphedema can be caused by a congenital defect in which there is a lack of lymphatic vessels, or it can be caused by surgery in which lymph nodes and vessels have been damaged or removed. Parasites, obstructing tumors, and injuries to the vessels are also known to cause lymphedema.

Lymphedema

In the classroom
....

Discuss the differences between edema (discussed in chapter 1) and lymphedema.

Cancer and the lymphatic and immune system

Cancer is the uncontrolled division of cells and it can develop within any tissue in the body. When cells become cancerous, the body can often recognize them as abnormal and so destroy them. However, if the immune system does not recognize the cells as cancerous, or is unable to destroy them, the cancerous cells can replicate to form a mass. This mass is called a tumor and is more difficult for the body to destroy.

Leukemia
Abnormal production of leucocytes. In other words, it is cancer of the white blood cells. Instead of forming a lump or tumor, leukemia cells remain as separate cancerous cells and crowd out healthy blood cells in the bloodstream. They also invade other organs such as the liver, spleen, and lymph nodes, and this results in an increased susceptibility to infection, bleeding, and anemia.

Lymphomas
Cancers of lymphocytes that can remain confined to a lymph node, spread to other lymphatic tissues such as the spleen or bone marrow, or spread to virtually any other organ in the body. The two main types of lymphoma are Hodgkin's disease and non-Hodgkin's lymphoma:

- **Hodgkin's disease (Hodgkin's lymphoma):** This is a malignant lymphoma characterized by the progressive, painless enlargement of the lymph nodes of the neck, armpits, groin, chest, or abdomen. Hodgkin's disease can sometimes be accompanied by fever, night sweats, weight loss, itching, and fatigue. The cause of Hodgkin's disease is unknown.
- **Non-Hodgkin's lymphoma:** This refers to a diverse group of lymphomas that are classified according to the type of cell involved and the degree of malignancy. They are found to be more common in elderly people and those whose immune systems are not functioning normally, and the main symptom is the painless enlargement of lymph nodes.

Metastasis
Although the function of the lymphatic system is to help protect the body from disease, it can sometimes be responsible for spreading diseases. An example of this is the **metastasis** of cancer. Cancer spreads from its origin to other sites via a process called metastasis, which occurs across body cavities, via the bloodstream, or via the lymphatic system.

Infectious diseases

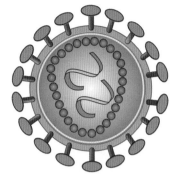

HIV virus

Acquired immunodeficiency syndrome (AIDS)

An unusual disorder in that the virus that causes it only lowers people's immunity and makes them more susceptible to other diseases. It is these other diseases that produce the fatal symptoms of AIDS.

AIDS is caused by the human immunodeficiency virus (HIV), and results in a lowered T4 lymphocyte count. Infected people then become susceptible to opportunistic infections, such as pneumonia or tuberculosis, which their immune system cannot fight. HIV is transmitted through bodily fluids such as blood, semen, vaginal secretions, and breast milk.

Glandular fever (infectious mononucleosis)

Contagious disease of the lymphatic system that results in large numbers of white blood cells in the bloodstream. It is caused by the Epstein-Barr virus and occurs mainly in children and young adults. It is often spread through kissing, and signs and symptoms include fatigue, headaches, dizziness, sore throat, enlarged and tender lymph nodes, and fever.

Tonsillitis

Inflammation of the tonsils. It can be caused by a virus or bacterium and is characterized by a sore throat, difficulty in swallowing, and fever.

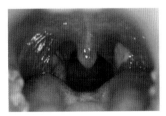

Tonsillitis

Autoimmune diseases and disorders

The role of the immune system is to attack foreign substances that have entered the body. Occasionally, however, the body does attack its own tissues. When this occurs a person is said to have an autoimmune disorder. Some autoimmune diseases and disorders that have already been discussed in other chapters of this book include rheumatoid arthritis, pernicious anemia, Addison's disease, Graves' disease, insulin-dependent (type 1) diabetes mellitus, myasthenia gravis, and multiple sclerosis. Systemic lupus erythematosus is also an autoimmune disease.

Systemic lupus erythematosus (SLE)

SLE or lupus is an autoimmune disease in which the body attacks its own connective tissue. Signs and symptoms vary but can include inflammation, painful joints, fever, fatigue, mouth ulcers, weight loss, hair loss, and an enlarged spleen. A "butterfly" rash across the nose and cheeks is common. The cause of lupus is unknown, but it affects young women more than any other group of people.

NEW WORDS	
Antibody	A specialized protein that is synthesized to destroy a specific antigen
Antigen	Any substance that the body recognizes as foreign
Inflammation	The body's response to tissue damage
Lymphocyte	A type of white blood cell involved in immunity; B cells and T cells are types of lymphocytes
Macrophage	A scavenger cell that engulfs and destroys microbes
Metastasis	The spread of cancer from its site of origin
Microbe (microorganism)	An organism that is too small to be seen by the naked eye; microbes include bacteria, viruses, protozoa, and some fungi
Pathogen	A disease-causing microorganism
Phagocyte	A cell that is able to engulf and digest microbes; phagocytes include macrophages and some types of white blood cells

Study Outline

Functions of the lymphatic system

Functions of the lymphatic system include drainage of interstitial fluid, transportation of dietary lipids, and protection against invasion.

Structure of the lymphatic system

1. Lymph is derived from interstitial fluid and is only found in lymphatic vessels. Lymph contains protein molecules, lipid molecules, foreign particles, cell debris, and lymphocytes.
2. Lymphatic capillaries are closed-ended vessels that permit fluid to flow into them but not out of them. They absorb lymph and transport it to lymphatic vessels.
3. Lymphatic vessels carry lymph from capillaries through nodes and into lymphatic trunks.
4. Lymphatic trunks empty lymph into the thoracic duct and the right lymphatic duct.
5. The thoracic duct drains lymph from the left side of the head, neck, and chest, as well as the left arm and the entire body below the ribs.
6. The right lymphatic duct drains lymph from the upper right side of the body only.
7. Lymph is moved through the lymphatic vessels by smooth muscle, skeletal muscle, and breathing movements. It is prevented from flowing backward by one-way valves.
8. Lymph flows through lymph nodes in only one direction. The vessels that bring lymph into the nodes are called afferent vessels and the vessels that take lymph away from the nodes are called efferent vessels.

Afferent = Arrive
Efferent = Exit

9. Lymph nodes filter lymph of potentially harmful substances and also produce lymphocytes.
10. Lymphatic organs include the thymus gland and the spleen.
11. The thymus gland produces hormones that help the development and maturation of T cells.
12. The spleen filters and cleans blood, destroys worn-out red blood cells, stores platelets and blood, and produces lymphocytes.

13. Lymphatic nodules (mucosa-associated lymphoid tissue) are strategically positioned to help protect the body from pathogens that have been inhaled or digested. They are found in mucous membranes lining body cavities.
14. Lymphatic nodules include the tonsils, Peyer's patches, and the appendix.

Resistance to disease and immunity

1. Defense mechanisms that give general protection against invaders are classified as non-specific mechanisms. These include mechanical and chemical barriers, natural killer cells and phagocytes, inflammation, and fever.
2. Defense mechanisms in which the body produces specific responses to particular organisms fall under the classification of immunity.
3. Immunity involves the body's ability to recognize microbes, respond to them appropriately, and remember them so that a secondary response will be quicker and more powerful.

Immunity

1. Immunocompetent cells include B cells and T cells.
2. B cells develop and mature in the red bone marrow and develop into plasma cells, which synthesize and secrete antibodies. B cells participate in antibody-mediated immune (AMI) responses.

B cells = anti**B**odies

3. In AMI responses, antibodies bind to antigens and destroy them.
4. T cells develop in red bone marrow and then migrate to the thymus gland where they mature. T cells participate in cell-mediated immune (CMI) responses.

T cells = **T**hymus

5. In CMI responses, killer cells attack and destroy antigens.
6. Acquired immunity is the body's ability to remember and recognize antigens that have previously caused an immune response.
   The primary response is slow while the secondary response is quick and more successful.

Review

1. Identify the functions of the immune system.
2. Compare blood plasma to lymph.
3. Compare blood capillaries to lymphatic capillaries.
4. Explain how lymph is moved through the lymphatic vessels.
5. Describe a lymph node.
6. Explain the function of Peyer's patches and describe where in the body they are found.
7. Explain the function of the thymus gland.
8. Explain the functions of the spleen.
9. Compare non-specific resistance to disease with immunity.
10. Explain how the body protects itself from general invasion.
11. Explain the inflammatory process.
12. Describe the immune response.

Multiple-Choice Questions

1. The axillary lymph nodes are located in the:
   a. Neck
   b. Shoulder
   c. Armpit
   d. Elbow

2. Which of the following statements is correct?
   a. After puberty the thymus gland begins to atrophy
   b. The thymus gland produces antibodies
   c. The thymus gland filters and stores blood
   d. The thymus continues to grow until old age

3. Lymphedema is:
   a. An accumulation of blood plasma in the tissues
   b. An accumulation of lymph in the tissues
   c. An accumulation of interstitial fluid in the lymphatic vessels
   d. None of the above

4. Where is the spleen located?
   a. Superior to the thymus
   b. Behind and to the left of the stomach
   c. Inferior to the large intestine
   d. In front of and to the right of the liver

5. Which of the following is not a lymph node of the pelvis and lower limbs?
   a. Popliteal
   b. Inguinal
   c. Iliac
   d. Supratrochlear

6. Where in the body are worn-out erythrocytes destroyed?
   a. Peyer's patches
   b. Appendix
   c. Axillary node
   d. Spleen

7. Which of the following is a function of the lymphatic system?
   a. Transportation of dietary lipids
   b. Transportation of hemoglobin molecules
   c. Transportation of carbon dioxide
   d. Transportation of bilirubin

8. Where in the body is mucosa-associated lymphoid tissue found?
   a. Liver
   b. Kidneys
   c. Urinary tract
   d. Ovaries

9. Where in the body do T cells mature?
   a. Liver
   b. Lungs
   c. Spleen
   d. Thymus

10. Bacteria, viruses, and fungi are all:
    a. Antibodies
    b. Lymphocytes
    c. Microbes
    d. Lacteals

The Digestive System

Introduction

An average person eats over 1,000 lb (approx. 454 kg) of food per year, and this food gets converted into energy that the body can use to move, breathe, function, and build and repair itself. Then the waste is excreted. This amazing transformation of food takes place in the gastrointestinal tract, a 25 feet (7.6 m) tube running from the mouth to the anus, and in this chapter we will follow the journey of our food through this tract.

Student objectives

By the end of this chapter you will be able to:

- Describe the functions of the digestive system
- Describe the organization of the gastrointestinal system
- Identify and describe the main organs and structures of digestion
- Explain the chemical breakdown of carbohydrates, proteins, and lipids
- Identify the common pathologies of the digestive system.

Functions of the Digestive System

The food we eat contains carbohydrates, fats, proteins, vitamins, and minerals—all essential nutrients for the life of every cell. However, none of these nutrients can be used by the body in the form in which they are eaten. They must be broken down into molecules that are small enough to cross the plasma membranes of cells. These foods also carry dangerous microbes and toxins that can harm our bodies and so they need to be prevented from passing into our cells. These are the primary functions of the digestive

Did you know?

Approximately 19 pints (9 liters) of fluid are secreted by the digestive system every day.

system: to break down the foods we eat and convert them into a usable form and to destroy or eliminate dangerous substances within them.

The functions of the digestive system can be broken down into the following six basic processes: **ingestion, secretion, mixing and propulsion, digestion, absorption,** and **defecation.**

Ingestion

Ingestion is the process of taking food into the mouth.

Secretion

Some organs and structures of the digestive system secrete mucus, water, acid, buffers, and enzymes. All of these secretions function in helping move and digest food.

Mixing and propulsion

The **gastrointestinal tract** is a tube that runs from the mouth to the anus and is where digestion and absorption take place. Food is mixed with digestive secretions and is propelled from the mouth to the anus.

Digestion

Digestion is the process by which large molecules of food are broken down into smaller molecules that can enter cells. Food is digested both mechanically and chemically:

- **Mechanical digestion:** In mechanical digestion, food is physically broken down and ground into smaller substances by the teeth, tongue, and physical movements such as peristalsis (to be discussed shortly). It is then mixed with fluids until it finally becomes a liquid. Once in a liquid state, it is easier for chemical digestion to take place.
- **Chemical digestion:** In chemical digestion, food molecules are broken down into smaller molecules by **enzymes.** The chart following outlines the breakdown of carbohydrates, fats, and proteins.

CHEMICAL DIGESTION OF CARBOHYDRATES, FATS, AND PROTEINS			
Nutrient	**Enzymes**	**From**	**To**
Carbohydrates	Amylases	Starches, polysaccharides, and disaccharides	Monosaccharides
Fats	Lipases	Triglycerides	Fatty acids and glycerol
Proteins	Proteases	Peptones and polypeptides	Amino acids

A closer look at enzymes

The digestion of food relies on the presence of enzymes. Enzymes are **catalysts**. They speed up reactions but do not actually become involved in the reactions themselves. Under optimal conditions, enzymes can increase the rates of reactions to up to 10 billion times faster than they would be without enzymes (Tortora and Derrickson, 2009).

Enzymes are very specific in what they catalyze and a particular enzyme can affect only a particular **substrate** (molecule on which the enzyme is acting). There are over a thousand known enzymes and each one of these has a specific three-dimensional shape with a uniquely shaped active site into which only its target substrate can fit. In other words, it can bond only to specific substrates that will fit its active site. In some cases, an enzyme's substrate is said to fit the enzyme like a key fits a lock; in other cases enzymes are said to surround the substrate.

Infobox

Anatomy and physiology in perspective

Scientists such as Emeran Mayer (2018) refer to the gut as the *second brain*. It has its own unique nervous system (the enteric nervous system, or ENS) containing as many nerve cells as there are in the spinal cord. There are more immune cells in the wall of the gut than in the bloodstream and bone marrow combined; it contains a huge number of endocrine cells, which release up to 20 different hormones; and it is the largest storage facility of serotonin in the body. No wonder what you eat affects your health and mood so much!

Organization of the Digestive System

Before studying the digestive system in detail, it will help you to have an overview of the basic structure and function of this system. As mentioned earlier, the digestive system is composed of a long tube that passes from the mouth to the anus. This is the gastrointestinal tract, or **alimentary canal**. This continuous tube forms the following organs and structures:

- Mouth
- Pharynx
- Esophagus
- Stomach
- Small intestine—composed of the duodenum, jejunum, and ileum
- Large intestine
- Anus.

In addition to the gastrointestinal tract, the digestive system includes accessory structures, which help

Absorption

Once the larger food molecules have been digested into smaller molecules, they enter the lining of the gastrointestinal tract by either active transport or passive diffusion (refer to chapter 2 to revise these processes). The molecules are absorbed into the bloodstream and lymphatic vessels and are then distributed to the rest of the body.

Defecation

Defecation is the process by which indigestible substances and some bacteria are eliminated from the body. They are eliminated as **feces** by the anus.

with the digestion of food. Most of them produce and/or store secretions that help with the chemical breakdown of food. These accessory structures are the:

- Teeth, tongue, and salivary glands—all located in the mouth
- Liver
- Gall bladder
- Pancreas.

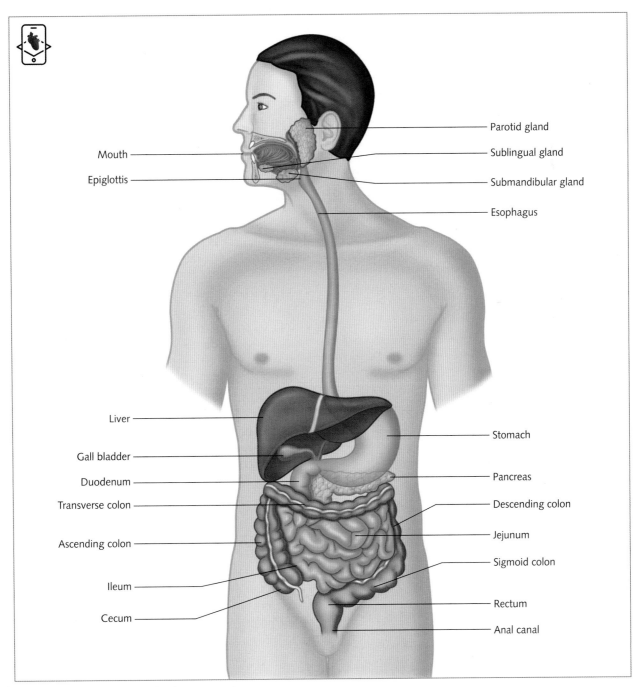

Figure 11.1 *Overview of the digestive system*

Wall of the gastrointestinal tract

The walls of the gastrointestinal tract (GI tract) are composed of four layers of tissue. This basic arrangement of tissue does differ slightly with some of the organs, but in general it is composed of the **mucosa**, **submucosa**, **muscularis**, and **serosa**.

- **Mucosa:** This is the deepest layer of the GI tract. Its inner lining is a **mucous membrane**, which functions in protection, secretion, and absorption. This mucous membrane is attached to the **lamina propria**, which is a loose connective tissue layer that supports the blood and lymphatic vessels into which digested molecules are absorbed. The lamina propria also contains mucosa-associated lymphoid tissue (MALT), which protects the body against the many microbes and toxins that may have been ingested. The third layer of the mucosa is the **muscularis mucosa**, which is a layer of smooth muscle.
- **Submucosa:** This is composed of areolar connective tissue and binds the mucosa to the muscularis layer. It contains many blood and lymphatic vessels and nerves, and houses the **submucosal (Meissner's) plexus**. This is a network of nerves that serves the smooth muscle cells of the mucosa and it forms part of the autonomic nervous system.

- **Muscularis:** This is a layer of muscle tissue. It includes some skeletal muscle tissue (especially in the mouth, pharynx, and upper portion of the esophagus, as these are the voluntary muscles of swallowing) and smooth muscle tissue. The smooth muscle tissue is composed of an inner sheet of circular fibers and an outer sheet of longitudinal fibers. These two sheets work together to physically break down and propel food along the GI tract. The muscularis also contains the **myenteric plexus (plexus of Auerbach)**. This is a major nerve supply to the GI tract.
- **Serosa:** This is the most superficial layer of the wall of the GI tract and it is a serous membrane. The esophageal portion of the serosa is called the **adventitia**, and it is composed of areolar connective tissue. The rest of the serosa is found below the diaphragm and is called the **visceral peritoneum**.

Peritoneum

The peritoneum is a large serous membrane lining the abdominal cavity. Like the pleural and pericardial serous membranes, the peritoneum has two layers:

- The **parietal peritoneum** lines the walls of the abdominopelvic cavity.
- The **visceral peritoneum** is also called the serosa, and it covers the organs of the digestive system. Between the two layers of the peritoneum is a space called the **peritoneal cavity**. This is filled with serous fluid.

However, unlike the pleural and pericardial serous membranes, which smoothly cover the lungs and heart, the peritoneum is composed of large folds. These folds weave between the organs, binding them to each other and to the walls of the abdominal cavity. These folds also contain many blood and lymphatic vessels and nerves, and include the:

- **Mesentery**, which binds the small intestine to the posterior abdominal wall
- **Mesocolon**, which binds the large intestine to the posterior abdominal wall
- **Falciform ligament**, which binds the liver to the anterior abdominal wall and diaphragm
- **Lesser omentum**, which links the stomach and duodenum with the liver

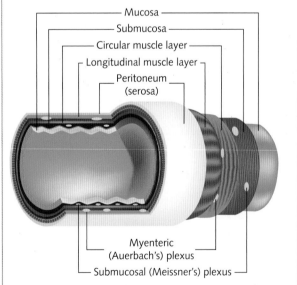

The wall of the gastrointestinal tract is composed of four layers: the inner mucosa lines the lumen of the tract, and layered on top of it are the submucosa, the muscularis, and the serosa.

Figure 11.2 *Structure of the wall of the gastrointestinal tract*

- **Greater omentum**, which covers the colon and small intestine.

Gastrointestinal Tract and Its Accessory Organs

The best way to learn the digestive system is to start by having something to eat. So go and get something to eat—make sure it includes carbohydrates, fats, and proteins! Now, let's follow the journey of your food.

Mouth (oral or buccal cavity)

Your food's journey begins in your mouth. You use your teeth to mechanically digest your food by biting and chewing it. Your tongue helps push the food around your mouth and also contains taste buds so that you can appreciate the food. Together with the sensation of the food in your mouth, your senses of taste, smell, and sight stimulate the release of saliva, which moistens the food in your mouth and begins the chemical breakdown of it.

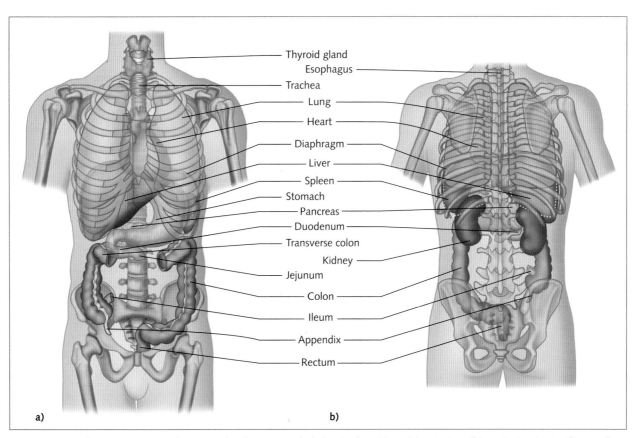

a)   b)

Figure 11.3 *The gastrointestinal tract in the thoracic and abdominal cavities, (a) anterior; (b) posterior (note: the small intestine and part of the transverse colon have been removed)*

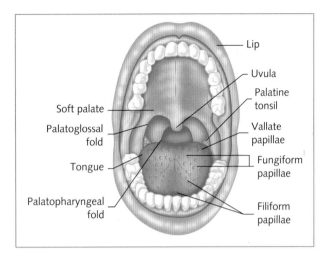

Figure 11.4 *Oral cavity*

Structure of the mouth

The mouth is a mucous-membrane-lined cavity formed by the cheeks, the hard and soft palates, and the tongue. The opening to the mouth is protected by the lips (**labia**). At the back of the mouth is a fingerlike projection hanging from the soft palate—this is called the **uvula** and, together with the soft palate, it closes off the nasopharynx during swallowing. Thus, food is directed into the esophagus rather than the respiratory tract.

The mouth includes the tongue, the teeth, and the salivary ducts and glands.

Tongue
- The tongue moves the food around the mouth.
- It is composed of skeletal muscle covered by a mucous membrane.
- It is attached to the hyoid bone, the styloid processes of the temporal bones, and the mandible, and is secured to the floor of the mouth by the **lingual frenulum**.

Infobox

Anatomy and physiology in perspective

Some babies are born "tongue-tied." This means that their frenulum is shorter than usual. If it is severe, the tongue-tie can easily be repaired by surgically cutting the frenulum.

- The tops and sides of the tongue are covered by small projections called **papillae**, and some of these papillae house the taste buds (for more information on the sense of taste, please refer to chapter 6).
- The surface of the tongue also contains glands that secrete the digestive enzyme **lingual lipase.** This enzyme begins the breakdown of fats.

Teeth (dentes)
- The teeth cut and chew food.
- They are composed of a calcified connective tissue called **dentine**, which encloses a cavity filled with **pulp.** Pulp is a connective tissue that contains blood and lymphatic vessels and nerves.
- They are located in sockets of the alveolar processes of the mandible and maxillae, and these sockets are covered with **gums** (**gingivae**) and lined by the **periodontal ligament**, which anchors the teeth in the gums and acts as a shock-absorber during chewing.
- Each tooth has three regions: a visible **crown**, one to three **roots** embedded in the socket, and a junction between the crown and roots called the **neck**.
- The dentine of the crown is covered by a layer of calcium phosphate and calcium carbonate. This is called **enamel**. Enamel is an extremely hard substance that protects the teeth from being worn down and also acts as a barrier against acids. The dentine of the root is covered by a substance called **cementum**. Cementum attaches the root to the periodontal ligament.
- In your life you have two sets of teeth. The first set is your **deciduous/primary/milk/baby teeth**. There are 20 in total and they start showing around the age of 6 months and then begin to fall out between 6 and 12 years. The second set is your **permanent/secondary teeth**. There are 32 in total.
- There are four types of teeth: **incisors** and **canines** are the sharp and pointed teeth used for cutting and biting, while **premolars** and **molars** are flatter, broader teeth used for grinding and chewing.

Salivary ducts and glands
- The salivary glands produce and secrete saliva.
- Saliva is an alkaline liquid that is continually secreted into the mouth. It helps keep the mouth moist, clean the mouth and teeth, lubricate food, and dissolve food molecules. It also contains an enzyme that begins the chemical digestion of

carbohydrates, and when it is swallowed it helps lubricate the esophagus. Saliva is:

- 99.5% water: Water acts as a dissolving medium
- 0.5% solutes: These solutes include ions, which buffer acidic foods; urea and uric acid, which help remove bodily wastes; mucus, which lubricates food; the chemical **lysozyme**, which helps destroy some bacteria; and the enzyme **salivary amylase**, which begins the breakdown of carbohydrates

- Saliva is secreted by the mucous membrane lining the mouth, the buccal glands, and the salivary glands. There are three pairs of salivary glands:
  - **The parotid glands:** These are located below and in front of the ear, near the masseter muscle. They secrete saliva into salivary ducts, which open into the mouth at the level of the second upper molar
  - **The submandibular glands:** These are located under the angle of the jaw and their ducts open into the mouth on either side of the lingual frenulum
  - **The sublingual glands:** These lie in front of the submandibular glands and have numerous ducts that open into the floor of the mouth

> ### Did you know?
>
> Enamel is the hardest substance in the body.

> ### Infobox
>
> #### Anatomy and physiology in perspective
>
> Mumps causes inflammation of the parotid salivary glands and because these glands are located near the masseter muscle it hurts to open the mouth or chew food when you have mumps.

> ### Did you know?
>
> Semi-solid food moves from the mouth to the stomach in approximately four to eight seconds, while very soft foods and liquids take only one second.

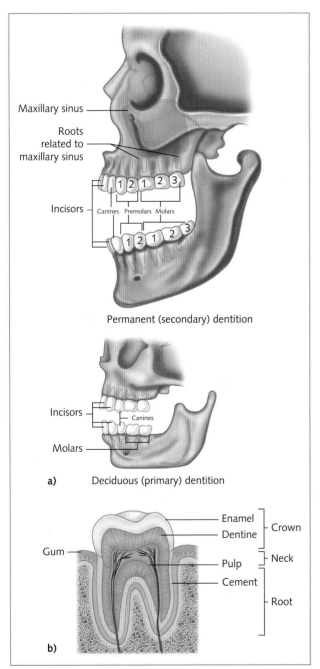

Figure 11.5 (a) The teeth of an adult and a child; (b) cross-section of a tooth

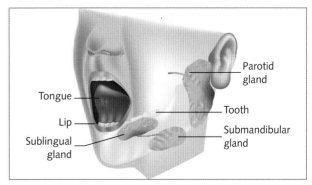

Figure 11.6 Salivary glands

DIGESTION IN THE MOUTH

Digestion/enzyme	Description
Mechanical digestion	
The mechanical digestion of food begins in the mouth	
Chewing (mastication)	The tongue moves food, the teeth grind it, and saliva mixes with the food and begins to dissolve it; finally, it is reduced to a soft, flexible mass called a **bolus**
Swallowing (deglutition)	Swallowing is the mechanical process by which the bolus is moved from the mouth into the stomach; it involves the mouth, pharynx, and esophagus: • The tongue forces the bolus to the back of the oral cavity and into the oropharynx • Breathing is then temporarily interrupted as the respiratory passages are closed by the upward movement of the soft palate and the uvula • As this movement occurs, the larynx comes forward and upward over the tongue and the epiglottis moves backward and downward, thus closing off the space between the vocal folds (**rima glottidis**) • This enables the bolus to pass through the laryngopharynx and into the esophagus without entering the respiratory tract • The entire process takes only 1–2 seconds and then the respiratory passage reopens and breathing continues as normal
Chemical digestion	
The digestion of both carbohydrates and lipids begins in the mouth. However, because the food is in the mouth for such a short time, the digestion of these continues in the stomach	
Salivary amylase (in saliva)	Salivary amylase begins the breakdown of large carbohydrate molecules such as starch or polysaccharides into disaccharides and then monosaccharides
Lingual lipase (secreted by glands on the tongue)	Lingual lipase begins the breakdown of fats (lipids) from triglycerides into fatty acids and glycerol

Esophagus

Having been swallowed, your food then travels down a long, collapsible tube running behind your trachea. This is your esophagus and it functions in transporting the bolus from the laryngopharynx to the stomach. No digestion takes place in the esophagus.

Structure and function of the esophagus

The esophagus is a muscular tube approximately 10 in (25 cm) long. It secretes mucus, which helps facilitate the movement of the bolus as it pushes it down toward the stomach through a process called **peristalsis**.

Peristalsis is a wave-like alternating contraction and relaxation of the involuntary circular and longitudinal fibers of the GI tract. The circular fibers above the bolus contract and constrict the walls of the tract. This squeezes the bolus downward.

Simultaneously, the longitudinal fibers of the tract beneath the bolus contract and shorten, pushing the walls of the tract outward and thus making room to receive the bolus.

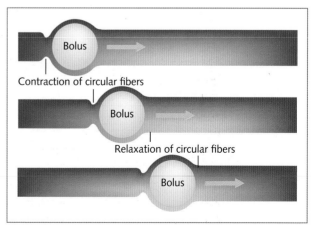

Figure 11.7 *Movement of a bolus through the gastrointestinal tract*

Stomach

Within seconds of biting into and chewing your food, it arrives in your stomach, where it accumulates in layers, the last bit you have eaten being layered on top of your previous mouthful. Once in your stomach, food is gradually churned and mixed with gastric juice, which contains a variety of substances that help digest it.

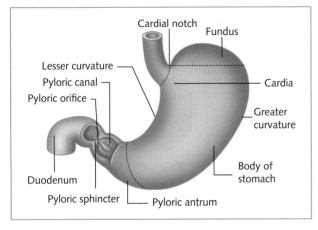

Figure 11.8   *Stomach and duodenum*

Structure of the stomach

The stomach is a J-shaped organ that is continuous with the GI tract. It lies below the diaphragm and in the left-hand side of the abdominal cavity, and is connected to the esophagus above it by the **cardiac** (**cardio-esophageal**) **sphincter** muscle and to the duodenum below it by the **pyloric sphincter** muscle. Because food is eaten more quickly than it can be digested, the stomach is specially structured to act as a mixing area and holding reservoir for food. The stomach can be divided into four regions:

- The **cardia** surrounds the superior opening to the stomach and receives food from the esophagus.
- The **fundus** is an expanded area to the side of the cardia where food can be held for up to one hour before it comes into contact with gastric juices.
- The **body** is the large, central mid-portion of the stomach.
- The **pylorus** is the area closest to the duodenum.

The stomach has an exceptional ability to stretch and when full it can hold up to 1 gallon (4 liters) of contents. When fully stretched, its walls are smooth; however, when empty, the stomach shrinks to about the size of a large sausage and its mucous membrane is thrown into large folds called **rugae.** The walls of the stomach have a similar arrangement of tissue to the rest of the GI tract. However, there are two differences:

- The inner lining of the mucosa is dotted with deep **gastric pits**, which are narrow channels containing gastric glands that secrete gastric juice.

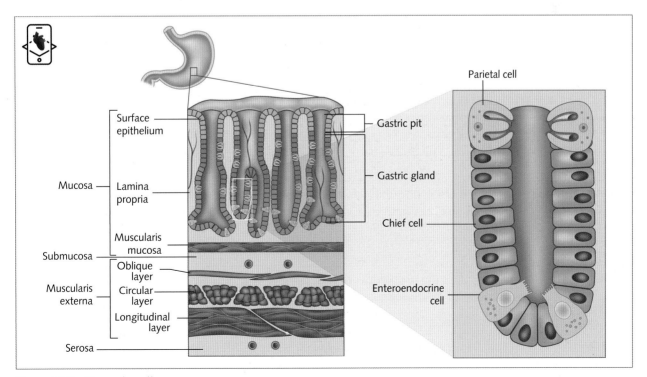

Figure 11.9   *Stomach wall*

Many different cells are also present in the mucosa that secrete a number of different digestive substances, which will be discussed shortly.

- The muscularis includes a third layer of involuntary muscle that is composed of obliquely arranged fibers. This enables the stomach to mix, pummel, and churn its contents and so reduce them to a liquid.

> **Did you know?**
>
> It takes approximately four hours for the stomach to be emptied after a meal, and if the meal had a very high fat content, then it can take up to six hours before the stomach is properly emptied.

DIGESTION IN THE STOMACH

Digestion/enzyme	Description
Mechanical digestion	
In the stomach food is mixed, pummeled, and churned into a thin liquid called **chyme**	
Mixing waves	Every 15–25 seconds a mixing wave passes over the stomach, pushing its contents backward and forward and compressing and pummeling it into a liquid state
Chyme is "squirted" into the duodenum	The pyloric sphincter muscle between the stomach and duodenum is never completely closed, and as the stomach contents are pushed against the muscle, small amounts of chyme (approximately 3 ml) are forced or squirted out of the stomach and into the duodenum
	The remaining contents continue to be mixed and churned until the next wave forces a little more chyme into the duodenum
Chemical digestion	
In the presence of food, endocrine cells in the walls of the stomach secrete the hormone **gastrin**, which stimulates the production of gastric juice. Gastric juice is secreted by gastric glands and contains: • **Water**—liquefies the food • **Hydrochloric acid** (HCl)—kills microbes that have been ingested, partially denatures proteins, stimulates the secretion of hormones that promote the flow of bile and pancreatic juice, stops the action of salivary amylase and lingual lipase, and is needed for the conversion of pepsinogen into pepsin • **Intrinsic factor**—necessary for the absorption of vitamin B12 from the ileum • **Pepsinogen**—an enzyme precursor that is converted into pepsin in the acidic environment of gastric juice; pepsin is an enzyme that begins the breakdown of protein • **Gastric lipase**—an enzyme that acts on lipids, breaking triglycerides down into fatty acids and monoglycerides A 1–3 mm layer of mucus forms a protective barrier between the acidic gastric juice and the stomach wall, and also protects the epithelial cells of the wall from pepsin, which digests proteins.	
Salivary amylase	The digestion of carbohydrates by salivary amylase continues in the stomach for about one hour before salivary amylase is denatured by hydrochloric acid
Lingual lipase	Similarly, the digestion of fats by lingual lipase continues for about one hour before the lingual lipase is denatured by hydrochloric acid
Gastric lipase	Continues the breakdown of fats; however, gastric lipase is soon denatured by the acidity of gastric juice
Pepsin	Pepsin begins the breakdown of proteins
Rennin	Rennin is an enzyme found only in the stomachs of infants; it begins the digestion of milk by converting the protein caseinogen into casein

From the stomach your food passes into the duodenum, the first part of your small intestine. However, before we look closely at the small intestine, we are going to take a detour in this journey and look at three accessory organs that secrete their substances into the duodenum. These are the pancreas, liver, and gall bladder.

Pancreas

The pancreas is a long, thin gland lying behind the stomach and connected to the duodenum by two ducts, the larger **pancreatic duct** (**duct of Wirsung**), which joins the common bile duct from the liver, and the smaller **accessory duct** (**duct of Santorini**). The pancreas has a head, body, and tail, and is 4¾–6 in (12–15 cm) long.

Exocrine cells comprise 99% of pancreatic cells, and they secrete **pancreatic juice**. This is a clear liquid composed of mostly water, some salts, sodium bicarbonate, and some enzymes. It is slightly alkaline and so buffers the acidic chyme coming from the stomach, stops the action of pepsin, and creates the correct pH in the small intestine in which the enzymes here can work. There are many different enzymes in pancreatic juice, including:

- **Pancreatic amylase:** Continues the breakdown of carbohydrates
- **Trypsin:** Continues the breakdown of proteins
- **Pancreatic lipase:** Continues the breakdown of lipids
- Enzymes that digest nucleic acids.

Did you know?

The stomach is not essential to life and a person can survive without it.

The remaining 1% of pancreatic cells are endocrine cells found in clusters called **pancreatic islets** (**islets of Langerhans**). These secrete hormones such as glucagon and insulin and are discussed in more detail in chapter 7.

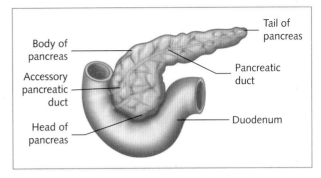

Figure 11.10   *Duodenum and pancreas*

Liver

Structure of the liver

The liver is a large organ located in the top-right portion of the abdominal cavity, below the diaphragm. It is composed of two lobes separated by the **falciform ligament.** The right lobe is larger than the left and both are covered by visceral peritoneum, under which is a layer of dense irregular connective tissue. Each lobe is composed of smaller functional units called **lobules**, and each lobule is made up of specialized epithelial cells called **hepatocytes.** These cells are arranged around a central vein.

Did you know?

The liver is the heaviest gland in the body, weighing approximately 3 lb (1.4 kg) in the average adult. It is also the second largest organ in the body, after the skin.

The liver does not contain capillaries. Instead, it has spaces through which blood passes. These spaces are called **sinusoids** and they are partly lined by phagocytes, which destroy microbes and potentially harmful foreign matter. The liver also has a unique double blood supply. It receives oxygenated blood via the **hepatic artery.** It also receives deoxygenated blood from the GI tract via the **hepatic portal vein.**

This blood contains newly absorbed nutrients as well as drugs, toxins, or microbes that may have been absorbed from the GI tract. This blood needs to be "cleaned," or "made safe," by the liver before

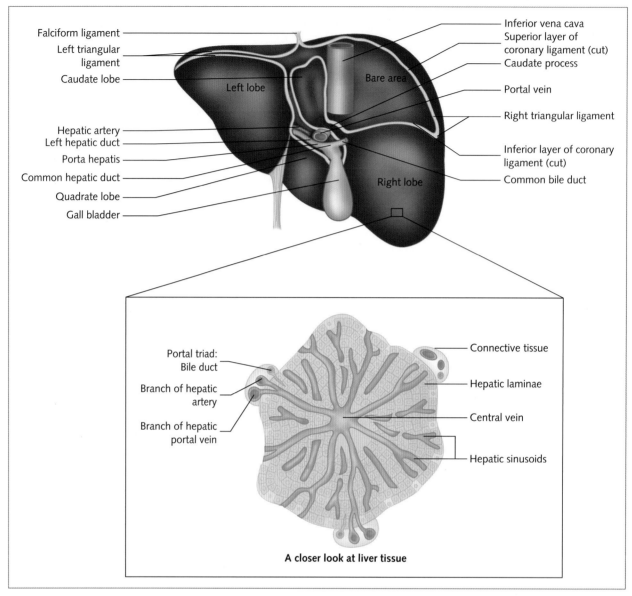

Figure 11.11 *Posterior view of the liver*

it can be circulated to the rest of the body (for more information on hepatic portal circulation, please refer to chapter 9).

Functions of the liver

The liver is a vital organ with many important functions in the body. These include:

- **Carbohydrate metabolism:** The liver maintains normal blood glucose levels.
  - If blood glucose levels are too low, the liver converts glycogen into glucose, which it then releases into the blood. If necessary, it can also convert some amino acids and lactic acid into glucose

  - If blood glucose levels are too high, the liver converts the excess glucose into glycogen and triglycerides, which it then stores
- **Lipid metabolism:** The liver stores fats and, when necessary, converts them into a form that can be used by the tissues. It also breaks down fatty acids; synthesizes lipoproteins, which are necessary for transporting fatty acids, triglycerides, and cholesterol; and synthesizes cholesterol.
- **Protein metabolism:** The liver synthesizes all the major plasma proteins. It also:
  - Converts one amino acid into another through a process called **transamination**
  - Removes the amino group, NH_2, from amino acids so they can be used for ATP production

or converted into carbohydrates or fats; this process is called **deamination**
  – Converts ammonia, which is a toxic by-product of deamination and is also produced by bacteria in the GI tract, into urea for excretion
- **Detoxification:** The liver removes and excretes alcohol and some drugs, and also chemically alters and excretes some hormones.
- **Storage of nutrients:** The liver stores glycogen; vitamins A, B12, D, E, and K; and the minerals iron and copper.
- **Phagocytosis:** Some liver cells phagocytize worn-out red blood cells, white blood cells, and some bacteria.
- **Activation of vitamin D:** Together with the skin and kidneys, the liver participates in activating vitamin D.
- **Production of bile:** The liver produces a brownish yellow (sometimes greenish) liquid called bile, which contains water, bile acids, bile salts, cholesterol, phospholipids, bile pigments, and some ions. The liver secretes bile into the gall bladder, where it is stored. The gall bladder then intermittently releases it into the duodenum, where it plays both excretory and digestive roles.
  – As an excretory product, bile contains **bilirubin**, which is a pigment from worn-out red blood cells that have been broken down
  – As a digestive product, bile contains **bile salts**, which function in the emulsification and absorption of fats. In this process, large lipid molecules are broken down into a suspension of droplets, which makes them more soluble and able to be absorbed

Infobox

Anatomy and physiology in perspective

Bile is broken down into a substance called **stercobilin**, which is excreted in feces and gives them their brown color.

Gall bladder

The gall bladder is a pear-shaped, green sac that is located behind the liver and attached to it by connective tissue. The gall bladder receives bile from the liver and concentrates and stores it. It then releases bile into the duodenum via the common bile duct.

Small intestine

From the stomach your food passes into a long, coiled and looped tube, where it spends the next three to five hours. This tube is the small intestine, and almost all the digestion and absorption of nutrients occurs here (bacteria in the large intestine complete the digestion of any nutrients that have not been fully broken down in the small intestine).

Structure of the small intestine

The small intestine is made up of three segments:

- **The duodenum:** This is the first segment of the small intestine and is also the shortest. It is approximately 10 in (25 cm) long and it receives

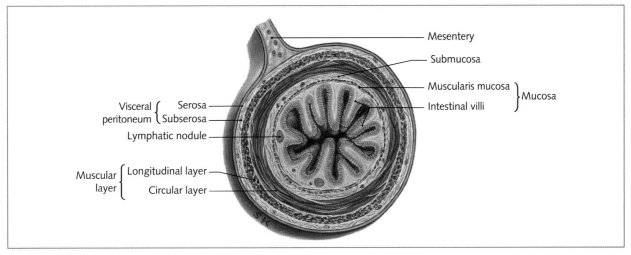

Figure 11.12 *Cross-section through the small intestine*

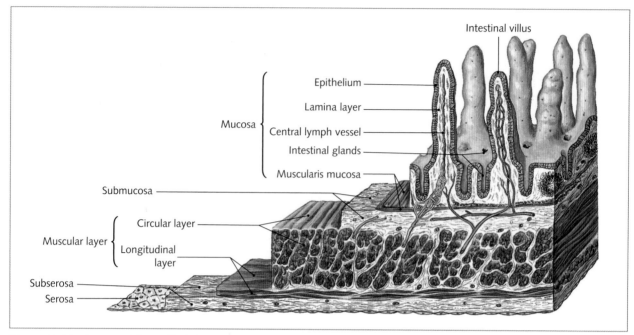

Figure 11.13 *Layers of the wall of the small intestine*

food from the stomach, bile from the gall bladder, and pancreatic juice from the pancreas.

- **The jejunum:** This is approximately 3 feet (1 m) long and lies between the duodenum and the ileum.
- **The ileum:** This is the longest segment of the small intestine at approximately 6½ feet (2 m) long. It receives food from the jejunum and passes it into the large intestine via the **ileocecal valve.**

> ### Did you know?
>
> Your small intestine is approximately 10 feet (3 m) long and has a diameter of 1 in (2.5 cm). However, the small intestine of a dead person has no muscle tone and is actually almost 21 feet (6.5 m) long.

The structure of the wall of the small intestine is similar to that of the rest of the GI tract in that it has the same basic four layers of tissue (mucosa, submucosa, muscularis, and serosa). However, because most digestion and absorption takes place in the small intestine, it is uniquely structured to ensure a large surface area.

- **Plicae circulares (circular folds):** The mucosa of the small intestine has ridges that are approximately 10 mm high. These ridges are called the plicae circulares, or circular folds, and

they increase the total surface area of the small intestine and also cause chyme to spiral through the intestine.
- **Villi:** The mucosa of the small intestine forms fingerlike projections called villi (singular = **villus**) that greatly increase the total surface area of the small intestine. These are 0.5–1 mm long and there are approximately 20–40 of them per square millimeter. Each villus contains an arteriole, venule, capillary network, and lacteal, and so enables absorbed nutrients to enter the bloodstream and lymphatic system.
- **Microvilli:** Every villus in the mucosa of the small intestine contains a variety of cells, including absorptive cells. Each absorptive cell has many tiny, membrane-covered projections called microvilli (singular = **microvillus**), which extend into the small intestine and further increase the surface area for absorption.
- **Brush border:** Together, the microvilli form the brush border across which large amounts of digestive nutrients diffuse into the absorptive cells. The brush border contains enzymes that have been secreted into the plasma membranes of the microvilli instead of into the lumen of the small intestine. Therefore, digestion also occurs at the surface of the cells and not just in the lumen.
- **Brush-border enzymes:** Brush-border enzymes continue the breakdown of disaccharides into monosaccharides, complete the digestion of

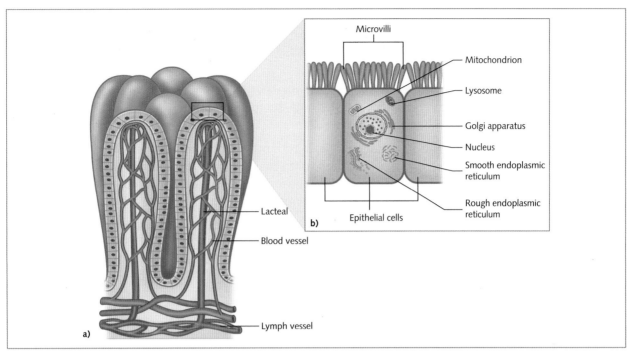

Figure 11.14 *Arrangement of (a) villi and (b) microvilli*

proteins and help digest nucleotides. These enzymes are:
- Alpha-dextrinase, maltase, sucrase, and lactase, which all act on carbohydrates
- Aminopeptidase and dipeptidase, which together are referred to as peptidases and which act on proteins
- Nucleosidases and phosphatases, which digest nucleotides
- **Intestinal glands (crypts of Lieberkühn):** The mucosa of the small intestine also contains cavities called the intestinal glands. They contain a number of specialized cells and secrete intestinal juice:
  - **Intestinal juice** is a clear yellow fluid that has a slightly alkaline pH of 7.6. It contains water and mucus and helps bring nutrient particles into contact with the microvilli
  - **Paneth cells** are specialized cells that secrete a bactericidal enzyme called **lysozyme**. Lysozyme also functions in phagocytosis
  - **Enteroendocrine cells** are another type of specialized cell, which secretes hormones into the intestinal glands. These hormones include **secretin** and **cholecystokinin**, which influence the release of pancreatic juice and bile, and **gastric inhibitory peptide**

- **Goblet cells** secrete mucus, which helps lubricate the small intestine
- **Peyer's patches:** The lamina propria of the mucosa of the small intestine contains many mucus-associated lymphoid tissues, including Peyer's patches.
- **Duodenal glands (Brunner's glands):** The submucosa of the duodenum contains duodenal glands, which secrete an alkaline mucus that helps to neutralize gastric acid in the chyme that has arrived from the stomach.

> **Did you know?**
> ··
> The many tiny villi lining the small intestine give it a velvety appearance.

> **Did you know?**
> ··
> It is estimated that there are about 200 million microvilli per square millimeter of small intestine.

DIGESTION IN THE SMALL INTESTINE

Digestion/enzyme	Description
Mechanical digestion	
In the small intestine, the thin liquid chyme is mixed with digestive juices and brought into contact with the villi and microvilli, where it can be further digested and absorbed. It is moved in and through the small intestine by two movements: segmentation and peristalsis:	
Segmentation	• Segmentation is the main movement in the small intestine • It involves localized contractions that move food back and forth and is a similar movement to squeezing opposite ends of a tube of toothpaste so that the paste is moved back and forth
Peristalsis	• Peristalsis in the small intestine is a weak movement compared to that in the esophagus or stomach • It slowly propels chyme forward toward the large intestine
Chemical digestion	
Chyme entering the small intestine contains partially digested nutrients, which are then broken down further by a combination of pancreatic juice, bile, intestinal juice, and brush-border enzymes. Digestion and absorption of most nutrients is usually completed in the small intestine:	
Carbohydrate digestion	
Pancreatic amylase	Pancreatic amylase present in pancreatic juice completes the breakdown of starches and glycogen; however, it does not digest cellulose, which passes into the large intestine as fiber
α-dextrinase	The brush-border enzyme α-dextrinase also acts on starches and breaks them down into glucose units
Maltase	The brush-border enzyme maltase breaks down maltose into glucose
Sucrase	The brush-border enzyme sucrase breaks down sucrose into glucose and fructose
Lactase	The brush-border enzyme lactase breaks down lactose into glucose and galactose
Protein digestion	
Trypsin, chymotrypsin, carboxypeptidase, elastase	These enzymes present in pancreatic juice break down proteins into peptides
Peptidases (aminopeptidase and dipeptidase)	These brush-border enzymes complete the breakdown of proteins into amino acids
Lipid digestion	
Bile salts	Bile salts emulsify lipids; i.e., they break down large globules of triglycerides into smaller droplets—this exposes a greater surface area to the enzyme pancreatic lipase
Pancreatic lipase	Pancreatic lipase present in pancreatic juice breaks down triglycerides into fatty acids and monoglycerides
Nucleic acid digestion	
Ribonuclease	Ribonuclease present in pancreatic juice breaks down RNA into nucleotides
Deoxyribonuclease	Deoxyribonuclease present in pancreatic juice breaks down DNA into nucleotides
Nucleosidases, phosphatases	These brush-border enzymes then break nucleotides down into pentoses, phosphates, and nitrogenous bases

Absorption in the small intestine

The process of digestion breaks large food particles into progressively smaller particles that can finally pass through the epithelial cells lining the small intestine and into the blood capillaries and lymphatic lacteals found in the villi. Absorption is this movement of digested nutrients, and 90% of all absorption takes place in the small intestine. The remaining 10% takes place in the stomach or large intestine.

Did you know?
....

Don't forget that all absorbed substances are transported in the blood to the liver, where the blood is "cleaned" before it can be circulated to the rest of the body.

Most substances are absorbed into the blood capillaries of the villi and are then carried in the bloodstream to the liver via the hepatic portal vein. Fatty acids, glycerol, and the fat-soluble vitamins (A, D, E, and K), however, are absorbed into lacteals (lymphatic vessels) in the villi, before being transported in the lymph to the bloodstream. The small intestine absorbs nutrients as well as water, electrolytes, and vitamins. Any remaining undigested or unabsorbed matter passes into the large intestine.

ABSORPTION IN THE SMALL INTESTINE	
Region of small intestine	**Nutrients absorbed**
Carbohydrates can only be absorbed as monosaccharides (glucose, fructose, galactose); proteins as amino acids, dipeptides, and tripeptides; and lipids as fatty acids, glycerol, and monoglycerides	
Duodenum	Microminerals
Jejunum	Water-soluble vitamins, amino acids, sugars, water, and some minerals
Ileum	Free fatty acids, cholesterol, fat-soluble vitamins, and bile

Large intestine

The journey of food from when you first ate it to when you eliminate it is almost over. It has passed through your mouth, esophagus, stomach, and small

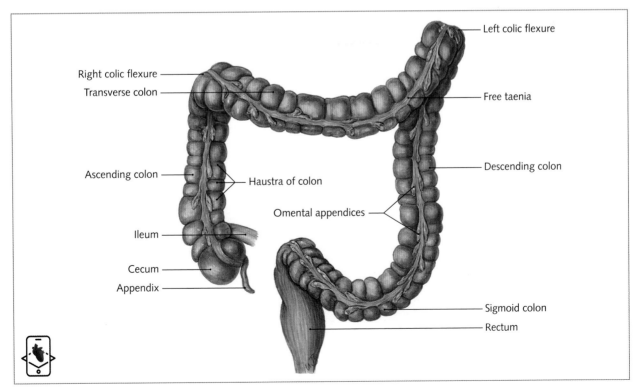

Figure 11.15 *Large intestine*

Right colic flexure
Transverse colon
Ascending colon
Haustra of colon
Ileum
Cecum
Appendix
Omental appendices
Left colic flexure
Free taenia
Descending colon
Sigmoid colon
Rectum

intestine and almost all of it has been broken down and absorbed into your bloodstream and lymphatic system. Now, any remaining material sits in your large intestine for anywhere from three to ten hours. Your large intestine is approximately 5 feet (1.5 m) long and 2½ in (6.5 cm) in diameter.

Structure of the large intestine

The large intestine is a wide tube running from the ileum to the anus. It is divided into four regions:

- **Cecum:** This is a 2½ in (6 cm) long pouch that receives food from the small intestine via the **ileocecal valve (ileocecal sphincter)**. Attached to the cecum is the **vermiform appendix**.
- **Colon:** This forms most of the large intestine and is a long tube made up of the:
  - **Ascending colon:** This part of the colon ascends from the cecum up the right side of the abdomen to just beneath the liver. Here it turns to the left, forming the **right colic (hepatic) flexure**
  - **Transverse colon:** The colon continues across the abdomen to beneath the spleen, where it curves downward at the **left colic (splenic) flexure**
  - **Descending colon:** The colon then descends to the level of the iliac crest, where it turns inward to form the last part of the colon

  - **Sigmoid colon:** This is the last part of the colon and it joins the rectum at the level of the third sacral vertebra
- **Rectum:** This is approximately 8 in (20 cm) long and lies in front of the sacrum and coccyx.
- **Anal canal:** The last ¾–1 in (2–3 cm) of the rectum is called the anal canal. Its external opening is called the **anus** and it is guarded by both internal and external sphincter muscles. These are usually closed except during defecation.

The structure of the wall of the large intestine is similar to that of the rest of the GI tract in that it contains all four tissue layers (mucosa, submucosa, muscularis, and serosa). However:

- The mucosa of the colon contains absorptive cells that absorb water, and goblet cells that secrete mucus to lubricate the contents of the large intestine.
- The muscularis has a unique arrangement of muscle fibers. Instead of forming a continuous layer of tissue, the longitudinal muscle fibers collect into three thickened bands at intervals along the colon. These are the **taeniae coli**, which are commonly called the "ribbons" of the colon. These taeniae coli are always slightly contracted (tonic) and so they gather the colon into pouches called **haustra**.

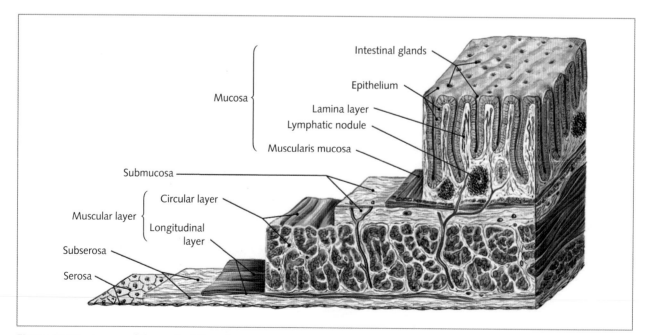

Figure 11.16 *Layers of the wall of the colon*

DIGESTION IN THE LARGE INTESTINE	
Digestion/enzyme	**Description**
Mechanical digestion	
Mechanical digestion in the large intestine is very slow and consists of three movements: haustral churning, peristalsis, and mass peristalsis:	
Haustral churning	The haustra, or pouches of the colon, are relaxed and distended until they are filled with matter, then they contract and squeeze their contents into the next haustrum. Thus, matter is slowly moved from haustrum to haustrum
Peristalsis	Peristalsis in the large intestine is a very weak, slow movement
Mass peristalsis	Three to four times a day, usually during or immediately after a meal, a very strong peristaltic wave begins in the middle of the transverse colon; it quickly travels across the rest of the colon, driving the colonic contents into the rectum
Chemical digestion	
As mentioned earlier, most digestion and absorption of nutrients is completed in the small intestine. However, small amounts of undigested nutrients do pass into the large intestine and these are digested by bacteria living in the lumen:	
Bacteria	Bacteria in the lumen prepare the chyme for elimination by: • Fermenting any remaining carbohydrates • Converting any remaining proteins into amino acids and breaking down amino acids into simpler substances • Decomposing bilirubin into simpler substances The bacteria also produce some B vitamins as well as vitamin K, which are absorbed in the colon

Absorption in the large intestine

The absorption of water and electrolytes takes place in the ascending and transverse colon.

Feces

Having spent 3–10 hours in the large intestine and having had most of its water content absorbed by the walls of the colon, the liquid chyme has now become a solid or semi-solid mass called **feces**. Feces contain water, inorganic salts, sloughed-off epithelial cells from the mucosa of the GI tract, bacteria, products of bacterial decomposition, and undigested foods. Feces are eliminated from the body by a process called **defecation**.

Did you know?

According to neuroscientist and gastroenterologist Emeran Mayer (2016, pp. 11–13), "There are 100,000 times more microbes in your gut alone as there are people on earth." These microbes not only assist in digesting food, they also help regulate metabolism, detoxify chemicals, and train the immune system.

Common Pathologies of the Digestive System

Red flags

- Abdominal pain accompanied by:
  - Signs of shock (tachycardia, low blood pressure, sweating, and confusion)
  - Fever, nausea, or vomiting
  - A distended (abnormally bloated) abdomen

- Diarrhea accompanied by:
  - Blood in the stool
  - Fever
  - Dehydration
- Nausea and vomiting accompanied by:
  - Headache, stiff neck, or changes in mental status
  - A distended (abnormally bloated) abdomen
  - Signs of shock (tachycardia, low blood pressure, sweating, and confusion)
- Severe constipation or diarrhea in elderly patients
- Blood or pus in the stool
- Jaundice
- Edema
- Chronic abdominal pain, constipation, or diarrhea accompanied by weight loss
- Iron-deficiency anemia in men can be suggestive of a gastrointestinal disorder.

Infobox

··

Anatomy and physiology in perspective: Stress and digestion

Embedded in the lining of the gut is the enteric nervous system. This system controls all digestive processes and is itself affected by the central nervous system. This gut–brain connection explains why you get "butterflies" in your stomach when you are nervous, or nausea when you are anxious or scared. In addition, simply thinking of, or smelling, food can trigger the release of digestive juices. It is no surprise, then, that when under emotional or mental stress we can develop functional bowel disorders such as pain, bloating, diarrhea, or constipation, even when there is no structural cause.

Pathologies of the mouth and teeth

Apical abscess (tooth abscess)
Collection of pus enclosed by damaged and inflamed tissue. It usually results from an infection that has spread from a tooth into the surrounding tissues.

Candida
Please refer to "Candidiasis" in the "Fungal infections of the skin" section, under "Common Pathologies of the Skin" in chapter 3.

Gingivitis
Inflammation of the gums and although not always painful, the gums become red and swollen and bleed easily. It is usually caused by poor oral hygiene, e.g., not

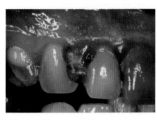
Gingivitis

flossing or brushing properly. However, it can also be a side effect of certain drugs, or caused by viral or fungal infections, vitamin deficiencies, an impacted tooth, pregnancy, or menopause.

Halitosis (bad breath)
Halitosis, or bad breath, has a wide range of causes. Most commonly, it is caused by poor oral hygiene; by eating foods that have volatile oils, such as garlic or onions; or by nose, throat, or lung infections. More extreme causes can include kidney failure, liver failure, or uncontrolled diabetes.

Pathologies of the esophagus and stomach

Dyspepsia (indigestion)
Commonly referred to as indigestion and characterized by pain or discomfort in the lower chest or upper abdomen. It usually occurs after eating and can be accompanied by nausea or vomiting. Dyspepsia has many causes, ranging from anxiety to gastritis (inflammation of the stomach) and stomach or duodenal ulcers.

Gastric ulcer
Please see "Peptic ulcers" under the section "Pathologies of the small and large intestines."

Gastritis
Inflammation of the lining of the stomach and is often symptom-free. If there are any signs and symptoms, they usually include pain, discomfort, nausea, and vomiting. Gastritis can be caused by bacterial, viral, or fungal infections, or by the excessive ingestion of irritants such as alcohol or drugs such as aspirin.

Gastroenteritis

Inflammation of the stomach and small intestine and it is characterized by diarrhea, cramping, vomiting, nausea, and a loss of appetite. Gastroenteritis has many different causes, including viral or bacterial infections that are transmitted from person to person or through contaminated utensils, food, or water. Gastroenteritis is often called "food poisoning."

Gastro-esophageal reflux disease (GERD)

Condition where the contents of the stomach flow back into the esophagus where they cause inflammation and pain. Signs and symptoms include heartburn and regurgitation, often provoked by bending forward, straining, or lying down. Causes of GERD include abnormalities of the esophageal sphincter muscle, delayed emptying of gastric contents, a hiatus hernia, certain foods (especially chocolate, fat, alcohol, and coffee), and increased intra-abdominal pressure due to pregnancy or obesity. It is important that GERD is treated, otherwise it can cause esophagitis or a pre-malignant condition called Barrett's esophagus.

Infobox

....

Anatomy and physiology in perspective

GERD and peptic ulcer disease are often treated with medications called proton pump inhibitors (PPIs). These inhibit the secretion of gastric acid.

Heartburn

Sensation of a burning discomfort or pain behind the breastbone. It is often accompanied by a bitter taste in the mouth due to the regurgitation of stomach contents.

Hiatus hernia

Condition where the stomach protrudes from the abdominal cavity through the diaphragm into the thoracic cavity. It can be accompanied by no symptoms at all, or symptoms of gastro-esophageal reflux and indigestion. The cause of hiatus hernia is unknown, although it is sometimes present at birth.

Hiccups (hiccoughs)

Abnormal spasms of the diaphragm accompanied by the quick and noisy closing of the rima glottidis (the space between the vocal folds). Their cause is not always known, but they can be triggered by laughing, talking, eating, or drinking.

Esophagitis

Inflammation of the esophagus, and signs and symptoms can range from mild redness and irritation to severe bleeding and ulceration. If left untreated, esophagitis can lead to iron-deficiency anemia or fibrous strictures. Esophagitis can be caused by gastro-esophageal reflux, infections, medications, or the swallowing of corrosives such as during suicide attempts.

Pernicious anemia

Please refer to the "Blood disorders" section in the "Common Pathologies" section of chapter 9.

Pathologies of the liver, gall bladder, and pancreas

Cholecystitis (inflammation of the gall bladder)

Characterized by severe upper abdominal pain, and usually accompanies gallstones.

Cirrhosis of the liver

Destruction of liver tissue and the replacement of it by scar tissue surrounding areas of healthy tissue. Signs and symptoms can include weakness, nausea, lack of appetite, and weight loss. Bile flow can sometimes be obstructed, which leads to signs and symptoms such as jaundice and itchiness. Cirrhosis is commonly caused by alcohol abuse or chronic hepatitis.

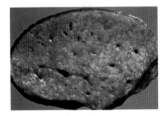

Cirrhosis of the liver

Gallstones

Hard masses of bile pigments, cholesterol, and calcium salts that form in the gall bladder. They do not always cause signs or symptoms. However, if they pass into the bile duct and obstruct the flow of bile this can lead to nausea and vomiting and sometimes infection.

Hepatitis

Inflammation of the liver and can be caused by viruses, chemicals, excessive alcohol intake, or the use of certain drugs. Hepatitis caused by viruses includes:

- **Hepatitis A:** This infectious form of hepatitis is caused by the hepatitis A virus and is transmitted via contaminated food, drink, feces, or utensils. It is characterized by a loss of appetite, nausea, diarrhea, fever, and chills, and most people recover from it within four to six weeks.
- **Hepatitis B:** This infectious hepatitis is caused by the hepatitis B virus, which is transmitted through sexual contact or contaminated syringes or infusion equipment. Hepatitis B is a chronic disease that can lead to cirrhosis of the liver.
- **Hepatitis C:** This infectious hepatitis is caused by the hepatitis C virus, which is usually transmitted through blood transfusions. It is also a chronic form of hepatitis that can lead to liver cirrhosis.

Other types of viral hepatitis exist, including hepatitis D and E.

Pancreatitis

Acute pancreatitis is sudden inflammation of the pancreas that is most often caused by gallstones or alcohol abuse. It is characterized by severe abdominal pain, which often penetrates to the back and which can be accompanied by nausea, vomiting, or retching. Chronic pancreatitis has similar symptoms to acute pancreatitis, but as it progresses and the cells of the pancreas are destroyed, the secretion of digestive enzymes decreases, and malabsorption and diabetes mellitus result. Chronic pancreatitis is often associated with inflammatory masses, cysts, or pancreatic cancer.

Pathologies of the small and large intestines

Appendicitis

Inflammation of the appendix usually characterized by abdominal pain that starts in the center and then moves to the lower right. This is then followed by a lack of appetite, nausea, and vomiting. Removal of the appendix is usually recommended.

Celiac disease

In celiac disease a person is intolerant to gluten, which is a protein found in wheat, rye, and barley. The consumption of gluten damages the lining of the small intestine and subsequently results in malabsorption. Signs and symptoms of celiac disease in adults include malnutrition, diarrhea, and weight loss, while in children it is characterized by painful abdominal bloating and light-colored, foul-smelling stools. Celiac disease is thought to be genetic.

Colitis

Inflammation of the colon and is characterized by lower abdominal pain and diarrhea. Blood or mucus can also be present in the stools. There are many different causes and types of colitis, including colitis caused by the use of antibiotics, which results in the overgrowth of certain bacteria in the colon; ulcerative colitis, which is thought to be genetic or linked to an overactive immune system; and mucous colitis, which is also called irritable bowel syndrome (discussed shortly).

Colon cancer (colorectal cancer)

Cancer of the large intestine. It usually develops from the lining of the large intestine and then begins to invade its wall as it grows. When the cancer metastasizes, it often spreads to the surrounding lymph nodes and liver. Colon cancer grows slowly and does not always cause any signs or symptoms until it is in its later stages. Signs and symptoms that can occur include fatigue, weakness, and sometimes blood in the stools.

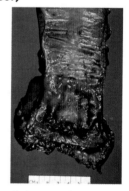

Colon cancer

Constipation

Condition in which bowel movements are infrequent or uncomfortable. Stools are usually hard and difficult to pass, and after passing them the person may feel that the rectum has still not been completely emptied. Constipation may be caused by drugs that slow the movement of matter through the large intestine, a lack of physical exercise, dehydration, a low-fiber diet, aging, depression, or obstruction of the large intestine.

Diarrhea

Frequent passing of abnormally soft or liquid stools, and it can be accompanied by abdominal cramping, large amounts of gas, or nausea. Diarrhea can be caused by infections, inflammation, stress, or irritable bowel syndrome (discussed shortly), and prolonged diarrhea can result in dehydration.

Diverticulosis and diverticulitis

Diverticula are small sac-like pouches that protrude through weak areas of the muscular layer of the GI tract (usually the large intestine).

- **Diverticulosis:** The development of diverticula is called diverticulosis, and although the causes of diverticulosis are not always known, they are thought to be related to a low-fiber diet or inadequate fluid intake. Diverticulosis has few signs or symptoms but can occasionally cause cramping, diarrhea, and bloody stools.
- **Diverticulitis:** Inflammation or infection of one or more diverticula, and is characterized by lower abdominal pain, tenderness, and fever. It is usually accompanied by either diarrhea or constipation.

Enteritis

Inflammation of the small intestine and usually characterized by diarrhea. Enteritis can be associated with Crohn's disease or gastroenteritis.

Flatulence

Presence of excess gas in the GI tract that is expelled via the mouth (belching) or the anus (flatulence). It is usually accompanied by abdominal pain and bloating. This excess gas may come from air that is swallowed while eating, may be produced by bacteria in the large intestine, or may be caused by deficiencies of certain digestive enzymes.

Hemorrhoids (piles)

Please refer to the "Heart and blood-vessel disorders" section in the "Common Pathologies" section of chapter 9.

Inflammatory bowel disease (IBD)

Ongoing, or chronic, inflammation of the bowel. Be careful not to confuse IBD with IBS, which is irritable bowel syndrome. The two most common types of IBD are Crohn's disease and ulcerative colitis, and they are thought to be genetic or autoimmune disorders.

- **Crohn's disease:** Chronic inflammation of the wall of the GI tract. It is characterized by irregular flare-ups or "attacks" of abdominal cramping, chronic diarrhea, fever, loss of appetite, and weight loss. Blood may be present in the stools.
- **Ulcerative colitis:** Chronic inflammation of the colon only. The main sign of ulcerative colitis is bloody diarrhea, and it does not usually have systemic or generalized signs or symptoms such as fever or loss of appetite.

Irritable bowel syndrome (IBS, spastic colon)

Condition characterized by recurring flare-ups of abdominal pain, constipation, and diarrhea in an otherwise healthy person. Other signs and symptoms can include fatigue, nausea, headaches, depression, anxiety, difficulty concentrating, abdominal bloating, and gas. The flare-ups are usually triggered by eating too quickly or too much, stress, diet, hormones, drugs, or minor irritants such as wheat, dairy, tea, coffee, or citrus fruits.

Peptic ulcers

Breaks in the mucous lining of the GI tract are called peptic ulcers because they are usually caused by the combined action of pepsin and hydrochloric acid. Together these two substances can digest the lining of the tract, causing pain and inflammation.

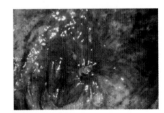

Peptic ulcer

Symptoms of peptic ulcers include feelings of gnawing, burning, aching, emptiness, or hunger, and they are usually caused by bacterial infection or the use of drugs that irritate the lining of the stomach (for example, aspirin, non-steroidal anti-inflammatory drugs, and corticosteroids). Peptic ulcers are named according to their location:

- **Duodenal ulcers** occur in the duodenum.
- **Gastric ulcers** occur in the stomach.

Eating disorders

Anorexia nervosa

Psychological disorder characterized by a distorted body image and a refusal to maintain a minimally healthy body weight. It is also accompanied by a fear of obesity and the absence of menstrual periods. Approximately 95% of people with anorexia nervosa are female.

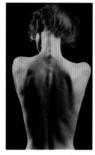

Anorexia nervosa

Bulimia nervosa

Psychological disorder characterized by bingeing and purging. When people with bulimia binge, they eat large amounts of food rapidly and often in secret. This gives them a sense of having lost control and so they purge themselves by making themselves vomit, taking laxatives, over-exercising, or dieting rigorously.

Obesity

Accumulation of excessive body fat, mostly in the subcutaneous tissues, and it is diagnosed by assessing one's body mass index (BMI). The BMI is a person's weight in kilograms divided by height in meters squared, and obesity is defined as a BMI of approximately 30 or more. Many factors influence a person's weight and, among other things, obesity can be linked to overeating, a lack of exercise, and sometimes genetics.

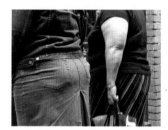

Obesity

NEW WORDS	
Absorption	The uptake of digested nutrients into the bloodstream and lymphatic system
Alimentary canal	*See* gastrointestinal tract
Catalyst	A substance that alters the rate of a chemical reaction without itself being changed by the reaction
Defecation	The process by which indigestible substances and some bacteria are eliminated from the body
Deglutition	The process of swallowing food
Digestion	The process by which large molecules of food are broken down into smaller molecules that can enter cells
Enzyme	A protein that speeds up a chemical reaction without itself being used up in the reaction
Feces	The waste material of the digestive system that is eliminated through the anus
Gastrointestinal (GI) tract	A tube that runs from the mouth to the anus where digestion and absorption take place
Ingestion	The process of taking food into the mouth
Mastication	The process of chewing food
Peristalsis	An involuntary wave-like movement that pushes the contents of the GI tract forward
Substrate	The substance on which an enzyme or catalyst acts

Study Outline

Digestion of carbohydrates

Polysaccharides such as starch are converted into monosaccharides such as glucose, fructose, and galactose. Digestion of carbohydrates begins in the mouth and is completed in the small intestine.

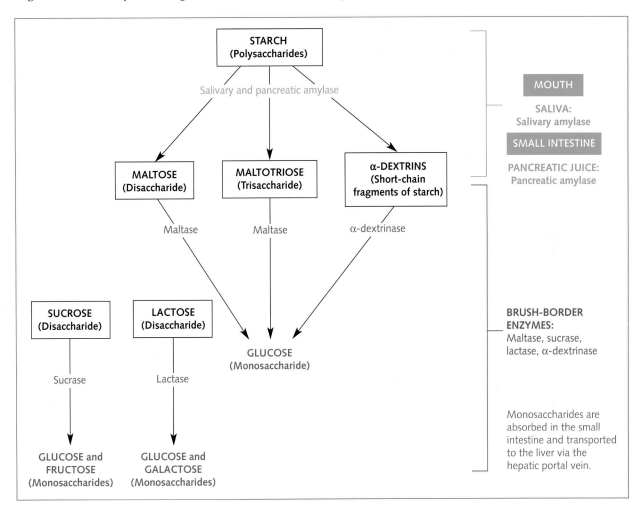

Digestion of proteins

Proteins are converted into amino acids. Digestion of proteins begins in the stomach and is completed in the small intestine.

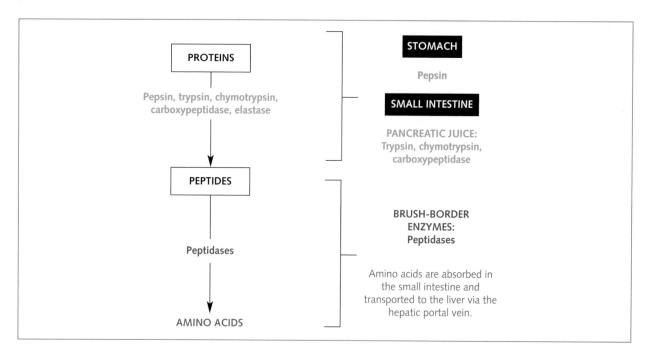

Digestion of lipids

Lipids are converted into fatty acids and monoglycerides. Minimal digestion of lipids begins in the mouth and stomach and most of the digestion of lipids takes place in the small intestine.

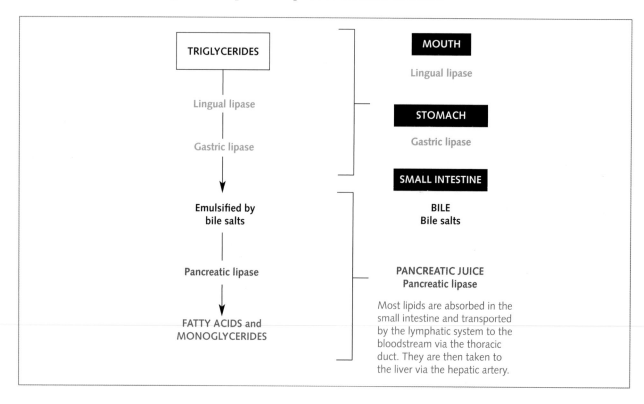

The journey of food

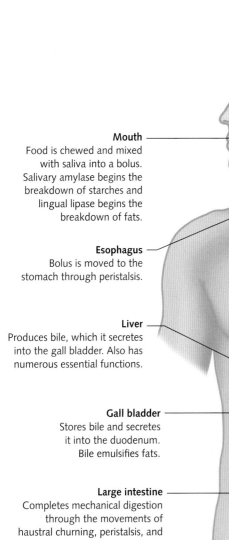

Mouth
Food is chewed and mixed with saliva into a bolus. Salivary amylase begins the breakdown of starches and lingual lipase begins the breakdown of fats.

Esophagus
Bolus is moved to the stomach through peristalsis.

Liver
Produces bile, which it secretes into the gall bladder. Also has numerous essential functions.

Gall bladder
Stores bile and secretes it into the duodenum. Bile emulsifies fats.

Large intestine
Completes mechanical digestion through the movements of haustral churning, peristalsis, and mass peristalsis. Bacteria complete all digestion and produce some B vitamins and vitamin K. Absorbs most of the water content of chyme and turns it into feces, ready for elimination.

Stomach
Bolus is churned and mixed with gastric juice until it becomes chyme. Salivary amylase and lingual lipase continue to act for about one hour until they are denatured by HCl. Gastric lipase continues the breakdown of fat until it is also denatured by HCl. Pepsin begins the breakdown of proteins and in infants rennin begins the digestion of milk.

Pancreas
Secretes pancreatic juice into the duodenum of the small intestine. Pancreatic juice contains pancreatic amylase, which continues the breakdown of carbohydrates; trypsin, which continues the breakdown of proteins; pancreatic lipase, which continues the breakdown of lipids; and enzymes that digest nucleic acids.

Small intestine
Moves chyme by the actions of segmentation and peristalsis. Completes the digestion of most nutrients by a combination of pancreatic juice, bile, intestinal juice, and brush border enzymes. Also absorbs most nutrients: the duodenum absorbs some micro-minerals; the jejunum absorbs water-soluble vitamins, amino acids, sugars, water, and some minerals; and the ileum absorbs free fatty acids, cholesterol, and fat-soluble vitamins.

Review

1. Identify the functions of the digestive system.
2. Explain the following terms:
   • Digestion
   • Absorption
   • Deglutition
   • Peristalsis
   • Enzyme.
3. Describe the organization of the gastrointestinal tract.
4. Explain the function of saliva.
5. Describe the digestion of carbohydrates.
6. Describe the digestion of proteins.
7. Describe the digestion of lipids.
8. Identify the functions of the liver.
9. Explain the following terms associated with the small intestine:
   • Villi
   • Microvilli
   • Brush border.
10. Identify the functions of the large intestine.

Multiple-Choice Questions

1. Which of the following enzymes is present in the mouth?
   a. Pepsin
   b. Trypsin
   c. Salivary amylase
   d. Pancreatic amylase

2. Where is bile manufactured?
   a. The pancreas
   b. The liver
   c. The gall bladder
   d. The duodenum

3. Which of the following are all parts of the small intestine?
   a. Duodenum, jejunum, ileum
   b. Duodenum, rugae, rectum
   c. Sigmoid, rectum, anus
   d. Sigmoid, rugae, rectum

4. Where are brush-border enzymes found?
   a. Mouth
   b. Stomach
   c. Small intestine
   d. Large intestine

5. Which of the following enzymes digest lipids?
   a. Salivary amylase, maltase
   b. Rennin, pepsin
   c. Lingual lipase, pancreatic lipase
   d. Trypsin, chymotrypsin

6. Which of the following statements is correct?
   a. Carbohydrates are broken down into glucose
   b. Proteins are broken down into lactose
   c. Fats are broken down into amino acids
   d. None of the above

7. What is the function of bile salts?
   a. They break down carbohydrates
   b. They convert proteins into peptides
   c. They emulsify fats
   d. They help mix all nutrients together

8. Where is the jejunum located?
   a. At the end of the esophagus
   b. Between the duodenum and the ileum
   c. Between the stomach and the small intestine
   d. At the end of the small intestine

9. Functions of the bacteria of the large intestine include:
   a. Producing some B vitamins and vitamin K
   b. Fermenting remaining lipids
   c. Decomposing minerals such as calcium
   d. None of the above

10. Which form of viral hepatitis is transmitted via contaminated food, drink, feces, or utensils?
    a. Hepatitis A
    b. Hepatitis B
    c. Hepatitis C
    d. Hepatitis D

The Urinary System

Introduction

Two small organs, each no bigger than a large bar of soap and buried in fat, filter and clean the blood of toxins, and control its volume, composition, pH, and pressure. In addition, these organs secrete essential hormones and can, in times of starvation, even manufacture glucose. These intricate organs are the kidneys, and each one is composed of around a million tiny filters that would stretch for more than 50 miles if unwound and placed end to end (Barnard, 1981).

The study of the urinary system is called **urology**, and in this chapter you will discover more about the invaluable role this system plays in your body.

Student objectives

By the end of this chapter you will be able to:

- Describe the functions of the urinary system
- Explain the organization of the urinary tract
- Describe the structure of the kidneys
- Explain how urine is produced and how the volume, composition, pH, and pressure of blood are regulated
- Describe the common pathologies of the urinary system.

Functions of the Urinary System

Water is vital to every cell in our bodies and without it we would not survive. It circulates in blood plasma, and as it circulates it gathers toxins, wastes, and any other substances that are not used by the cells. Blood, therefore, needs to be continually cleaned and its water content regulated, otherwise tissue cells would "drown" in their own water, and blood would become a river of circulating toxins and waste products.

This vital role of cleaning and regulating blood is carried out by the two kidneys. They function in controlling the composition, volume, and pressure of blood, and in doing this they help to maintain homeostasis of the entire body. The other organs of

the urinary system (the ureters, bladder, and urethra) transport, store, and excrete urine.

Regulation of blood composition and volume

The kidneys filter blood and remove from it any substances that the body no longer needs. For example, waste products, toxic substances, and excess essential materials such as water. During this filtering process, the kidneys also restore certain amounts of water and solutes to the blood if and when it needs them. Thus, the composition and volume of blood are constantly regulated.

Infobox

Anatomy and physiology in perspective

There are many accounts of people on hunger strikes, who refuse to eat as a form of non-violent protest. Mahatma Gandhi is one such example. Some strikers have been known to survive for many weeks if they have received fluids, but anyone who tries to refuse water cannot survive even a few days. Why is water so vital to our bodies?

After oxygen, water is the most important substance to our survival:

- Every cell in our bodies contains water.
- The size and shape of every cell is maintained by water.
- Our blood is mainly water (91.5% of blood plasma is water).
- Water is the solvent in all body fluids.
- Water is the medium for all biochemical processes in the body.
- More than half our body weight comes from water.
- Every day we lose about 3–3.6 pints (1.5–1.7 liters) of water through our urine, sweat, feces, and the air we exhale.

Regulation of blood pH

In addition to regulating the composition and volume of blood, the kidneys also filter out and excrete differing amounts of hydrogen (H^+) ions from the blood. This helps to regulate its pH.

Regulation of blood pressure

The kidneys secrete an enzyme called **renin**, which causes an increase in blood pressure and blood volume. Thus, they help to regulate blood pressure.

Other regulatory functions

The kidneys also have other functions in the body:

- **Synthesis of calcitriol:** The kidneys help synthesize the hormone calcitriol, which is the active form of vitamin D.
- **Secretion of erythropoietin:** The kidneys secrete the hormone erythropoietin, which stimulates the production of red blood cells.
- **Synthesis of glucose:** During periods of starvation the kidneys can synthesize new glucose molecules in a process called gluconeogenesis.

> **Study tip**
>
> Don't confuse the digestive enzyme **rennin** with the renal enzyme **renin**.

Organization of the Urinary System

The urinary system is composed of:

- **Two kidneys:** These are the functional organs of the urinary system and are the site where blood is filtered and its composition, volume, and pressure are regulated.
- **Two ureters:** These are long, thin tubes that transport urine from the kidneys to the bladder. One ureter leaves each kidney.
- **The urinary bladder:** This is a collapsible muscular sac where urine is temporarily stored.
- **The urethra:** This is a thin-walled tube that transports urine from the bladder to the outside of the body.

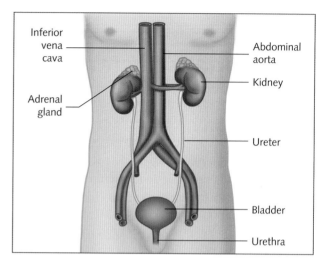

Figure 12.1 *The urinary system*

Kidneys

The kidneys are a pair of reddish, kidney-bean-shaped organs located slightly above the waistline, between the levels of the last thoracic and third lumbar vertebrae. They are partially protected by the eleventh and twelfth pairs of ribs, and the right kidney is slightly lower than the left because the liver occupies such a large area on the right side of the abdominopelvic cavity.

> **Study tip**
>
> *Nephros* and *renalis* are different names for the kidneys. So if you see any words that are derived from these names, remember that they will be related to the kidneys. For example, "renal," "nephron," or "nephritis."

Anatomy of the kidneys

The kidneys are approximately 4–4¾ in (10–12 cm) long, 2–2¾ in (5–7 cm) wide and 1 in (2.5 cm) thick, and are uniquely structured to filter blood and produce urine. Each kidney is encapsulated in and protected by three layers of tissue:

- **Renal fascia:** This outer, superficial layer of dense irregular connective tissue holds the kidneys in place, binding them to their surrounding structures and the abdominal wall.
- **Adipose capsule (perirenal fat):** This intermediate layer of fatty tissue protects the kidneys and also holds them firmly in place.

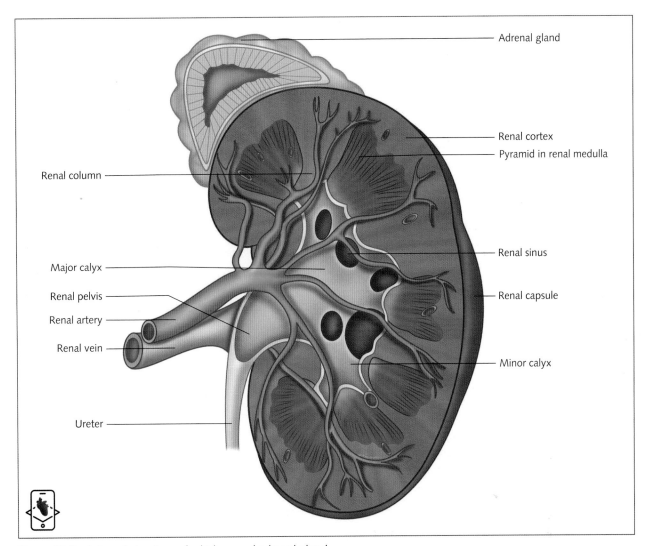

Figure 12.2 *Internal structure of a kidney and adrenal gland*

- **Renal capsule:** This inner, deep layer is composed of a smooth, transparent, fibrous membrane that is continuous with the outer coat of the ureters and that protects the kidneys and helps to maintain their shape.

Above each kidney sits an **adrenal (suprarenal) gland**.

Each kidney is shaped like a bean, with its concave border facing inward, toward the vertebral column. In this concave border is a deep fissure where the ureter leaves the kidney and where blood vessels, lymphatic vessels, and nerves enter and exit the kidneys. This fissure is called the **renal hilum** and is the entrance to the **renal sinus**, a cavity within the kidney.

Did you know?

Although the adrenal glands sit on top of the kidneys, they are part of the endocrine and not the urinary system.

Study tip

The word *cortex* means "rind or bark," the word *medulla* means "inner," and the word *pelvis* means "basin."

If you cut a kidney lengthwise in a frontal (coronal) section, you will see that it has three distinct regions:

- **Renal cortex:** The outer, reddish region of the kidney is called the renal cortex. Parts of the cortex extend into their neighboring region and these extensions are called **renal columns**.
- **Renal medulla:** The middle, reddish-brown region is the renal medulla. It is composed of cone-shaped structures called **renal (medullary) pyramids,** whose broad bases face the cortex and thin tips (apexes) point toward the center of the kidney.
- **Renal pelvis:** The inner, whitish cavity connected to the ureter is called the renal pelvis.

Together, the renal cortex and renal pyramids form the functional part of the kidney. They are composed of approximately one million microscopic structures called **nephrons**. These are the functional units of the kidney and are where urine is formed.

Once urine has been formed in the nephron it drains into a large duct, the **papillary duct**, which transports urine into a cuplike structure known as a **minor calyx** (plural = **calyces**). The minor calyx collects urine and delivers it to a **major calyx**, which then empties the urine into the renal pelvis. From here the ureter carries urine to the bladder.

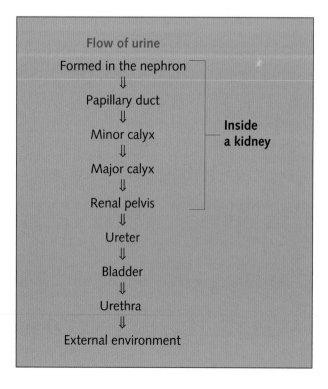

Did you know?

You are born with all your nephrons, and if you lose them through injury or disease they cannot be replaced. However, the remaining nephrons can increase their workload to compensate for the ones you lose.

Nephrons: The functional units of the kidney

Nephrons function in maintaining homeostasis of the blood by:

- Filtering blood through a process called **glomerular filtration**
- Secreting substances that were not originally absorbed during glomerular filtration and reabsorbing useful materials that the body may need—these processes are called **tubular secretion** and **tubular reabsorption**.

These functions will be discussed in more detail shortly.

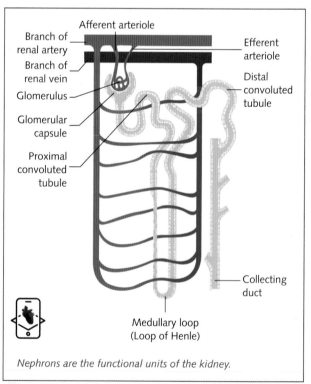

Nephrons are the functional units of the kidney.

Figure 12.3   A nephron and associated blood vessels

Structure of a nephron

In order to carry out its functions of filtering, secreting, and reabsorbing materials, a nephron is composed of:

- A **renal corpuscle**, which filters blood plasma
- A **renal tubule**, in which secretion and reabsorption take place.

Renal corpuscle

Renal corpuscles lie in the renal cortex and are composed of:

- A knotted network of capillaries called the **glomerulus**
- A cuplike structure surrounding the glomerulus called the **glomerular (Bowman's) capsule**, which is the closed end of the renal tubule.

Blood flows through the capillaries in the glomerulus and water and most solutes filter from the blood into the glomerular capsule across a membrane called the **filtration membrane**. However, large plasma proteins and formed elements such as red and white blood cells are too big to filter through the walls of the glomerulus and so remain in the blood.

Renal tubule

Filtered fluid passes from the glomerular capsule into the renal tubule, which is composed of three sections:

- **Proximal convoluted tubule (PCT):** This is the area closest to the glomerular capsule. It is a coiled tubule lying in the renal cortex and is the section of the renal tubule where the reabsorption of most substances takes place (this will be discussed shortly).
- **Loop of Henle (nephron loop):** From the proximal convoluted tubule, the renal tubule extends into the renal medulla where it makes a sharp turn and then returns to the cortex. This section of the tubule is called the loop of Henle, and water and salts are reabsorbed here.
- **Distal convoluted tubule (DCT):** This is the area furthest from the glomerular capsule and is the section of the tube where "fine-tuning" of the filtrate occurs. Like the proximal convoluted tubule, it also lies in the renal cortex.

Distal convoluted tubules empty their contents into collecting ducts that drain into papillary ducts, which then drain into the minor calyces. You will shortly learn about how nephrons function in filtering and regulating the blood. However, before doing this we need to take a quick look at the blood supply to the kidneys and nephrons.

Blood supply to the kidneys and nephrons

The kidneys clean and regulate blood and so it is not surprising that they have an exceptionally rich supply of it: although they make up only 1% of the total body mass, they receive a quarter of total resting cardiac output.

Blood is brought to the kidneys by the right and left **renal arteries** and, once inside the kidneys, these divide into **segmental arteries**, which supply segments of the kidney. These arteries then branch into **interlobar arteries**, which are found in the renal columns between the renal pyramids. The interlobar arteries then arch at the base of the renal pyramids, where they are referred to as the **arcuate arteries**, before becoming the interlobular arteries. They finally branch into **afferent arterioles** in the renal cortex.

Each nephron receives an afferent arteriole, which divides into the knot of capillaries known as the **glomerulus**. The glomerular capillaries then reunite to form an **efferent arteriole**, which takes blood out of the glomerulus. The efferent arteriole then divides into a secondary capillary network called the **peritubular capillaries**. These capillaries supply the rest of the nephron with oxygen and nutrients.

Did you know?

The kidneys receive approximately 2½ pints (1200 milliliters) of blood per minute.

Peritubular capillaries drain into **peritubular venules**, which drain into **interlobular veins, arcuate veins, interlobar veins,** and finally **segmental veins.** Segmental veins drain into the right and left **renal veins**, which transport blood away from the kidneys.

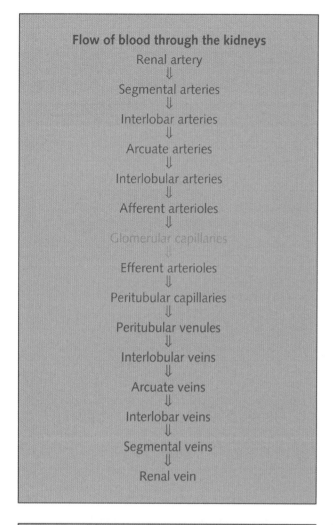

Flow of blood through the kidneys

Renal artery
⇓
Segmental arteries
⇓
Interlobar arteries
⇓
Arcuate arteries
⇓
Interlobular arteries
⇓
Afferent arterioles
⇓
Glomerular capillaries
⇓
Efferent arterioles
⇓
Peritubular capillaries
⇓
Peritubular venules
⇓
Interlobular veins
⇓
Arcuate veins
⇓
Interlobar veins
⇓
Segmental veins
⇓
Renal vein

Study tip

Note that although blood usually drains out of capillaries into **venules**, blood draining from the glomerulus drains into **arterioles** again.

Physiology of the kidneys
Urine

Urine is a clear to pale yellow fluid that is produced in the kidneys and excreted from the body via the urethra. Although the kidneys filter approximately 316 pints (180 liters) of fluid every day, only 1¾–3½ pints (1–2 liters) is excreted as urine and the rest is reabsorbed into the blood. The chart below identifies the characteristics and content of normal urine in a healthy person.

Infobox

Anatomy and physiology in perspective

The analysis of urine gives many clues to the internal state of the body, and substances that should not normally be present in urine include glucose, proteins, pus, red blood cells, hemoglobin, and bile pigments. The presence of any of these substances needs to be investigated further.

As mentioned earlier, nephrons have three functions (filtration, secretion, and reabsorption) and it is through these functions that the composition and volume of blood are regulated and urine is produced. The remaining areas of the kidneys function as passageways and storage areas.

We will now take a closer look at how nephrons function.

ANALYSIS OF NORMAL URINE	
Characteristic	**Description**
Volume	1¾–3½ pints (1–2 liters) every 24 hours
Color	• Clear to pale yellow • The color of urine is due to the presence of pigments and can vary depending on the concentration of the urine and on one's diet and health
Odor	• Initially slightly aromatic but quickly becomes ammonia-like upon standing • As with color, the odor of urine can vary depending on the concentration of the urine and one's diet and health

ANALYSIS OF NORMAL URINE	
Characteristic	**Description**
pH	• Varies considerably according to diet, and ranges between 4.6 and 8.0 • Diets high in protein produce more acidic urine, while vegetarian-based diets produce more alkaline urine
Solute	**Description**
Urea	The main product of protein metabolism
Creatinine	Product of muscle activity
Uric acid	Product of nucleic acid metabolism
Urobilinogen	Bile pigment derived from the breakdown of hemoglobin
Inorganic ions	These vary with one's diet

Urine production

There are three steps involved in urine production:

1. **Glomerular filtration:** In this initial step of urine production, water and solutes move from the blood into the glomerular capsule and then into the renal tubule.
2. **Tubular reabsorption:** As the fluid moves through the renal tubule, some of it is reabsorbed by the tubule cells and returned to the blood.
3. **Tubular secretion:** Also, as the fluid moves through the renal tubule, wastes, drugs, and excess ions that are still in the blood are secreted by the tubule cells into the tubule fluid so that they can be removed from the body via the urine.

Glomerular filtration

As blood passes through the capillaries of the glomerulus, fluid and small solutes pass through the filtration membrane into the glomerular (Bowman's) capsule. This fluid is now called the **glomerular filtrate**.

Filtration is assisted by specific structural features of the renal corpuscles:

- The filtration membrane is thin and porous.
- Glomerular capsules have a large surface area.
- Afferent arterioles bringing blood to the glomerulus have a larger diameter than efferent arterioles draining blood away from the glomerulus. This means that the pressure in the glomerulus, called the **glomerular hydrostatic pressure**, is higher than the pressure in the glomerular capsule. Thus, fluid is forced into the

glomerular capsule. However, there is still some pressure in the glomerular capsule that opposes the capillary hydrostatic pressure. If there were no opposing pressure, fluid would simply stream into the glomerular capsule. This opposing pressure is made up of **blood osmotic pressure** and **capsular hydrostatic pressure**, which combine to form the pressure within the capsule.

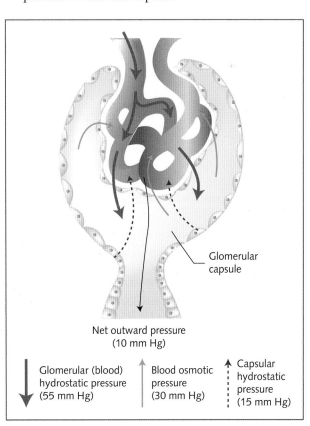

Net outward pressure
(10 mm Hg)

Glomerular (blood) hydrostatic pressure (55 mm Hg)

Blood osmotic pressure (30 mm Hg)

Capsular hydrostatic pressure (15 mm Hg)

Glomerular capsule

Figure 12.4 *Glomerular filtration*

Did you know?

Glomerular filtrate contains all the materials present in blood except the large plasma proteins and formed elements.

Tubular secretion

Blood filters through the glomerulus quite quickly, so there is not enough time for all substances to be filtered into the glomerular capsule. Therefore, the cells of the tubule secrete these remaining substances into the filtrate as it passes through the convoluted tubules. This is to ensure that the blood is cleared of all foreign materials and substances that it no longer needs.

Tubular reabsorption

Once blood plasma has been filtered into the glomerular capsule, the glomerular filtrate travels through the renal tubule, where 99% of it is reabsorbed into the bloodstream. The remaining 1% is excreted from the body as urine.

Reabsorption is carried out by the epithelial cells lining the renal tubule and most reabsorption occurs in the proximal convoluted tubule, which is lined by microvilli that greatly increase the surface area for absorption. The distal convoluted tubule functions more in "fine-tuning" the remaining filtrate.

Substances that are reabsorbed into the bloodstream include glucose, amino acids, small proteins, and some ions. Other substances that the body no longer needs or cannot use—for example, urea and uric acid—remain in the tubules to form urine. The reabsorption of some substances is regulated by hormones, as shown in the following chart.

Functions of the nephron in a nutshell

It is easy to remember the functions of a nephron if you think about what happens to your household waste: waste disposal vehicles (your blood) transport your household waste (cellular waste products and foreign substances) to a central sorting station (a nephron). At the station it is put onto a conveyor (renal tubule), and as it travels along the belt workers remove recyclable materials such as cans (reabsorption) and, at the same time, add any additional trash that may be on the floor (secretion). What is left on the conveyor (urine) is finally put into another vehicle and transported to a landfill site.

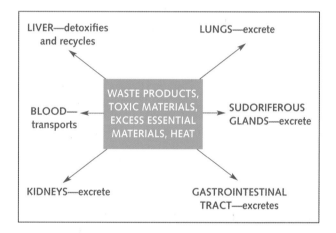

In the classroom

Discuss the different ways in which the body deals with its waste products, toxic materials, excess essential materials, and excess heat.

HORMONAL REGULATION OF TUBULAR REABSORPTION		
Endocrine gland	**Hormone**	**Regulation**
Parathyroid glands	Parathyroid hormone (parathormone)	Increases blood calcium and magnesium levels and decreases blood phosphate levels
Thyroid gland	Calcitonin	Lowers blood calcium levels
Adrenal cortex	Aldosterone	Increases blood levels of sodium and water and decreases blood levels of potassium

Did you know?

At least half of your body weight is made up of water:

- Females are approximately 50% water.
- Males are approximately 60% water.
- Babies are approximately 75% water.
- The elderly are approximately 45% water.

Fluid and electrolyte balance

In the process of producing urine, the kidneys also regulate the fluid and electrolyte balance of the blood and control its pH and pressure.

Water makes up at least 50% of our total body weight and is found in two "fluid compartments" in the body. Two-thirds of the fluid in the body is found in **intracellular fluid (ICF)**. This is the fluid inside cells. The remaining third is found in **extracellular fluid (ECF)**, which is the fluid outside the cells. This includes blood plasma, interstitial fluid, cerebrospinal fluid, serous fluid, aqueous humor, and lymph.

Study tip

Electrolytes are ions (charged particles) that when dissolved in water can conduct an electrical current. Examples of electrolytes in the body include calcium ions, which are necessary for muscular contraction (see chapter 5), and sodium and potassium ions, which are necessary for the propagation of nerve impulses (see chapter 6).

Because water is the universal solvent in the body and electrolytes such as calcium, sodium, and potassium dissolve in water, it is vital that the amount of water in each compartment remains constant. This essential role is carried out by the kidneys, which regulate the amount of fluids and electrolytes in the body by reabsorbing them or excreting them when necessary. This ensures that the total volume of fluid in the body remains stable despite fluctuating fluid intake.

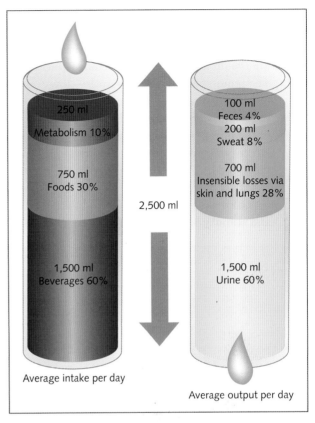

250 ml
Metabolism 10%

750 ml
Foods 30%

1,500 ml
Beverages 60%

2,500 ml

100 ml
Feces 4%
200 ml
Sweat 8%

700 ml
Insensible losses via skin and lungs 28%

1,500 ml
Urine 60%

Average intake per day

Average output per day

Figure 12.5 *Water intake and output*

Two hormones help regulate the reabsorption of water and electrolytes by the kidneys:

- **Antidiuretic hormone (ADH; vasopressin):** Specialized cells in the hypothalamus, called **osmoreceptors**, detect a decrease in water or an increase in solutes in the blood. They send a message to the posterior pituitary gland, which then releases antidiuretic hormone. A diuretic is a substance that stimulates an increase in urine production. Thus, "anti"-diuretic hormone has the opposite effect and it decreases the secretion of urine by causing the collecting ducts of the kidneys to reabsorb more water. When this additional water is returned to the bloodstream, it increases the volume, and therefore pressure, of the blood.
- **Aldosterone:** This is a hormone secreted by the adrenal cortex. It regulates the reabsorption of sodium ions back into the bloodstream and the secretion of potassium ions into the filtrate. Because sodium is responsible for the osmotic flow of water, aldosterone helps regulate the

amount of water in the blood. The release of aldosterone is stimulated by:

- Decreased sodium levels or increased potassium levels in the extracellular fluid
- The renin-angiotensin mechanism—low blood pressure in the afferent arterioles of the kidneys or changes in the solute content of the filtrate stimulate the release of **renin** (an enzyme produced by the kidneys) into the bloodstream; renin catalyzes a series of reactions that produce **angiotensin II**, which causes vasoconstriction of blood vessels and stimulates the release of aldosterone

---

Infobox

....

Anatomy and physiology in perspective

Some of the drugs used to treat hypertension (high blood pressure) include diuretics and ACE inhibitors. Both these drugs act on the urinary system. Diuretics decrease blood pressure by increasing the volume of urine excreted by the kidneys, while ACE inhibitors inhibit the conversion of angiotensin I to angiotensin II and thereby decrease blood pressure by causing vasodilation.

Ureters

The ureters are two 10–12 in (25–30 cm) long tubes that carry urine from the kidneys to the bladder. Each ureter drains the renal pelvis of a kidney and inserts into the posterior aspect of the bladder.

The ureters do not have a physical valve that prevents the backflow of urine from the bladder into the ureters. However, when the bladder is full, pressure from within it compresses the ureter openings. This, coupled with the force of gravity, prevents any urinary backflow.

The walls of the ureters are composed of three layers of tissue:

- The **adventitia** (outer layer) consists of areolar connective tissue and contains the blood vessels, lymphatic vessels, and nerves that supply the ureters. This tissue also holds the ureters in place.
- The **muscle** (intermediate layer) consists of both longitudinal and circular smooth muscle fibers that move urine via the action of peristalsis.
- The **mucosa** (inner layer) is lined with a mucous membrane of transitional epithelium. These transitional epithelial cells give the ureters their ability to stretch and to be watertight.

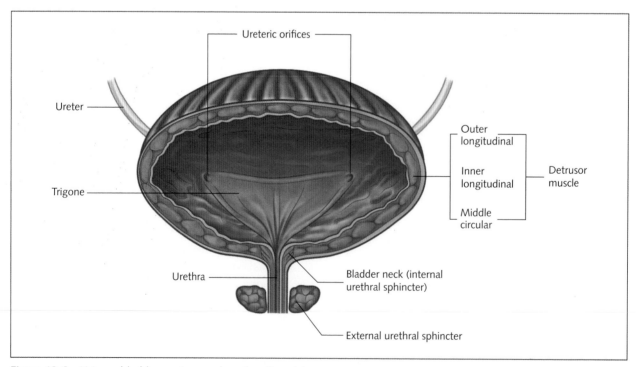

Figure 12.6 *Urinary bladder, ureters, and urethra (female)*

Urinary bladder

The urinary bladder, which is more commonly referred to as the bladder, is a freely movable, hollow muscular organ that is held in its place by folds of the peritoneum. The bladder acts as a reservoir, storing urine until it is excreted out of the body.

The bladder changes its shape depending on how much urine it is holding: when empty it is pear-shaped, while when full it is more oval in shape. The location of the bladder also varies depending on one's sex: in females the bladder lies in front of the vagina and below the uterus, while in males it lies in front of the rectum. Furthermore, the size of the bladder varies depending on one's sex: females have a smaller bladder than males because of the uterus above it.

On the floor of the bladder is a triangular area called the **trigone**. The openings to the ureters are located in the posterior two corners of the trigone, and the urethral opening, the **internal urethral orifice**, is located in the anterior corner.

Similar to the walls of the ureters, the walls of the bladder consist of three layers of tissue: the **adventitia** (outer layer), the **detrusor** muscle, including the outer longitudinal, inner longitudinal, and middle circular muscles (intermediate layer), and the **mucosa** (inner layer). The bladder also has two sphincter muscles that regulate **micturition**, which is the emptying or voiding of the bladder:

- The **internal urethral sphincter** is composed of smooth muscle fibers. When the bladder is approximately half full, stretch receptors in the wall of the bladder send messages to the spinal cord. From here a reflex arc returns to the sphincter causing it to relax and empty the bladder. This is known as the **micturition reflex**.
- The **external urethral sphincter** is composed of striated muscle fibers and, although emptying the bladder is a reflex action, the external urethral sphincter is controlled voluntarily. Thus, emptying the bladder becomes a learned, voluntary action.

Urethra

At the end of the urinary system is a passageway that functions in discharging urine from the body. This passageway is the urethra, and it is a small tube leading from the internal urethral orifice in the bladder to the external environment.

Just as the size and location of the bladder differ according to one's sex, so do the size and location of the urethra differ. In females the urethra is a 1½ in (4 cm) tube lying behind the pubic symphysis and opening to the outside between the clitoris and vaginal opening. In males the urethra is a 6–8 in (15–20 cm) tube that runs through the prostate gland (prostatic urethra), then through the urogenital diaphragm (membranous urethra), and finally through the penis (spongy urethra), at the head of which it opens to the outside. The urethra also differs between sexes in what it transports: in females the urethra transports only urine, while in males it transports urine and reproductive secretions.

Common Pathologies of the Urinary System

Changes in urination patterns or urine composition, color, and odor are symptomatic of pathologies of the urinary system, while common features of renal disease are hypertension, proteinuria, and edema. Be aware of the following symptoms, which are suggestive of urinary tract disorders:

- **Anuria:** This is failure of the kidneys to produce urine. It should be investigated immediately.
- **Dysuria:** This is painful or uncomfortable urination. Common causes of dysuria include urinary tract infections and sexually transmitted infections.
- **Hematuria:** This is the presence of red blood cells in the urine. This may present as blood in the urine or it may only be discovered during urinalysis. It is important to have the urine tested for red blood cells as certain diseases, foods, food colorings, or drugs may also cause a reddish brown discoloration. Hematuria is most commonly caused by a urinary tract infection, prostatitis, or the presence of renal calculi. In patients aged over 50 years it can suggest cancer or prostate disease.
- **Nocturia:** This is the need to urinate regularly during the night. It is more common in pregnant women, the elderly, and men with enlarged prostate glands.

- **Oliguria:** This is the production of unusually small amounts of urine and can occur after heavy sweating, diarrhea, or blood loss. It may also result from kidney disease, edema, or poisoning.
- **Polyuria:** This is the excretion of more than three liters of urine per day and is most commonly caused by uncontrolled diabetes mellitus.
- **Proteinuria (albuminuria):** This is the presence of protein in the urine and it is often associated with kidney or heart disease.
- **Renal colic:** This is a severe cramping pain that occurs in the lower back region and often radiates to the groin. It is a symptom of many kidney and urinary tract disorders.
- **Urinary frequency:** This is the need to urinate many times during the day but in normal or less than normal volumes (be aware of the difference between polyuria and urinary frequency). Urinary frequency accompanies many conditions, including urinary tract infections, urinary incontinence, prostate disorders, and urinary tract calculi.

Red flags

- Anuria
- Dysuria accompanied by:
  - Fever
  - Flank pain, back pain, or weakness of the legs
- Hematuria, especially if:
  - Person is over 50 years of age
  - Accompanied by hypertension and edema
- Polyuria, especially if:
  - Sudden onset
  - In a young child
  - Accompanied by night sweats and weight loss
- The cause of any unusual urinary symptoms in children should be investigated, especially if there are other signs or concerns of sexual abuse.

Aging and the urinary system

As we age we become more prone to urinary disorders, especially incontinence and urinary tract infections. This is because renal blood flow, glomerular filtration, and urea clearance all decrease with age, and the filtering mechanism of a healthy 70-year-old is half as effective as that of a healthy 40-year-old.

Elderly men also often suffer with prostate gland problems, which lead to urinary retention and difficulties in urinating. Postmenopausal women, on the other hand, suffer more with incontinence due to a thinning of the urethral lining and a weakening of the urinary sphincters caused by the decrease in estrogen.

Calculi (kidney, bladder, and ureteral stones)

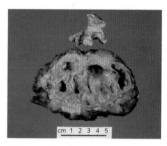

Kidney stones

Hard masses that can form in the urinary tract (as well as in the gall bladder) and, depending on where they are located, they are commonly referred to as kidney, bladder, or ureteral stones. Stones are composed mainly of calcium salts and can form either from an excess of salts in the urine or from a lack of stone inhibitors in the urine. They are more common in the elderly, men, and people who eat a high protein diet and have a low water intake. Signs and symptoms of stones include renal colic, back pain, nausea, vomiting, fever, and blood in the urine.

Enuresis (bed-wetting)

This is normal in young children. However, after the age of five or six years, it may be symptomatic of an infection, narrowing of the urethra, inadequate nerve control, or a psychological problem.

Nephritis (Bright's disease)

Inflammation of the kidneys characterized by impaired kidney function, fluid and urea retention, and blood in the urine. Nephritis can be caused by a variety of factors, including bacterial infection of the kidneys, exposure to toxins, and even abnormal immune reactions. It can occur anywhere in the kidneys.

- **Glomerulonephritis (glomerular nephritis):** This is inflammation of the glomeruli, and when the glomeruli are damaged they are unable to selectively filter blood. Thus, substances such as large proteins and red and white blood cells can pass into the filtrate and be excreted in urine. Urine production also declines and metabolic waste products accumulate in blood. Eventually, scarring of the kidney tissue and impaired kidney function can result.

- **Pyelonephritis:** This is a bacterial infection of the kidneys and is characterized by fever, shivering, and pain.

Nephroblastoma (Wilms' tumor)

Malignant cancer that is usually found only in young children. Signs and symptoms include a rapidly enlarging abdomen, abdominal pain, fever, loss of appetite, nausea, and vomiting. High blood pressure and blood in the urine may also occur. The cause is unknown, although genetic abnormalities may sometimes be involved.

Prostate cancer

Please see chapter 13.

Pyelitis

Inflammation of the pelvis of the kidney and it is characterized by pain, shivering, and fever. Pyelitis is usually caused by a bacterial infection.

Renal failure (kidney failure)

Renal failure is the kidneys' inability to filter blood efficiently and regulate its composition and volume properly. A rapid decline in kidney function is termed acute renal failure, and can be caused by kidney disease or any condition that reduces renal blood flow or that obstructs urine flow. Chronic renal failure (also called chronic kidney disease, or CKD) is a slower, more gradual decline in the functioning of the kidneys and is caused either by acute kidney failure that has been left to develop or by diseases such as diabetes mellitus or hypertension.

> ### Did you know?
> ....
> It is estimated that up to 40% of end-stage renal failure is caused by diabetes mellitus (Colledge et al., 2010).

Signs and symptoms of renal failure vary depending on the cause, progression, and severity of the disorder. They can include edema of the feet, ankles, face, and hands; dark urine; minimal to no urination; fatigue; lack of concentration; loss of appetite; nausea; and an overall itchiness. In chronic renal failure, blood pressure usually rises and the kidneys' inability to produce sufficient erythropoietin (the hormone that stimulates the production of red blood cells) results in anemia. If renal failure is caused by an obstruction in the urinary tract, then pain may be an additional symptom.

> ### Infobox
> ....
> **Anatomy and physiology in perspective**
>
> Even if the kidneys are damaged, blood still needs to be cleaned. This can be done through the mechanical process of **kidney dialysis**.

Uremia

Presence of unusually large amounts of nitrogenous wastes, such as urea, in the blood. Signs and symptoms include drowsiness, lethargy, nausea, and vomiting. Uremia is usually caused by renal failure and it can be fatal if left untreated.

Urinary incontinence

Urinary incontinence, more commonly referred to as incontinence, is the involuntary passing of urine. It is more common in the elderly and also more common in women than in men. Incontinence can be caused by weakened pelvic-floor muscles after childbirth or pelvic surgery, menopause, an enlarged prostate, prostate surgery, obesity, constipation, or a variety of psychological factors.

Urinary tract infection (UTI)

An infection anywhere along the urinary tract is called a urinary tract infection (UTI), and it is usually caused by microbes (most commonly bacteria) that enter the urinary tract either via the urethra or via the bloodstream. UTIs are more common in women as they have a shorter urethra than men. UTIs are generally classified as upper or lower UTIs. Upper UTIs are infections of the kidneys (pyelonephritis) or ureters (ureteritis). Lower UTIs are infections of the urethra (urethritis) or bladder (cystitis).

- **Cystitis** is inflammation of the urinary bladder. It is characterized by frequent, burning urination.
- **Pyelonephritis** is inflammation of the kidneys.
- **Ureteritis** is inflammation of the ureters. It often accompanies cystitis.
- **Urethritis** is inflammation of the urethra. It is characterized by painful or difficult urination.

NEW WORDS	
Diuretic	A substance that increases urine production
Electrolyte	A charged particle (ion) that conducts an electrical current in an aqueous solution
Micturition	Urination
Urology	The study of the urinary system

Study Outline

Functions of the urinary system

1. The kidneys are the functional organs of the urinary system and they regulate the volume and composition of blood and produce urine.
2. The kidneys also regulate and balance the pH and pressure of the blood.
3. They secrete calcitriol and erythropoietin and, in times of starvation, produce glucose.
4. They also reabsorb amino acids, small proteins, and glucose.

Organization of the urinary system

The urinary system is made up of two kidneys, two ureters, one urinary bladder, and one urethra.

Kidneys

The kidneys are paired organs located between the levels of the last thoracic and third lumbar vertebrae.

Anatomy of the kidneys

1. Each kidney is encapsulated in three layers of tissue: the outer renal fascia, the intermediate adipose capsule, and the inner renal capsule.
2. Each kidney is shaped like a bean with its concave border facing medially, and it has the following structures:
   - Renal hilum: This is a deep fissure where the ureter leaves the kidney and the blood vessels, lymphatic vessels, and nerves enter and exit
   - Renal sinus: This is a cavity within the kidney
3. Internally, a kidney has three regions:
   - The outer renal cortex, whose renal columns extend into the neighboring region
   - The middle renal medulla, which consists of renal pyramids
   - The inner renal pelvis, which drains into the ureter

Nephrons: The functional units of the kidneys

1. The functional units of the kidneys are nephrons. These are where urine is formed.
2. Once the nephrons have produced the urine it drains into papillary ducts, then minor and major calyces, then the renal pelvis, and eventually into the ureters, which carry it to the bladder.
3. Nephrons consist of a renal corpuscle, which filters blood plasma, and a renal tubule, where secretion and reabsorption take place.
4. Renal corpuscles are composed of a network of capillaries called the glomerulus and a cuplike structure called the glomerular capsule. This is the closed end of the renal tubule.
5. The renal tubule can be divided into three regions: the proximal convoluted tubule, the loop of Henle, and the distal convoluted tubule.

Blood supply to the kidneys and nephrons

1. Blood is brought to the kidneys by the right and left renal arteries and, once inside the kidneys, these divide into a series of arteries that eventually branch into afferent arterioles in the renal cortex.
2. Each nephron receives an afferent arteriole, which divides into the knot of capillaries known as the glomerulus.
3. The glomerular capillaries then reunite to form an efferent arteriole, which takes blood out of the glomerulus.

> Afferent = Arrive
> Efferent = Exit

4. The efferent arteriole then divides into a secondary capillary network called the peritubular capillaries. These capillaries supply the rest of the nephron with oxygen and nutrients.
5. Peritubular capillaries drain into peritubular venules, which then drain into a series of veins until they finally drain into the right and left renal veins, which transport blood away from the kidneys.

Physiology of the kidneys
Urine
Normal constituents of urine include urea, creatinine, uric acid, urobilinogen, and varying quantities of inorganic ions.

Urine production
1. Nephrons regulate the volume and composition of blood through the production of urine.
2. Urine is produced through glomerular filtration, tubular secretion, and tubular reabsorption.
3. In glomerular filtration, blood passes through the capillaries of the glomerulus and fluid and small solutes pass through the filtration membrane into the capsular space. This fluid is now called the glomerular filtrate.
4. In tubular secretion, the cells of the tubule secrete any remaining substances into the filtrate as it passes through the convoluted tubules.
5. In tubular reabsorption, the tubules reabsorb any substances that the body may need and most of the fluid in the filtrate. What is left passes out of the kidneys as urine.
6. Hormones that regulate tubular secretion include parathyroid hormone, calcitonin, and aldosterone.

Fluid and electrolyte balance
1. The kidneys also regulate the fluid and electrolyte balance of the blood and control its pH and pressure.
2. The hormones that help regulate the reabsorption of water and electrolytes by the kidneys are antidiuretic hormone (vasopressin) and aldosterone.
3. Antidiuretic hormone is secreted by the posterior pituitary gland in response to a decrease in water or an increase in solutes in the blood.

4. Antidiuretic hormone decreases the secretion of urine by causing the collecting ducts of the kidneys to reabsorb more water.
5. Aldosterone is secreted by the adrenal cortex and its release is stimulated by either fluctuations in sodium and potassium levels or the renin-angiotensin mechanism.
6. In the renin-angiotensin mechanism, the enzyme renin (produced by the kidneys) catalyzes a series of reactions that produce angiotensin II. Angiotensin II is a molecule that causes vasoconstriction of blood vessels and stimulates the release of aldosterone.

Ureters, bladder, and urethra
1. The ureters are long tubes that carry urine from the kidneys to the bladder.
2. The bladder acts as a reservoir, storing urine until it is excreted out of the body.
3. The urethra is a passageway that functions in discharging urine from the body.

Review

1. Explain the functions of the urinary system.
2. Describe the organization of the urinary system.
3. Describe the structure of the kidneys.
4. Identify the flow of urine from its formation in the nephrons to the external environment.
5. Describe the nephron and explain its functions.
6. Identify two differences between afferent arterioles and efferent arterioles.
7. Describe how urine is produced.
8. Explain the differences between tubular secretion and tubular reabsorption.
9. Identify the hormones that help regulate the reabsorption of water and electrolytes by the kidneys.
10. Describe the following disorders of the urinary system:
    - Renal failure
    - Nephritis
    - Incontinence.

Multiple-Choice Questions

1. The renal hilum is:
   a. The outer protective tissue layer of the kidney
   b. A deep fissure where the ureter leaves the kidney and the blood vessels, lymphatic vessels, and nerves enter and exit
   c. A cavity within the kidney
   d. None of the above

2. Where in the kidneys is urine produced?
   a. The ureters
   b. The calyces
   c. The nephrons
   d. The urethra

3. What is the term used to describe the fluid in the renal tubules?
   a. Filtrate
   b. Solvent
   c. Solution
   d. Solute

4. Another term for kidney failure is:
   a. Nephrotic failure
   b. Oliguria
   c. Renal failure
   d. Renal colic

5. Which of the following statements is correct?
   a. The pancreas functions in controlling the composition, volume, and pressure of blood
   b. The spleen functions in controlling the composition, volume, and pressure of blood
   c. The liver functions in controlling the composition, volume, and pressure of blood
   d. None of the above

6. Functions of the kidneys also include the synthesis of:
   a. Bilirubin
   b. Calcitriol
   c. Vitamin K
   d. Lingual lipase

7. Which of the following statements is correct?
   a. The renal cortex is the outer region of the kidney, the renal pelvis is the middle region of the kidney, and the renal medulla is the inner region
   b. The renal pelvis is the outer region of the kidney, the renal medulla is the middle region of the kidney, and the renal cortex is the inner region
   c. The renal cortex is the outer region of the kidney, the renal medulla is the middle region of the kidney, and the renal pelvis is the inner region
   d. The renal medulla is the outer region of the kidney, the renal cortex is the middle region of the kidney, and the renal pelvis is the inner region

8. Which of the following is the correct sequence of the flow of urine?
   a. Papillary ducts, minor calyces, nephrons, major calyces, bladder, renal pelvis, ureter, urethra, external environment
   b. Nephrons, papillary ducts, minor calyces, major calyces, renal pelvis, urethra, bladder, ureter, external environment
   c. Papillary ducts, minor calyces, nephrons, major calyces, renal pelvis, ureter, bladder, urethra, external environment
   d. Nephrons, papillary ducts, minor calyces, major calyces, renal pelvis, ureter, bladder, urethra, external environment

9. Pyelitis is:
   a. Inflammation of the pelvis of the kidney
   b. Bed-wetting, which is normal in young children
   c. The presence of unusually large amounts of nitrogenous wastes, such as urea, in the blood
   d. The involuntary passing of urine

10. What is the name of the cuplike structure surrounding the glomerulus?
    a. Distal convoluted tubule
    b. Glomerular capsule
    c. Renal medulla
    d. Papillary duct

The Reproductive System

Introduction

Although it is the last system to be discussed, the reproductive system is one of the most fascinating of all. It is the only system in the body that does not work continually from birth. Instead, it waits until puberty, when it bursts into action. It is the only system that is structurally and functionally different in men and women, and it is also the only system in which a unique type of cellular division occurs, creating cells with half the number of chromosomes of all other cells in the body.

Student objectives

By the end of this chapter you will be able to:

*   Describe the functions of the reproductive system
*   Describe meiosis, spermatogenesis, and oogenesis
*   Identify the organs and structures of the male reproductive system
*   Identify the organs and structures of the female reproductive system
*   Explain the female reproductive cycle
*   Explain the effects aging has on the reproductive system
*   Identify some of the common pathologies of the reproductive system.

Functions of the Reproductive System

Reproduction occurs in all living organisms and is the process by which a new member of a species is produced. In humans, the reproductive system is unique in that it is the only system in the body that produces cells that have 23 chromosomes instead of 46 chromosomes. These cells are called reproductive cells.

Reproductive cells are called **gametes** and are produced in the gonads (testes or ovaries) of

men and women. Female gametes are produced through the process of **oogenesis** in the ovaries of a woman and are called **ova** (eggs). Male gametes are produced through the process of **spermatogenesis** in the testes of a man and are called **spermatozoa**, or sperm.

> ### In the classroom
>
> Before continuing with this chapter, it may help to revise somatic cell division (chapter 2). Somatic cell division occurs in most body cells and its function is to replace dead and injured cells or produce new cells for growth. Somatic cell division occurs through a process of nuclear division called **mitosis**, in which a single diploid (containing 46 chromosomes) parent cell duplicates itself to produce two identical diploid daughter cells.

Reproductive cell division occurs through a process of nuclear division called **meiosis**. Unlike in mitosis, in which a cell divides only once to produce two identical diploid daughter cells, in meiosis a cell divides twice to produce four daughter cells. These daughter cells are not identical, and each has only one set of chromosomes (23 chromosomes) instead of the usual two sets (46 chromosomes) that diploid cells have. These new cells, containing only one set of chromosomes, are referred to as **haploid** cells.

A male gamete formed in the male reproductive system then enters the female reproductive system through sexual intercourse. The male and female gametes unite and fuse in a process called **fertilization**. This produces a **zygote**, which is a new cell that now contains two sets of chromosomes (46 chromosomes)—one set from the mother and one from the father. The zygote then begins to divide by mitosis and develops into a new organism.

A REMINDER OF THE KEY DIFFERENCES BETWEEN MITOSIS AND MEIOSIS		
Characteristic	Mitosis	Meiosis
Description	Somatic cell division	Reproductive cell division
Function	For growth and repair of cells	For reproducing a new organism and the continuation of the species
Number of daughter cells produced	Two	Four
Are daughter cells identical?	Yes—exact copies	No—allows for genetic variation
Number of chromosomes in each daughter cell	46 = two sets, diploid number	23 = one set, haploid number

Male Reproductive System

The male reproductive system consists of the testes, which are the gonads where sperm are formed, a system of ducts for transporting and storing sperm, and accessory organs that produce supporting substances.

Scrotum

Structure of the scrotum

The word *scrotum* means "bag," and the scrotum is a sac of loose skin and superficial fascia in which lie the testes. The scrotum hangs from the root of the penis and is divided internally into two sacs. Each sac contains one testis.

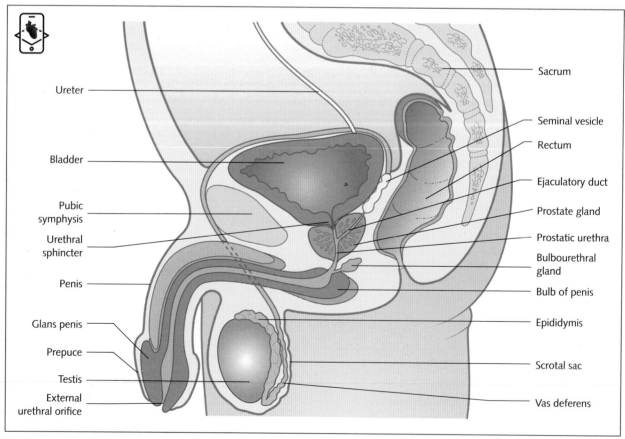

Figure 13.1   *Overview of the male urinary and genital systems (mid-sagittal view)*

Function of the scrotum

The function of the scrotum is to house the testes and maintain a temperature approximately 5°F (3°C) cooler than normal body temperature.

Did you know?

A urologist is a specialist who deals with both the urinary system and the male reproductive system.

Infobox

Anatomy and physiology in perspective

The internal temperature of the body is too high for the functioning of the testes. Thus, they are kept in a small sac hanging outside the body, where it is cooler. This sac is the scrotum.

Testes (testicles)

Structure of the testes

The testes (singular = testis), or testicles, are a pair of oval glands located in the scrotum. They are the gonads of the male reproductive system.

- Each testis is enclosed by a dense, white, fibrous capsule called the **tunica albuginea**, which itself is covered by a serous membrane called the **tunica vaginalis**.
- Extensions of the tunica albuginea divide the testis into 200–300 internal compartments called **lobules**.
- Each of these lobules contains tightly coiled tubules called **seminiferous tubules**. It is here, in these seminiferous tubules, that spermatogenesis occurs and sperm are formed.
  - Specialized cells called **sustentacular cells** are also located in the seminiferous tubules. These cells protect, support, and nourish the sperm and produce the fluid in which sperm are transported. In addition, these cells help regulate the effects of testosterone and follicle-stimulating hormone (FSH)
  - In the spaces between the seminiferous tubules are small clusters of highly specialized cells that secrete **testosterone**. These cells are called **interstitial endocrinocytes (Leydig cells)**

Study tip

The testes produce male sex hormones called **androgens**. The principal androgen is **testosterone**, which:

- Stimulates the development of masculine secondary sex characteriztics such as the development of pubic, axillary, facial, and chest hair; a general thickening of the skin; the skeletal and muscular widening of the shoulders and narrowing of the hips; an increase in sebaceous-oil-gland secretion; and the enlargement of the larynx and subsequent deepening of the voice
- Promotes growth and maturation of the male reproductive system and sperm production
- Promotes male sexual behavior and stimulates libido (sex drive)
- Stimulates anabolism, which is protein synthesis, resulting in heavier muscle and bone mass.

Did you know?

Women also produce androgens, which contribute to their libido. However, they are produced in far smaller quantities than in men and are produced by the adrenal cortex and not by the female gonads.

Did you know?

Over 300 million sperm cells mature every day.

Function of the testes: Spermatogenesis

The testes produce sperm through the process of spermatogenesis. Sperm are highly specialized cells that are able to travel the long journey from the testes, through the male reproductive ducts, into the female reproductive system, and finally into an ovum. They are composed of a **head**, which contains the cell's DNA as well as powerful enzymes that help to penetrate into the ovum; a **midpiece** containing many energy-producing mitochondria; and a **tail**, which propels the sperm toward the ovum.

Epididymis

Structure of the epididymis

From the seminiferous tubules in each testis, sperm travel down a series of tubules and ducts into a comma-shaped organ lying along the posterior border of each testis. This is the epididymis and is composed of a series of coiled ducts that empty into a single tube called the **ductus epididymis**.

Function of the epididymis

The epididymis is the site of sperm maturation. It stores sperm until they are fully mature and then helps propel them via peristaltic contractions.

Vas deferens (ductus deferens, seminal duct)

Structure of the vas deferens

The end of the ductus epididymis straightens and widens and continues as the vas deferens. This is a very long duct that runs from the epididymis into the pelvic cavity, where it loops over the ureter and then over the side and down the posterior surface of the bladder. It finally ends in the urethra.

Function of the vas deferens

The vas deferens transports sperm via peristaltic contractions from the epididymis to the urethra.

Did you know?

The ductus epididymis is so tightly coiled that it appears to be only approximately 1½ in (4 cm) long. However, when uncoiled, it measures up to 20 feet (6 m).

Infobox

Anatomy and physiology in perspective

A vasectomy is the surgical removal of a portion of the vas deferens, and it results in sterility.

Spermatic cord

Running alongside the vas deferens is a supporting structure consisting of blood vessels, lymphatic vessels, nerves, and muscles. This structure is called the spermatic cord.

Urethra

Structure of the urethra

The urethra is the terminal duct of both the reproductive and urinary systems and is made up of three sections:

- The **prostatic urethra** runs through the prostate gland (to be discussed shortly).
- The **membranous urethra** runs through the urogenital diaphragm.
- The **spongy** (**penile**) **urethra** runs through the penis and terminates in the external urethral orifice.

Function of the urethra

The urethra transports both semen and urine to the exterior of the body.

Did you know?

Between ½–1 tsp (2.5 and 5 ml) of semen is ejaculated at one time and usually contains 50–150 million sperm per milliliter. However, only one sperm will get to fertilize an egg.

Accessory sex glands and semen

The word *semen* means "seed," and **semen** is the fluid in which sperm, their nutrients, and other supporting substances are transported. It is a slightly alkaline, milky substance that is sticky to touch.

Closely associated with the urethra are a number of glands whose secretions enter the urethra via small ducts. The fluids of these glands combine with sperm to produce semen:

- **Seminal vesicles:** These are paired pouch-like structures located at the base of the bladder. They secrete a viscous alkaline fluid that helps neutralize the acidity of the vagina. This fluid contains fructose, which the sperm use for energy production; prostaglandins, which help sperm mobility and also stimulate muscular contractions of the female reproductive tract; and clotting proteins that coagulate sperm after ejaculation.
- **Prostate gland:** This is a doughnut-shaped gland that surrounds the prostatic urethra. It secretes a milky, slightly acidic fluid that contributes to sperm mobility and viability.

- **Bulbourethral (Cowper's) glands:** These are paired pea-sized structures located on either side of the membranous urethra. They secrete a lubricating mucus and an alkaline substance that neutralizes the acidity of urine in the urethra and lubricates the end of the penis and the lining of the urethra. Together, this protects sperm from being damaged during ejaculation.

Penis

Structure of the penis

The penis is a cylindrical organ composed of erectile tissue permeated by blood sinuses. When sexually stimulated, arteries supplying the penis dilate and large quantities of blood enter the sinuses, which then expand. In expanding, these sinuses compress any veins that normally drain the penis and so the blood in the penis becomes trapped. This is an erection of the penis.

Three regions make up the penis:

- The **root** is the region attached to the trunk of the body.
- The **shaft (body)** is the main cylindrical region of the penis.
- The **glans penis** is the highly sensitive, acorn-shaped enlargement at the distal end of the penis and it contains a slit-like opening called the **external urethral orifice**. Enclosing the glans penis is a loosely fitting fold of tissue called the **prepuce (foreskin)**.

Infobox

Anatomy and physiology in perspective

Circumcision is the surgical removal of the prepuce (foreskin).

Functions of the penis

The functions of the penis are to excrete urine and ejaculate semen. During ejaculation, the sphincter muscle at the base of the urinary bladder closes to prevent any urine passing into the urethra.

Female Reproductive System

The female reproductive system is specially structured not only to produce gametes, but also to house, nourish, and nurture a growing fetus. It consists of the ovaries, which are the gonads where ova are formed; the Fallopian tubes, where an ovum is fertilized and, once fertilized, becomes a zygote; the uterus, where a zygote develops into a fetus; and the vagina, through which the fetus enters into the world.

Did you know?

A gynecologist is a specialist who deals with the female reproductive system.

Ovaries

Structure of the ovaries

The female gonads, or ovaries, are paired almond-shaped organs located in the superior portion of the pelvic cavity on either side of the uterus. They are held in place by a series of ligaments and a fold of the peritoneum called the **broad ligament**. Inside the ovaries are small sac-like structures called **ovarian follicles**.

- Each follicle houses an **oocyte** (an immature ovum) in its differing stages of development. The follicle also contains cells that nourish the oocyte and begin to secrete estrogens as it enlarges.
- The follicle enlarges as the oocyte matures and eventually develops into a mature **Graafian follicle (vesicular ovarian follicle)**. This is a large, fluid-filled follicle that soon ruptures and expels the ovum in a process called **ovulation** (to be discussed later in this chapter).
- After expelling the ovum, the now empty follicle develops into a glandular structure called the **corpus luteum**. For the first 10–14 days after ovulation the corpus luteum produces the female hormones **progesterone, estrogen, relaxin,** and **inhibin**.
- The corpus luteum finally degenerates into a white fibrous tissue called the **corpus albicans**.

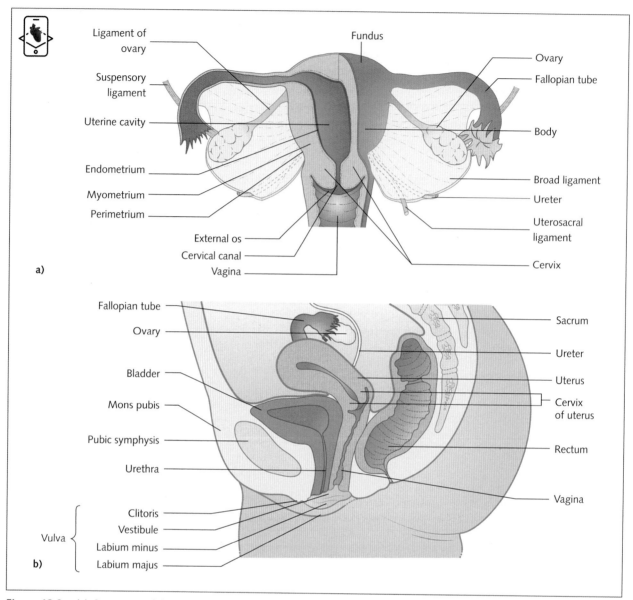

Figure 13.2 *(a) Overview of the female reproductive organs (anterior view); (b) overview of the female urinary and genital systems (mid-sagittal view)*

Study tip

···

Estrogens and **progesterone** are the principal female sex hormones and are produced mainly by the ovaries, although small amounts are also produced by the adrenal cortex, testes, and placenta.

Estrogens are secreted mainly by the follicle cells that nourish the oocyte, and they:

- Stimulate the development and maintenance of feminine secondary sex characteriztics such as enlarged breasts, the pattern of hair growth on the head and body, a broadened pelvis, and the distribution of adipose tissue over the abdomen and hips
- Help regulate the fluid and electrolyte balance and lower blood cholesterol levels
- Increase protein anabolism.

Progesterone is secreted mainly by the corpus luteum and works together with estrogens to prepare the uterus for pregnancy and the mammary glands for lactation.

Inhibin is a hormone that inhibits the secretion of follicle-stimulating hormone (FSH), and relaxin is a hormone that is produced by both the ovaries and placenta during pregnancy. It helps dilate the cervix and increase the flexibility of the pubic symphysis during childbirth.

Functions of the ovaries: Oogenesis and ovulation

The ovaries have two functions: oogenesis and ovulation.

Oogenesis is the process through which the ovaries produce ova, or eggs. This occurs in two stages.

- Firstly, during fetal development germ cells differentiate into millions of immature eggs called **primary oocytes**, and at birth a woman has all the oocytes she will ever have.
- Secondly, the release of gonadotropic hormones at puberty stimulates meiosis of a primary oocyte. This occurs in one oocyte, in one follicle, each month after puberty. The primary oocyte develops into a **secondary oocyte**, or **ovum**, and the follicle in which this development occurs is the mature Graafian follicle.

Ovulation is the process by which a mature Graafian follicle releases an ovum. The released ovum then travels down the Fallopian tube toward the uterus. Ovulation will be discussed in more detail later in the chapter.

Did you know?

A baby girl is born with between 200,000 and 2 million oocytes in each ovary. However, many of these degenerate and only about 400 will actually mature and be viable for ovulation.

Fallopian (uterine) tubes

Structure of the Fallopian tubes

The Fallopian tubes are two thin tubes running from the ovaries to the uterus. They are composed of:

- An outer **serous membrane**.
- An intermediate **muscularis** consisting of both circular and longitudinal smooth muscle fibers, which contract rhythmically to move the ovum via peristalsis.
- An internal **mucosa** lined with cilia that help move a fertilized ovum toward the uterus; the mucosa also contains secretory cells, which provide nutrition for the ovum during its journey.

Functions of the Fallopian tubes

The Fallopian tubes have two functions:

- They are the site of fertilization, when sperm and ovum unite and fuse to form a zygote.
- They transport the zygote to the uterus. It takes approximately seven days for the zygote to travel down a tube and into the uterus.

Uterus (womb)

Structure of the uterus

The uterus, or womb, is a muscular sac located between the bladder and rectum. It is approximately the size and shape of an inverted pear and is divided into three regions:

- The **fundus** is the dome-shaped region superior to the Fallopian tubes.
- The **body** is the central portion of the uterus.
- The **cervix** is the inferior portion, or neck, of the uterus, which forms the narrow opening to the vagina. It is lined with mucus-secreting cells that produce a mixture of water, proteins, lipids, enzymes, and inorganic salts. This is called **cervical mucus** and approximately 4–12 tsp (20–60 ml) is produced each day.

Infobox

Anatomy and physiology in perspective

Cervical cancer is often called the "quiet killer" because it has few symptoms until it is in its later stages. However, it can be detected early in its development through a **Pap smear**. In this procedure, cells are removed from the cervix and from the vaginal area surrounding the cervix and then examined microscopically. Malignant cells have a characteristic appearance that can be easily identified.

The walls of the uterus are composed of three layers of tissue:

- **Outer perimetrium (serosa):** This is continuous with the visceral peritoneum and extends laterally to become the broad ligaments, which attach the uterus to the pelvic cavity.
- **Intermediate myometrium:** This is the muscular layer forming the bulk of the uterine wall. It is composed of layers of circular,

longitudinal, and oblique smooth muscle fibers that, under the influence of the hormone oxytocin, contract powerfully to expel the fetus during childbirth.

- **Inner endometrium:** This is a highly vascularized layer of tissue that forms the lining of the uterus. It is divided into two layers:
  - **Stratum functionalis:** This is the functional layer of the endometrium and is the layer closest to the uterine cavity. The stratum functionalis is shed during menstruation (to be discussed later in this chapter)
  - **Stratum basalis:** This is the permanent base layer of the endometrium. It produces a new stratum functionalis after each menstruation

Functions of the uterus

Before fertilization, the uterus acts as a pathway through which sperm travel into the Fallopian tubes, where they attempt to fertilize an ovum.

If fertilization is successful, then the uterus becomes the site of implantation of a zygote and houses the developing fetus throughout pregnancy. It then contracts forcefully during labor to expel the fetus.

If, however, fertilization is not successful, the uterus becomes the site of **menstruation**. This is the process by which the lining of the uterus, the stratum functionalis, is shed and discarded. Menstruation will be discussed in more detail later in this chapter.

Vagina

Structure of the vagina

The vagina is a muscular tube located between the bladder and rectum and attached to the uterus. The walls of the vagina are composed of three layers:

- **Outer adventitia:** This is composed of areolar connective tissue and it anchors the vagina to its adjacent organs.
- **Intermediate muscularis:** This comprises layers of circular and longitudinal smooth muscle fibers that are able to stretch immensely during childbirth.
- **Inner mucosa:** This is continuous with that of the uterus and it lies in a series of transverse folds called **rugae**. It secretes an acidic mucus, which retards microbial growth but which also harms sperm.

The opening of the vagina to the external environment is called the **vaginal orifice**. It is protected by a thin mucous membrane called the **hymen**, which partially occludes it. The hymen is usually ruptured during one's first sexual intercourse. Occasionally, the hymen completely occludes the vaginal orifice. This condition is called an imperforate hymen.

Functions of the vagina

The vagina acts as a passageway for:

- Blood during menstruation
- Semen during sexual intercourse
- The fetus during childbirth.

Vulva (external female genitalia)

The word *volvere* means "to wrap around" and the vulva are the fleshy folds surrounding the opening to the vagina. They are also referred to as the female external genitalia, and consist of the:

- **Mons pubis:** This is an elevation of adipose tissue that cushions the pubic symphysis. It is covered by skin and protected by coarse pubic hair.
- **Labia majora:** These are two longitudinal folds of skin that are covered by pubic hair and contain adipose tissue, sebaceous glands, and sudoriferous glands. They extend inferiorly and posteriorly from the mons pubis.
- **Labia minora:** These are two smaller folds of skin running medially to the labia majora. They contain many sebaceous glands but no adipose tissue and very few sudoriferous glands. They are not covered by hair.
- **Clitoris:** This is a small, cylindrical mass of erectile tissue and nerves. It enlarges on tactile stimulation and is found at the anterior junction of the labia minora.
- **Vestibule:** This is the entire region between the labia minora and it consists of the vaginal orifice and external urethral orifice. It also houses the openings to several ducts, including those from:
  - The mucus-secreting **paraurethral (Skene's) glands** located on either side of the urethral orifice

- The mucus-secreting **greater vestibular (Bartholin's) glands** located on either side of the vaginal orifice
- Several lesser vestibular glands

Perineum

The perineum is a diamond-shaped area that contains the external genitals and the anus. It is located between the thighs and buttocks and is present in both males and females.

Mammary glands

Structure of the mammary glands

The mammary glands, or breasts, are two modified sudoriferous glands. They are located over the pectoralis major muscles and are attached to them by a layer of dense irregular connective tissue.

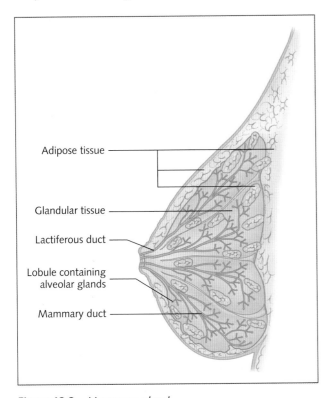

Adipose tissue

Glandular tissue

Lactiferous duct

Lobule containing alveolar glands

Mammary duct

Figure 13.3 *Mammary gland*

Internally, a breast is supported by strands of connective tissue called **suspensory (Cooper's) ligaments** and is composed of compartments separated by adipose tissue. These compartments are called **lobes,** and inside each lobe are smaller compartments called **lobules.** Lobules contain grape-like milk-secreting glands called **alveolar glands,** which secrete milk into secondary tubules, which drain into the **mammary ducts.** It is then stored temporarily and excreted externally through **lactiferous ducts,** via the nipple. Externally, each breast has:

- **A nipple:** This is a pigmented projection of tiny openings leading from lactiferous ducts.
- **An areola:** This is a circular area of pigmented skin surrounding the nipple and contains modified sebaceous oil glands.

Functions of the mammary glands

The mammary glands synthesize and secrete milk through the process of **lactation.**

The production of milk is stimulated by the hormone **prolactin** (with smaller contributions from progesterone and estrogens) and the ejection of milk is stimulated by the hormone **oxytocin,** whose release is stimulated by the suckling action of the baby on the breast.

Female reproductive cycle

Every month after the onset of puberty a woman's body prepares itself for possible pregnancy through a series of events called the **reproductive cycle.** The reproductive cycle lasts anywhere from 24 to 35 days and involves:

- An **ovarian cycle,** in which an oocyte matures until it is ready for ovulation
- A **uterine (menstrual) cycle,** in which the endometrium of the uterus is prepared for the arrival of a fertilized ovum.

If fertilization does not occur, the stratum functionalis of the endometrium is then shed and **menstruation** occurs. The chart following highlights the major phases of these two cycles and is based on an average 28-day reproductive cycle.

Female hormones in a nutshell

- **Estrogens**—necessary for reproductive and sexual development
- **Progesterone**—prepares the body for pregnancy
- **Testosterone**—increases bone and muscle strength as well as sexual desire
- **Follicle-stimulating hormone (FSH)**—stimulates ovarian follicles to grow

- **Luteinizing hormone (LH)**—stimulates rupture of the mature Graafian follicle and development of the corpus luteum
- **Inhibin**—inhibits secretion of FSH
- **Relaxin**—helps prepare a pregnant woman's body for childbirth

FEMALE REPRODUCTIVE CYCLE

Hormonal regulation	Ovarian cycle	Uterine (menstrual) cycle

Menstrual phase (menstruation, menses)

The word *menses* means "month" and menstruation marks the beginning of a woman's monthly cycle. Menstruation normally lasts approximately 5 days and the first day of menstruation is termed day 1 of a woman's cycle

Before menstruation begins, a woman's uterus, especially the stratum functionalis of the endometrium, is prepared to receive a fertilized ovum. If it does not receive a fertilized ovum, levels of estrogens and progesterone decline and the stratum functionalis dies and is discharged from the body via menstrual flow

Hormonal regulation	Ovarian cycle	Uterine (menstrual) cycle
- Declining levels of estrogens and progesterone cause uterine arteries to constrict and endometrial cells to become deficient in blood - These cells eventually die and the entire stratum functionalis of the endometrium is sloughed off	Approximately 20 small follicles, some in each ovary, begin to enlarge	Menstrual flow (consisting of blood, tissue fluid, mucus, and epithelial cells derived from the endometrium) is discharged from the vagina

Preovulatory phase

The preovulatory phase is the time between menstruation and ovulation. In a 28-day cycle it is usually 6–13 days in length. In this phase a mature Graafian follicle forms and the endometrium proliferates

Hormonal regulation	Ovarian cycle	Uterine (menstrual) cycle
- Follicle-stimulating hormone (FSH) from the anterior pituitary gland stimulates follicles to grow - These growing follicles then secrete higher levels of estrogens and inhibin, which in turn decrease FSH secretion	- The follicles continue to develop and around day 6, one follicle in one ovary outgrows the other follicles - This becomes the dominant follicle, which is now called the mature Graafian follicle (vesicular follicle) and which continues to enlarge until ovulation - The other follicles begin to degenerate - The menstrual and preovulatory phases are called the **follicular phase** of the ovarian cycle	- Estrogen secreted by the follicles stimulates the repair of the endometrium, which now thickens and proliferates - This phase is also called the **proliferative phase** of the uterine cycle

FEMALE REPRODUCTIVE CYCLE

Hormonal regulation	Ovarian cycle	Uterine (menstrual) cycle

Ovulation

Ovulation usually occurs around day 14 of a 28-day cycle and involves the rupture of the mature Graafian follicle and the release of an ovum into the pelvic cavity. It is during this phase that a woman can now become pregnant

• High levels of estrogens stimulate the hypothalamus to release gonadotropin-releasing hormone (GnRH), which stimulates the anterior pituitary gland to release FSH and luteinizing hormone (LH) • Note that progesterone levels are now low	• LH stimulates the rupture of the mature Graafian follicle and the release of the ovum into the pelvic cavity • The follicle then develops into the corpus luteum, which, under the influence of LH, secretes progesterone, estrogens, relaxin, and inhibin	The prepared endometrium waits for the arrival of a fertilized ovum

Postovulatory phase

The 14 days after ovulation form the postovulatory phase. This is a "waiting time" in which the endometrium awaits the arrival of a fertilized ovum. It is now thickened, highly vascularized, and secreting tissue fluid and glycogen. Thus, this phase is also called the **secretory phase** of the uterine cycle or the **luteal phase** of the ovarian cycle

If fertilization has occurred, the ovum takes approximately a week to arrive at the endometrium, where it becomes embedded and develops into a fetus. At this stage a woman is now pregnant

If fertilization has not occurred, menstruation and the reproductive cycle begin again

- The corpus luteum survives approximately two weeks and secretes increasing amounts of progesterone and some estrogens
- If fertilization has occurred, the corpus luteum (and the hormones it secretes) remains longer than two weeks and is maintained by human chorionic gonadotropin (hCG), a hormone produced by the embryo approximately 8–12 days after fertilization
- Once the embryo is implanted in the endometrium, the hormones of pregnancy come into effect
- If fertilization has not occurred, the corpus luteum degenerates and the lack of progesterone and estrogens causes menstruation

Study tip

It is easy to become confused when learning about the female reproductive cycle, so it helps to remember that this cycle actually involves two smaller cycles: the ovarian cycle and the uterine cycle:

	Before ovulation	OVULATION	After ovulation
Uterine cycle	Menstrual AND proliferative phases		Secretory phase
Ovarian cycle	Follicular phase		Luteal phase

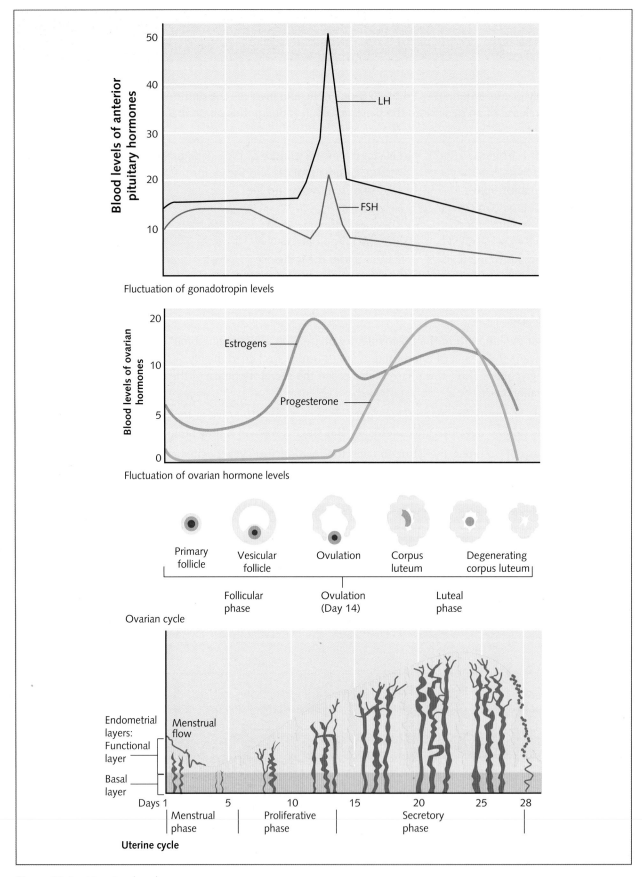

Figure 13.4 *Menstrual cycle*

Aging and the Reproductive System

Unlike any other system in the body, the reproductive system appears to be dormant until a child reaches approximately 10 years of age. From this age, hormone-directed changes occur and the child goes through **puberty**. The word *puber* means "marriageable age" and puberty is the time in which a person develops secondary sexual characteriztics and becomes able to reproduce.

Aging and the male reproductive system

Puberty

Before puberty, which occurs around the age of 14, a boy has low levels of LH, FSH, and testosterone, and it is only at puberty that the levels of these hormones begin to increase under the influence of GnRH from the hypothalamus. Sustentacular cells in the testes mature and secrete testosterone, and spermatogenesis begins.

Increased levels of testosterone bring about the development of secondary sexual characteriztics, the enlargement of the reproductive glands, and both muscular and bone growth.

Old age

From around the age of 55 years, testosterone levels begin to decline and men lose their muscular strength. Their sperm also become less viable and their libido decreases. However, healthy men are still able to reproduce into their eighties and sometimes even their nineties.

Aging and the female reproductive system

Puberty

Before puberty, a girl has low levels of LH, FSH, and estrogens. However, under the influence of GnRH at the onset of puberty, LH and FSH stimulate the ovaries to produce estrogens and girls then develop secondary sexual characteriztics and begin menstruating. This event is marked by **menarche**, which is a girl's first menses around the age of 12 years.

Pregnancy

Once a woman has begun to menstruate, she is capable of falling pregnant. Pregnancy is the sequence of fertilization, implantation, embryonic growth, and fetal growth.

An average pregnancy lasts 40 weeks from the first day of the woman's last menstrual period (approximately 38 weeks from conception) and is divided into three trimesters, each trimester being made up of approximately three months.

Trimester 1, months 0–3
During the first trimester the embryo implants and secures itself in the uterus. It grows from a single cell into a fully formed fetus in only 12 weeks, and by the end of the first trimester it has all its organs, muscles, limbs, and bones.

Trimester 2, months 4–6
The fetus is now fully formed and just growing and maturing. During the second trimester it develops its individual fingerprints, its toe- and fingernails, its eyebrows and lashes, and a firm hand grip. It is in this trimester that it even starts grimacing and frowning.

Trimester 3, month 7–birth
During the third trimester the fetus develops its sense of hearing, practices its breathing motions, and learns to focus and blink its eyes. It is fully formed and puts on a great deal of weight in the last few weeks.

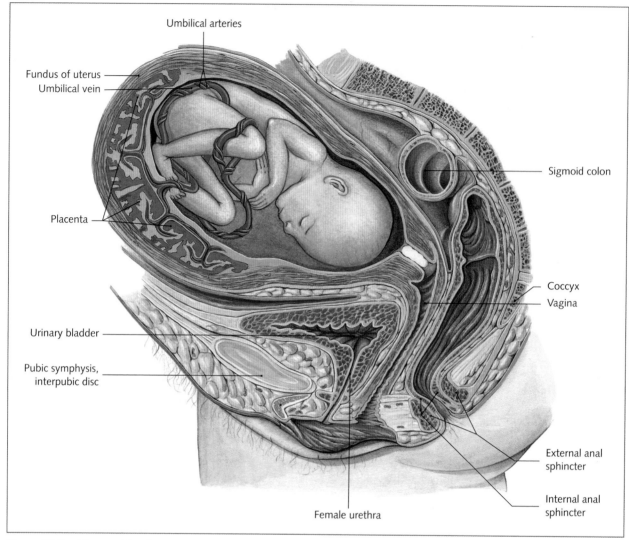

Figure 13.5 *Uterus with a fetus*

Menopause

Although men are capable of reproducing well into old age, women are only capable of reproducing into their forties or fifties. At this age they go through **menopause**, which is the cessation of the menses. Menopause is often called the "change of life" and can be accompanied by a number of signs and symptoms, including hot flushes, headaches, thinning of hair and skin, sweating, vaginal dryness, decreased bone density, insomnia, weight gain, and mood swings. After menopause, a woman's reproductive organs begin to atrophy.

Infobox

····································

Anatomy and physiology in perspective

The symptoms of menopause can sometimes be unbearable for a woman and one form of treatment for these symptoms is hormone replacement therapy (HRT). Estrogenic hormones, or a combination of estrogens and progestin (a drug similar to the hormone progesterone), can be used. HRT has a number of benefits, but it also has risks and it is up to a woman and her doctor to decide on the best course of treatment for her menopausal symptoms.

Common Pathologies of the Reproductive System

Male reproductive system—red flags

- Isolated swellings, nodules, or cysts (not necessarily painful)
- Painful swellings or scrotal pain, especially if accompanied by tenderness, warmth, redness, or discoloration
- Sores that do not heal
- Purulent urethral discharge or bleeding
- Blood in the semen for more than one month
- Erectile dysfunction accompanied by numbness or paresthesia in the groin/saddle area
- Persistent abnormal erection without sexual desire (priapism), especially if accompanied by pain, fever, and night sweats, or following a recent trauma
- The cause of any unusual genito-urinary symptoms or any sexually transmitted infections in children should be investigated, especially if there are other signs or concerns of sexual abuse.

Benign prostatic hyperplasia (BPH)

Benign (non-cancerous) enlargement of the prostate gland. This enlargement leads to a difficulty in urination, incomplete urination, and a consequent susceptibility to kidney stones and urinary tract infections. BPH is more common in older men and is thought to be linked to changes in testosterone levels.

Epididymitis

Inflammation of the epididymis commonly caused by a groin injury or an infection such as a sexually transmitted bacterium or mumps. Chemical epididymitis occurs when urine flows backward in the epididymis because of heavy lifting or straining. Signs and symptoms of epididymitis can include testicular pain, swelling, inflammation, penile discharge, or bleeding. There may also be discomfort or pain in the lower abdomen, and urination may be accompanied by pain, urgency, or increased frequency.

Impotence (erectile dysfunction)

Continual inability to either achieve or maintain an erection. It is sometimes caused by diseases affecting the circulation—for example, atherosclerosis or diabetes—or it can be due to nerve damage or illness, fatigue, or stress.

Penile cancer

Condition where malignant cells form in the tissues of the penis. Signs of penile cancer can include thickening of skin, a change in skin color, a lump, a sore, or a rash. Bleeding or discharge may also occur. Risk factors for penile cancer are human papillomavirus (HPV) infection, human immunodeficiency virus (HIV) infection, poor hygiene, and cigarette smoking. Circumcision is thought to help protect against penile cancer.

Prostate cancer

Very slow growing cancer that begins as a small bump in the prostate gland. It usually causes no symptoms until it is in its advanced stages, and then signs and symptoms can include difficulty in urinating, the need to urinate frequently or urgently, and, in advanced cases, blood in the urine or the inability to urinate. The causes of prostate cancer are not yet known.

Prostatitis

Inflammation of the prostate gland and characterized by spasms of the muscles in the bladder and pelvis; pain in the lower back, perineum, penis, and testes; and the urge to urinate frequently and burning or painful urination. Prostatitis is usually caused by a bacterial infection.

Testicular cancer

Cancer of the testes characterized by an irregularly shaped testis with a solid, growing lump either in the testis or, sometimes, elsewhere in the scrotum. The cause of testicular cancer is not known, but it is more common in men whose testes did not descend into the scrotum in early childhood.

Female reproductive system—red flags

- Vaginal discharge that is accompanied by changes in color (white or clear is normal), itching, pain, or a strong smell
- Pain during sexual intercourse (dyspareunia)

- Bleeding
  - During or after sexual intercourse
  - Between menstrual periods
  - After menopause
- Absence or cessation of menstrual periods for no known reason
- Pelvic or lower abdominal pain for no apparent reason—especially if pain is deep and persistent
- Lymphadenopathy of inguinal nodes
- Urinary incontinence
- Development of male-pattern hair growth and other masculine physical traits (virilization)
- Vaginal bleeding or pelvic pain accompanied by fever, chills, nausea, vomiting, low blood pressure, tachycardia, or fainting
- The cause of any unusual genito-urinary symptoms or any sexually transmitted infections in children should be investigated, especially if there are other signs or concerns of sexual abuse.

The following breast symptoms should be examined by a medical professional as they are suggestive of breast cancer:

- Solid lumps (these can be painless)
- Tissue and skin changes such as dimpling, pitting, or thickening (tissue may resemble "orange peel")
- Sores that do not heal
- Swelling, warmth, tenderness
- Redness or discoloration of the breast
- Eczema of the nipple or areola
- Development of an indrawn nipple
- Bleeding or discharge from the nipple.

Breast cancer
Malignant tumor of the breast that is far more common in women than men. There are different types of breast cancer, but they usually present with a lump in one breast that feels distinctly different from the surrounding tissue. If the cancer is in its more advanced stages, signs and symptoms can also include swollen bumps and sores developing on the breasts, and the skin over the lump taking on a dimpled and leathery appearance. Some of the risk factors for developing breast cancer include old age, a family history of breast cancer, and never having had a baby.

Candidiasis (candidosis, thrush, yeast infection)
Please refer to chapter 3.

Cervical cancer
Cancer of the cervix caused by the human papillomavirus (HPV), which is transmitted through sexual intercourse. Thus, women at risk of cervical cancer are those who have had a number of different sexual partners. Cervical cancer begins on the surface of the cervix and does not usually have any signs or symptoms until it is in its later stages. Signs can then include unusually heavy bleeding during menstruation, bleeding between periods, or bleeding after intercourse.

Ectopic (extrauterine) pregnancy
In an ectopic pregnancy, a fetus develops outside the uterus. The most usual location of an ectopic pregnancy is a Fallopian tube, and it usually occurs if the Fallopian tube in which the ovum was fertilized is narrowed or blocked and the ovum becomes stuck. The fetus of an ectopic pregnancy cannot survive. Risk factors for an ectopic pregnancy include having a disorder of the Fallopian tubes, a history of pelvic inflammatory disease, or a previous ectopic pregnancy, and signs and symptoms include cramping with unexpected vaginal bleeding.

Endometriosis
Disorder in which endometrial tissue—usually found only lining the uterus—develops outside the uterus on other pelvic organs, such as the ovaries or large intestine. Signs and symptoms of endometriosis include lower abdominal and pelvic pain, an irregular menstrual cycle, and often severe bleeding and cramping during menstruation. Its cause is still unknown.

Fibroids
Non-cancerous (benign) tumors consisting of muscle and fibrous tissue. One or more fibroids can develop in the muscular wall of the uterus and cause signs and symptoms such as pain, a sense of pressure or heaviness in the pelvic area, and excessive menstrual bleeding.

Infertility
Inability of a couple to conceive a baby after trying for at least one year. Either the man or the woman may be infertile and infertility can be caused by a number of factors, including problems with ovulation, sperm or the Fallopian tubes. If a couple are infertile they can try to conceive with the help of fertility drugs or fertilization techniques such as in

vitro fertilization (IVF). In IVF, eggs are taken out of a woman's body and fertilized in a laboratory. Once they have been fertilized successfully, the resultant embryos are implanted into the woman's uterus.

Infobox

Anatomy and physiology in perspective

The aim of oral fertility medications is to increase pituitary secretion of FSH and LH in order to stimulate egg growth. Clomiphene achieves this by blocking estrogen receptors, while letrozole blocks an enzyme necessary for estrogen synthesis.

Mastitis

Inflammation of the breast usually caused by a bacterial infection. It is rare except for around the time of childbirth or after an injury or surgery to the breast. Signs and symptoms of mastitis include swelling, redness, warmth, and tenderness.

Menstrual disorders

Although every woman has a slightly different menstrual cycle, it is not normal to have extremely heavy or painful periods or to have no periods at all. There are many different menstrual disorders, including:

- **Abnormal uterine bleeding:** Includes menstruation of excessive duration or amount, diminished menstrual flow, intermenstrual or too-frequent menstrual bleeding, and postmenopausal bleeding. Abnormal uterine bleeding can be caused by a number of factors, including hormonal disorders, emotional factors, or fibroids.
- **Amenorrhea:** Absence of a menstrual period and can be due to obesity or extreme weight loss, or abnormal levels of estrogens due to deficiencies of pituitary or ovarian hormones.
- **Dysmenorrhea:** Severe pain associated with menstruation. It can also be accompanied by headaches, nausea, diarrhea, or constipation, and the urge to urinate frequently. Dysmenorrhea is often caused by another disorder, such as pelvic inflammatory disease, endometriosis, or fibroids.
- **Menorrhagia:** Abnormally heavy bleeding during menstruation. It is usually associated with other conditions, such as fibroids, pelvic inflammatory disease, or endometriosis.
- **Premenstrual syndrome (PMS), premenstrual tension (PMT):** Common syndrome that affects many women. It refers to both a physical and an emotional distress that occurs late in the postovulatory phase of the menstrual cycle and sometimes extends into the menstrual phase. Signs and symptoms can include edema, weight gain, breast swelling and tenderness, abdominal distension, backache, joint pain, constipation, skin eruptions, fatigue and lethargy, depression or anxiety, irritability, mood swings, food cravings, headaches, and poor coordination and clumsiness.

Pelvic inflammatory disease (PID)

Collective term for any infection of the pelvic organs. It is usually caused by bacteria and is more common in sexually active women. Signs and symptoms of PID tend to be cyclical, usually occurring around the end of menstruation, and can include fever, abdominal pain, irregular vaginal bleeding, and a foul-smelling vaginal discharge.

Polycystic ovary syndrome (PCOS) (Stein–Leventhal syndrome)

Hormonal disorder in which follicles fail to ovulate and collect as cysts over the ovaries. Women with PCOS have unusually high levels of androgens and often develop male secondary 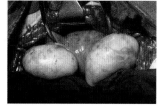 sexual characteriztics such as chest and facial hair, a decrease in breast size, and an increase in muscle size. Other signs can include acne, weight gain, and irregular vaginal bleeding.

Polycystic ovary syndrome

Postnatal (postpartum) depression

Depression that can occur in the first few weeks or months after childbirth. A few weeks of "baby blues" is normal after giving birth, but a feeling of extreme sadness that lasts for weeks or even months is not normal and is referred to as depression. The exact causes of postnatal depression are unknown, but it is linked to the sudden change in hormone levels, the lack of sleep, and the stresses of having to care for a newborn baby.

Pre-eclampsia

Pregnancy-related complication that can arise after 20 weeks' gestation, and because it is asymptomatic it is important that pregnant women are regularly screened by their doctor. Pre-eclampsia is characterized by high blood pressure accompanied by protein in the urine, and it can develop into seizures (eclampsia) if not controlled.

Prolapsed uterus

Uterus that has dropped downward from its normal position. Either only the cervix may have dropped downward, or the entire uterus may have dropped down through the vagina. The most common symptom of a prolapsed uterus is a feeling of heaviness or pressure in the vagina. A prolapsed uterus can be caused by weakness or injury to the ligaments, connective tissue, and muscles of the pelvis, and it can result from pregnancy, vaginal delivery of a fetus, chronic coughing, obesity, straining during bowel movements, or even lifting an extremely heavy object.

Toxic shock syndrome

State of shock due to poisoning, usually caused by toxins produced by staphylococci bacteria on foreign objects, such as tampons, that have been put into the body. The signs and symptoms of toxic shock syndrome are sudden and severe and include a high fever, headache, fatigue, sore throat, red eyes, confusion, low blood pressure, vomiting, and diarrhea.

Vaginitis

Inflammation of the lining of the vagina characterized by itching, painful urination, and increased vaginal discharge. Vaginitis can be caused by a bacterial or fungal infection, and can also be the result of poor hygiene, not cleaning the genital area properly, or wearing tight and non-absorbent underwear.

Sexually transmitted infections (STIs, STDs, venereal disease)

Encompasses all diseases that are transmitted through sexual intercourse, and these can affect both men and women. Many STIs may be asymptomatic and can therefore be passed from one partner to another with neither of them knowing. Certain STIs don't have genital signs or symptoms but affect other organs in the body. For example, hepatitis B virus affects the liver, and HIV affects the immune system. Generalized signs and symptoms suggesting a possible STI include:

- Discharge from the penis, vagina, or anus, especially if it is purulent
- Pain during sexual intercourse, urination, or bowel movements
- Lower abdominal or pelvic pain
- Genital lumps or ulceration
- Genital itching, irritation, or odor
- Bleeding between menstrual periods or after sexual intercourse.

Chlamydia

Common sexually transmitted infection caused by the bacterium *Chlamydia trachomatis*. Signs and symptoms are similar to those of gonorrhea but much milder. Infected women are often asymptomatic or may present with pain during intercourse, frequent and painful urination, and vaginal discharge. Infected men may experience frequent and painful urination and a clear or purulent urethral discharge.

Gonorrhea

Sexually transmitted infection caused by the bacterium *Neisseria gonorrheae*. Transmission is via vaginal, anal, or oral sex, and infected mothers may pass the bacterium to their babies during childbirth, resulting in gonococcal conjunctivitis. There are no signs or symptoms in 80% of infected women (Colledge et al., 2010), although some women can present with frequent and painful urination, vaginal discharge, and fever. Men, on the other hand, usually have a purulent urethral discharge and pain on urination. Symptoms of rectal infection include discomfort around the anus and rectal discharge.

Human papillomavirus (HPV) infection

There are more than 100 types of human papillomavirus and they produce epithelial tumors such as warts. Sexually transmitted strains of HPV cause anogenital warts and also play a significant role in the development of cervical, penile, and anal cancers.

Syphilis

Sexually transmitted infection caused by the bacterium *Treponema pallidum*. It has an incubation period of 14–28 days and then progresses through four different stages:

- **Primary syphilis:** This is characterized by the development of a painless sore (called a chancre) at the site of infection.
- **Secondary syphilis:** A skin rash develops six to eight weeks after the chancre. This is often accompanied by mild fevers, headaches, and a sense of malaise.
- **Latent syphilis:** The infection continues but there are no signs or symptoms. This stage may last for many years.
- **Tertiary syphilis:** The infected person is no longer contagious. There are three main types of tertiary syphilis:
  - **Benign:** In benign tertiary syphilis a person develops slow-growing lumps called gummas that heal slowly and cause scars
  - **Cardiovascular:** This form of tertiary syphilis is characterized by disorders such as aneurysms of the aorta. It can be fatal if there is no surgical intervention
  - **Neurosyphilis:** This causes serious neurological problems and can coexist with cardiovascular syphilis

A pregnant woman can pass the treponemal infection to her unborn child, and this is known as **congenital syphilis**. If the pregnancy does not end in a miscarriage, stillbirth, or premature birth, the child will be born very ill with signs such as hepatosplenomegaly, pneumonia, and a bullous rash.

Did you know?

Famous historical figures diagnosed with or strongly suspected of having syphilis include Oscar Wilde, Friedrich Nietzsche, Al Capone, Casanova, Eduard Manet, Paul Gauguin, Vincent van Gogh, Ludwig van Beethoven, Robert Schumann, and Franz Schubert (Tampa et al., 2014).

Trichomoniasis

Common STI caused by the parasitic protozoan *Trichomonas vaginalis*. Infected men are usually asymptomatic but women develop a greenish-yellow, frothy discharge and may experience pain during sexual intercourse and/or frequent, painful urination. The vulva may also be inflamed, irritated, and sore.

NEW WORDS	
Fertilization	The union and fusion of an ovum and a spermatozoon to form a zygote
Gamete	A mature sex cell (ovum or spermatozoon)
Gonad	A male or female reproductive organ in which gametes are produced
Haploid cell	A cell with a single set of chromosomes (23 chromosomes)
Lactation	The secretion of milk by the mammary glands
Meiosis	Reproductive cell division in which four haploid daughter cells are produced
Menopause	The time in a woman's life when she stops menstruating and ovulating and is no longer able to bear children
Oogenesis	The production of mature ova in the ovaries
Ova (singular = **ovum**)	Mature female sex cells (commonly called eggs)
Puberty	The time of life when people become capable of reproducing children and their bodies develop secondary sexual characteriztics
Semen (seminal fluid)	Fluid containing sperm and a mixture of fluids secreted by the reproductive glands
Spermatogenesis	The production of spermatozoa in the testes
Spermatozoa (singular = **spermatozoon**)	Mature male sex cells (commonly called sperm)

Study Outline

Functions of the reproductive system

1. The human reproductive system functions in reproducing life and continuing the species.
2. Reproductive cells are produced through a type of cell division called meiosis.
3. Meiosis results in four daughter cells that each have only one set of chromosomes (23 chromosomes).
4. Reproductive cells are called gametes and are produced in reproductive organs called gonads.
5. Female gonads are ovaries and they produce ova through the process of oogenesis.
6. Male gonads are testes and they produce spermatozoa through the process of spermatogenesis.
7. The male reproductive system functions in producing spermatozoa and ejaculating them into a woman's reproductive tract.
8. The process in which an ovum and spermatozoon unite and fuse is called fertilization and it results in a zygote.
9. The female reproductive system functions in producing ova, receiving spermatozoa, being the site of fertilization, and housing the fertilized zygote so that it can grow and develop into a fetus. This is called pregnancy. The female reproductive system also functions in delivering the fetus into the external world through the process of childbirth (labor).

Male reproductive system

The male reproductive system consists of the:

1. Scrotum: This is a paired sac of loose skin hanging externally and housing the testes and epididymis. It functions in maintaining the correct temperature of the testes.
2. Testes: These are a pair of oval glands located in the scrotum. They are the gonads where sperm are formed through spermatogenesis. They also secrete testosterone.
3. Epididymis: This is a series of ducts that are the site of sperm maturation.
4. Vas deferens: This is a long duct that transports sperm from the epididymis to the urethra. It is supported by a structure called the spermatic cord.

5. Urethra: This is the terminal duct of both the reproductive and urinary systems. It transports semen and urine out of the body.
6. Accessory glands: These are the seminal vesicles, prostate gland, and bulbourethral glands, which all produce fluids that combine with sperm to form semen.
7. Penis: This is a cylindrical organ that excretes urine and ejaculates sperm.

Female reproductive system

The female reproductive system consists of the:

1. Ovaries: These are a pair of almond-shaped organs that are the gonads where ova are produced through oogenesis. They also function in ovulation.
   - The ovaries contain small sac-like structures called ovarian follicles. Each follicle houses an immature ovum called an oocyte.
   - One follicle becomes the dominant follicle and is called the mature Graafian follicle. At ovulation this follicle expels the ovum into the uterine cavity.
   - The now empty follicle develops into the corpus luteum, a glandular structure that secretes female hormones.
   - The corpus luteum finally degenerates into the corpus albicans.
2. Fallopian tubes: These are two thin tubes running from the ovaries to the uterus. They are the site of fertilization and they transport a zygote to the uterus.
3. Uterus: This is a muscular sac composed of three layers of tissue: the outer perimetrium, the middle myometrium, and the inner endometrium. The endometrium contains the stratum functionalis, which is shed during menstruation. The uterus is a passageway for sperm traveling to an ovum. If fertilization then occurs, the uterus houses a fetus until birth. If fertilization does not occur, the uterus is the site of menstruation.
4. Vagina: This is a muscular tube that acts as a passageway for menstrual flow, semen, and a fetus.
5. Vulva: This is the external genitals of a woman and includes the mons pubis, labia majora, labia minora, clitoris, and vestibule.
6. Mammary glands: These are modified sudoriferous glands that function in lactation.

Female reproductive cycle

1. A woman's reproductive cycle lasts anywhere from 24 to 35 days and involves both:
   - An ovarian cycle in which an oocyte matures until it is ready for ovulation
   - A uterine (menstrual) cycle in which the endometrium of the uterus is prepared for the arrival of a fertilized ovum.
2. The reproductive cycle consists of a menstrual phase in which the stratum functionalis of the endometrium is shed via menstrual flow, a preovulatory phase in which the Graafian follicle forms and the endometrium proliferates, ovulation, and the postovulatory phase, which is a "waiting time." If fertilization has occurred the zygote implants in the uterus and a woman becomes pregnant. If it has not occurred, the cycle returns to the menstrual phase.

Aging and the reproductive system

1. Puberty is the time in which a person develops secondary sexual characteriztics and becomes able to reproduce.
2. Girls reach puberty when they begin to menstruate. From their first period until they go through menopause they are able to become pregnant. Menopause is the end of menstruation and a woman's capability to bear children.

Review

1. Explain the functions of the reproductive system.
2. Describe the organization of the male reproductive system.
3. Identify the functions of the following:
   - Testes
   - Epididymis
   - Urethra.
4. Identify the principal male hormone.
5. Describe the organization of the female reproductive system.
6. Identify the functions of the following:
   - Ovaries
   - Fallopian tubes
   - Vagina.
7. Explain the structure of the uterus.
8. Describe the female reproductive cycle.
9. Identify the main female hormones.
10. Describe the following disorders:
    - Pelvic inflammatory disease
    - Breast cancer
    - Prostatitis.

Multiple-Choice Questions

1. The principal male hormone is:
   a. Estrogen
   b. Progesterone
   c. Progestin
   d. Testosterone

2. Which of the following is not an STI?
   a. AIDS
   b. Chlamydia
   c. Endometriosis
   d. Syphilis

3. The function of the epididymis is to be:
   a. The site of spermatogenesis
   b. The site of sperm maturation
   c. The site of oogenesis
   d. The site of ova maturation

4. Which of the following statements is correct?
   a. The mature Graafian follicle ruptures to release an ovum into the pelvic cavity
   b. The mature Graafian follicle secretes estrogen, progesterone, relaxin, and inhibin
   c. The mature Graafian follicle is the site of fertilization
   d. The mature Graafian follicle is found as part of the menstrual flow

5. How many chromosomes are found in a haploid cell?
   a. 13
   b. 23
   c. 43
   d. 46

6. How many trimesters are in a pregnancy?
   a. 1
   b. 3
   c. 6
   d. 9

7. Which of the following is the correct definition of a gamete?
   a. An organ where sex cells are produced
   b. A fertilized ovum
   c. A cell derived through somatic cellular division
   d. A mature sex cell

8. Which of the following statements is correct?
   a. Fibroids are benign tumors consisting of muscle and fibrous tissue
   b. Fibroids are malignant tumors consisting of muscle and fibrous tissue
   c. Fibroids are cancerous tumors consisting of muscle and fibrous tissue
   d. None of the above

9. What is menopause?
   a. The time in which a person becomes capable of reproducing
   b. The time in which a girl has her first menstrual period and becomes capable of bearing children
   c. The time in which a man stops producing sperm
   d. The time in which a woman stops menstruating and becomes incapable of bearing children

10. Which layer of the uterus is shed during menstruation?
   a. Perimetrium
   b. Myometrium
   c. Stratum basale
   d. Stratum functionalis

Answers to Multiple-Choice Questions

Chapter 1
1. b
2. d
3. b
4. c
5. d
6. b
7. c
8. a
9. b
10. c
11. a
12. b
13. a
14. d
15. b

Chapter 2
1. c
2. a
3. c
4. c
5. b
6. a
7. d
8. b

9. c
10. a
11. b
12. d
13. b
14. a
15. d
16. d
17. b
18. c
19. a
20. c

Chapter 3
1. b
2. c
3. b
4. c
5. b
6. a
7. d
8. d
9. b
10. a
11. b
12. b

13. c
14. d
15. b

Chapter 4
1. c
2. a
3. b
4. b
5. d
6. a
7. c
8. d
9. a
10. b

Chapter 5
1. b
2. a
3. c
4. d
5. b
6. c
7. d
8. c
9. a

10. b
11. c
12. d
13. c
14. a
15. c

Chapter 6
1. c
2. c
3. a
4. a
5. d
6. c
7. d
8. a
9. b
10. a

Chapter 7
1. c
2. b
3. a
4. d
5. a
6. d

7. b
8. d
9. d
10. c

Chapter 8
1. b
2. d
3. a
4. b
5. a
6. d
7. a
8. b
9. d
10. c

Chapter 9
1. c
2. a
3. c
4. a
5. c
6. c
7. a
8. d

9. c
10. a

Chapter 10
1. c
2. a
3. b
4. b
5. d
6. d
7. a
8. c
9. d
10. c

Chapter 11
1. c
2. b
3. a
4. c
5. c
6. a
7. c
8. b
9. a
10. a

Chapter 12
1. b
2. c
3. a
4. c
5. d
6. b
7. c
8. d
9. a
10. b

Chapter 13
1. d
2. c
3. b
4. a
5. b
6. b
7. d
8. a
9. d
10. d

Appendix

VITAMINS AND MINERALS			
Vitamin	Major dietary sources	Major functions	Signs of deficiency
A **Retinol and beta-carotene**	• Animal sources of retinol: liver, eggs, cheese, butter, and milk • Plant sources of beta-carotene: orange or yellow vegetables, fruit, and dark green leafy vegetables	• Known as the "vision vitamin" or the "anti-infection" vitamin • Promotes healthy skin, eyes, and bones • Protects against infections and boosts the immune system • Essential for night vision • Antioxidant	Skin problems such as dry flaky skin and dandruff, mouth ulcers, poor night vision, acne, frequent colds or infections
B1 **Thiamine**	• In general, nuts, whole grains, and pork • Also organ meats, yeast extract, wheatgerm, sunflower seeds, peanuts, legumes	• Energy production • Brain function and maintenance of the nervous system	Fatigue, poor memory, lack of concentration, and depression
B2 **Riboflavin**	• In general, organ meats and yeast extract • Also almonds, wheatgerm, dairy products, wholegrain products	• Helps turn fats, sugars, and protein into energy • Important for the skin, hair, nails, and eyes	Burning or gritty eyes, sensitivity to bright lights, cracked skin around the mouth, sore tongue, and burning lips
B3 **Niacin**	• In general, meat and fish • Also yeast extract, raw peanuts, chicken, eggs, brown rice, and seeds	• Energy production • Brain function and a healthy nervous system • Healthy skin • Helps balance blood sugar and lower cholesterol levels	Lack of energy, insomnia, memory loss, muscle weakness, and skin problems
B5 **Pantothenic acid**	• In general, organ meats, eggs, and yeast extracts • Also whole grains, nuts, seeds, pulses, broccoli, and cauliflower	• Energy production • Essential for the brain and nerves and helps one cope with stress • Promotes healthy skin and hair and boosts the immune system	Poor skin, depression, fatigue, loss of appetite, and poor coordination

VITAMINS AND MINERALS

Vitamin	Major dietary sources	Major functions	Signs of deficiency
B6 **Pyridoxine**	Seeds, whole grains, pulses, yeast extract, bananas, nuts, potatoes, broccoli, cauliflower	• Essential for a healthy immune system and the formation of red blood cells • Helps relieve the symptoms of PMS and menopause and necessary for a healthy pregnancy • Natural antidepressant • Functions in the metabolism of fats and proteins	Disorders of the nervous system, fluid retention, oily scaling skin, muscular spasms, and PMS
B12 **Cyanocobalamin**	• Mainly in animal products such as liver, oysters, and sardines • Rare in plant-based foods • Vegetarians can obtain B12 from fermented soybean curd or fermented milks	• The feel-good vitamin • Essential for a healthy nervous system, memory, and concentration • Helps the blood carry oxygen • Essential for energy	Fatigue, exhaustion, anemia, menstrual disorders, poor hair condition, and a lack of energy
Biotin	• In general, organ meats, soybeans, and whole grains • Also in cauliflower, eggs, mushrooms, nuts, and pulses	• Vital for cell growth and replication • Particularly important in childhood • Helps the body use essential fats and maintain healthy skin, hair, and nerves	Dry skin, poor hair condition, premature graying hair, tender or sore muscles, poor appetite, nausea, eczema, dermatitis
C **Ascorbic acid**	• In general, green vegetables, fruits, and fruit juices • Also in tomatoes and potatoes	• Strengthens the immune system and fights infection • Makes collagen to keep bones, skin, and joints firm and strong • Antioxidant • Detoxifies pollutants	Weakness, frequent colds, lack of energy, frequent infections, bleeding or tender gums, easy bruising, nose bleeds, slow wound healing, red pimples on skin
D **Ergocalciferol** **Cholecalciferol**	• Formed by the action of sunlight on the skin • Also present in fatty fish, cottage cheese, and eggs	• The "sunshine vitamin" • Essential for strong and healthy bones	Joint pain or stiffness, backache, tooth decay, muscular weakness and spasm, hair loss

VITAMINS AND MINERALS			
Vitamin	Major dietary sources	Major functions	Signs of deficiency
E D-alpha tocopherol	• In general, nuts, seeds, and their oils • Also soybeans, whole grains, and a wide variety of fruits and vegetables	• Primary antioxidant in the body • Essential for immune function • Slows aging and protects against pollution • Good for the skin	Lack of sex drive, exhaustion after light exercise, easy bruising, slow wound healing, varicose veins, loss of muscle tone, infertility
Folic acid	• In general, green leafy vegetables • Also wheatgerm, peanuts, sprouts, asparagus, seeds, and nuts • Poor in animal foods	• Critical during pregnancy and also essential for brain and nerve function • Needed for utilizing protein and red-blood-cell formation	Weakness, lethargy and fatigue, irritability, insomnia, recurrent miscarriages, and problems with lactation
K Phylloquinone	• Produced by bacteria in the large intestine • Also present in dark green leafy vegetables, oats, and wholewheat	• Controls blood clotting • Necessary for the formation of strong bones	Heavy menstrual bleeding, poor blood clotting, osteoporosis
Calcium	• Dark green vegetables, nuts, seeds, bean curd • Also dairy products and brewer's yeast	• Essential for healthy skin, bones, and teeth • Maintains healthy nerves and necessary for muscular contraction	Muscle cramps or tremors, insomnia, nervousness, joint pain, arthritis, tooth decay, high blood pressure, osteoporosis, and osteomalacia
Chromium	• In general, whole grains, eggs, and meat • Fruits and vegetables are low in chromium	Helps control blood sugar levels and therefore normalize hunger and reduce cravings	Hypoglycemia, fatigue, mood swings, and obesity
Iron	• In general, animal products such as liver, kidney, and meat • Plant products include brewer's yeast, kelp, blackstrap molasses, and pumpkin seeds	• As a component of hemoglobin, iron transports oxygen and carbon dioxide to and from cells • Component of enzymes • Vital for energy production and the immune system	Anemia, pale skin, sore tongue, fatigue, listlessness, loss of appetite, sensitivity to cold

VITAMINS AND MINERALS

Vitamin	Major dietary sources	Major functions	Signs of deficiency
Magnesium	• In general, whole grains, nuts, seeds, and bean curd • Also green leafy vegetables • Fish, meat, and milk are low in magnesium	• Strengthens bones and teeth • Necessary for the normal functioning of muscles and nerves • Activates many enzymes	Muscle cramps, PMS, sugar cravings, fatigue, nervousness, difficulty relaxing
Manganese	• In general, whole grains, nuts, and avocados • Also tea, fruits, and vegetables	• Important for blood sugar balance, bone formation, and detoxification • Activates several enzymes	Blood sugar imbalances, muscle twitches, childhood growing pains, dizziness or poor sense of balance, fatigue
Molybdenum	In general, pulses and whole grains	• Helps rid the body of the protein breakdown products and detoxifies the body • Essential for the metabolism of iron, amino acids, and fats	Irritability
Phosphorus	Present in almost all foods	• Forms and maintains bones and teeth • Essential for the structure of cell membranes • Aids metabolism and energy production	• Deficiency is unlikely, but may occur with long-term antacid use or with stresses such as bone fracture • Signs and symptoms include general muscle weakness, loss of appetite, mental confusion, and osteomalacia
Potassium	Raisins, potatoes, avocados, bananas, and a diet generally rich in vegetables and fruit and low in sodium	• Promotes healthy nerves and muscles • Maintains fluid balance • Involved in metabolism, the control of acid/alkali levels in the blood, the functioning of the heart, and general health	Muscle weakness, pins and needles, irritability, nausea, water retention, depression, and fatigue

VITAMINS AND MINERALS			
Vitamin	Major dietary sources	Major functions	Signs of deficiency
Selenium	Tuna, oysters, molasses, mushrooms, herrings, cottage cheese, cabbage, liver, courgettes, cod, chicken	• Antioxidant • Slows premature aging • Reduces inflammation • Stimulates the immune system • Promotes a healthy heart • Important in male potency and libido	Premature aging, cataracts, frequent infections, poor detoxification
Sodium	Table salt, cured meats, pickles, soy sauce, olives	• Maintains water balance in body • Helps nerve functioning • Used in muscle contraction • Utilized in energy production • Helps move nutrients into cells	Weakness, dizziness, heat exhaustion, low blood pressure, and headaches
Zinc	• In general, shellfish, fish, and red meats • Also seeds, nuts, pulses, and whole grains	• Essential for the immune system and the structure and function of cell membranes • Essential for growth and healing, hormones, a healthy nervous system, bones and teeth, energy, and healthy hair • Helps one cope with stress	Regular infections, poor sense of taste or smell, white marks on nails, stretch marks, acne, greasy skin, low fertility, pale skin, tendency for depression, loss of appetite

Bibliography

Agur, A., A. Dalley, and K. Moore (2010). *Clinically Oriented Anatomy*. 6th ed. Baltimore: Lippincott Williams & Wilkins.

Alcamo, I. (2003). *Anatomy Colouring Workbook*. 2nd ed. New York: Random House.

Allen, R. (1990). *The Concise Oxford Dictionary of Current English*. Oxford: Clarendon.

Arnould-Taylor, W. (1998). *A Textbook of Anatomy and Physiology*. 3rd ed. Cheltenham: Stanley Thornes.

Bakalar, N. (2015). 'Take a number. 37.2 Trillion: Galaxies or Human Cells?' *New York Times*, 19 June 2015. Available at: https://www.nytimes.com/2015/06/23/science/37-2-trillion-galaxies-or-human-cells.html.

Barnard, C. (ed.) (1981). *The Body Machine*. Willemstad: Multimedia Publications.

Beers, M. (ed.) (2003). *The Merck Manual of Medical Information*. 2nd Home ed. New Jersey: Merck.

Blakey, P. (1992). *The Muscle Book*. Stafford: Bibliotek Books.

Cancer Research UK (2018a). 'Cancer Mortality for Common Cancers'. Last updated 2 May 2018. Available at: https://www.cancerresearchuk.org/health-professional/cancer-statistics/mortality/common-cancers-compared.

Cancer Research UK (2018b). 'Tobacco Statistics'. Last updated 23 July 2018. Available at: https://www.cancerresearchuk.org/health-professional/cancer-statistics/risk/tobacco.

Cheshire, E. (1998). *Gastrointestinal System*. Barcelona: Mosby International.

Chrousos, G. (2009). 'Stress and Disorders of the Stress System'. *Nature Reviews Endocrinology* 5(7): 374–81.

Colledge, N., B. Walker, and S. Ralston (eds) (2010). *Davidson's Principles and Practice of Medicine*. 21st ed. Edinburgh: Elsevier.

Davidson, E., A. Foulkes, M. Longmore, A. Mafi, and I. Wilkinson (2010). *Oxford Handbook of Clinical Medicine*. 8th ed. Oxford: Oxford University Press.

Douglas, G., F. Nicol, and C. Robertson (eds) (2009). *Macleod's Clinical Examination*. 12th ed. Edinburgh: Elsevier.

Drake, R., A. Vogl, and A. Mitchell (2015). *Gray's Anatomy for Students*. 3rd ed. London: Elsevier.

Dreyer, A., M. Dreyer, E. Hattingh, and Y. Thandar (2012). *Pharmacology for Nurses and Other Health Workers*. 3rd ed. Cape Town: Pearson Education South Africa.

Genetic Science Learning Center (2010). 'The Evolution of the Cell'. Learn.Genetics (accessed 18 February 2019). Available at: https://learn.genetics.utah.edu/content/cells/organelles/.

Gould, F. (2005). *Anatomy and Physiology*. Cheltenham: Nelson Thornes.

Homeier, B., J. Kaplan, and R. Porter (2008). *The Merck Manual of Patient Symptoms*. West Point: Merck.

Hull, R. (2019). *Anatomy, Physiology and Pathology Colouring and Workbook*. Chichester: Lotus.

Jarmey, C. (2022). *The Pocket Atlas of Human Anatomy*. Chichester: Lotus.

Jarmey, C. (2018). *The Concise Book of Muscles*. 4th ed. Chichester: Lotus.

Marieb, E. (2003). *Essentials of Human Anatomy and Physiology*. 7th ed. San Francisco: Benjamin Cummings.

Mayer, E. (2018). *The Mind-Gut Connection*. Digital ed. Harper Wave.

McFerran, T. (ed.) (1998). *Minidictionary for Nurses*. 4th ed. Oxford: Oxford University Press.

McGuinness, H. (2006). *Anatomy and Physiology Therapy Basics*. 3rd ed. London: Hodder Arnold.

Miranda, J. (ed.) (1992). *Milady's Art and Science of Nail Technology*. 2ⁿᵈ ed. New York: Milady.

Mortimore, D. (2001). *The Complete Illustrated Guide to Vitamins and Minerals*. London: Harper Collins.

National Sleep Foundation (n.d.). 'Melatonin and Sleep'. SleepFoundation.org (accessed 26 February 2019). Available at: https://www.sleepfoundation.org /articles/melatonin.

Neighbors, M., and R. Tannehill-Jones (2000). *Human Diseases*. New York: Delmar Thomson Learning.

Nilsson, L. (1987). *The Body Victorious*. London: Dell.

Parsons, T. (2002). *An Holistic Guide to Anatomy and Physiology*. London: Thomson.

Presbury, D. (2000). *Know Your Skin*. Randburg: Medpress.

Pugliese, P. (1991). *Advanced Professional Skin Care*. Bernville: APSC.

Putz, R., and R. Pabst (eds) (2008). *Sobotta Atlas of Human Anatomy*. Munich: Elsevier.

Rippey, J. (1994). *Illustrated Lecture Notes General Pathology*. Johannesburg: Witwatersrand University Press.

Shen, H. (2018). 'Does the Adult Brain Really Grow New Neurons?' *Scientific American*, 7 March 2018. Available at: https://www.scientificamerican.com /article/does-the-adult-brain-really-grow-new-neurons/.

Tampa, M., I. Sarbu, C. Matei, V. Benea, and S. R. Georgescu (2014). 'Brief History of Syphilis'. *Journal of Medicine and Life* 7(1): 4–10.

Telegraph reporters (2018). 'Stephen Hawking Greatest Quotes: "Remember to look up at the stars and not down at your feet."' *Telegraph*, 14 March 2018. Available at: https://www.telegraph.co.uk /science/2018/03/14/stephen-hawking-greatest-quotes-without-imperfection-would-not/.

The Stephen Hawking Foundation (n.d.). 'Brief Biography'. Hawking.org, accessed 26 February 2019. Available at: http://www.hawking.org.uk /about-stephen.html.

Tortora, G., and B. Derrickson (2009). *Principles of Anatomy and Physiology*. 12ᵗʰ ed. Hoboken: John Wiley & Sons (Asia).

Tortora, G., and S. Grabowski (1996). *Principles of Anatomy and Physiology*. 8ᵗʰ ed. New York: Harper Collins College Div.

Underwood, J. (ed.) (2000). *General and Systematic Pathology*. London: Harcourt.

Walker, R. (1994). *Atlas of the Human Body*. London: Quarto Children's Books.

Walker, R. (2001). *Human Body*. London: Dorling Kindersley.

Waugh, A., and A. Grant (2001). *Anatomy and Physiology in Health and Illness*. 9ᵗʰ ed. London: Harcourt.

Wingate, P. (1976). *Medical Encyclopedia*. 2ⁿᵈ ed. Harmondsworth: Penguin Books.

World Health Organization (2018). 'Diabetes'. 30 October 2018. Available at: https://www.who.int /news-room/fact-sheets/detail/diabetes.

Glossary

A

Abdomen
Region of the body between the diaphragm and pelvis

Abduction
Movement away from midline of body

Abrasion
Damaged area of the skin caused by the skin being scraped or worn away

Absorption
Uptake of digested nutrients into the bloodstream and lymphatic system

Acetylcholine
Neurotransmitter found in both the peripheral and central nervous systems

Acid mantle
Film of sebum and sweat on the surface of the skin that protects against bacteria

Actin
Protein that functions in muscle contraction

Action potential
Electrical charge that occurs on the membrane of a muscle cell in response to a nerve impulse

Active transport
Movement of a substance across a cellular membrane that involves the release of energy; takes place against a concentration gradient

Adduction
Movement toward the midline of the body

Adenosine triphosphate (ATP)
Main energy-transferring molecule in the body

Adipocyte
Fat cell

Adrenaline
See epinephrine

Adrenocorticotropic hormone (ACTH)
Hormone secreted by the anterior pituitary gland that stimulates and controls the adrenal cortex

Aerobic
Requiring oxygen

Afferent
Carrying toward a center

Afferent neurons
See sensory neurons

Agonist
See prime mover

Agranulocytes
Group of white blood cells that do not contain granules in their cytoplasm (includes lymphocytes and monocytes)

Albuminuria
Presence of albumin (protein) in urine

Aldosterone
Hormone secreted by the adrenal cortex that regulates the reabsorption of sodium and water in the kidneys

Alimentary canal
See gastrointestinal tract

Alveoli
Air sacs inside the lungs

Amphiarthroses
Slightly movable joints that permit a minimal amount of flexibility and movement

Anaerobic
Not requiring oxygen

Anagen
Active growing stage of the hair cycle

Anal canal
Last ¾–1⅕ in (2–3 cm) of the rectum that opens to the exterior

Anaphylaxis
Exaggerated reaction of organism to a foreign protein, an extreme allergic reaction

Anatomical position
Position in which the body is standing erect with the feet parallel, the arms hanging down by the side, and the face and palms facing forward

Anatomy
Study of the structure of the body

Anemia
Reduction in the oxygen-carrying capacity of the blood

Aneurysm
Sac formed by localized dilatation of blood vessel

Anoxia
The absence of oxygen in an area

Antagonist
Muscle that opposes the movement caused by the prime mover, or agonist

Anterior
At the front of the body, in front of

Antibody
Specialized protein that is synthesized to destroy a specific antigen

Antidiuretic hormone (ADH)
Hormone released by the posterior pituitary gland that has an antidiuretic effect and raises blood pressure

Antigen
Any substance that the body recognizes as foreign

Antioxidant
Substance that combats or neutralizes free radicals

Anuria
Failure of kidneys to produce urine

Apocrine gland
Type of sweat gland located in the armpits, pubic region, and the areolae of the breasts

Aponeurosis
Flat, sheet-like tendon that attaches muscles to bone, skin, or another muscle

Apoptosis	The normal, ordered death and removal of cells as part of tissue development, maintenance, and renewal
Appendicular skeleton	Part of the skeleton consisting of the upper and lower limbs and their girdles
Appendix (vermiform)	Sac attached to the cecum of the large intestine
Aqueous humor	Fluid that nourishes the lens and cornea and helps produce intraocular pressure
Arachnoid	Middle meninx (covering) of the brain and spinal cord
Areola	Circular area of pigmented skin surrounding the nipple
Arrector pili muscles	Smooth muscles attached to hairs that contract to pull the hairs into a vertical position
Arteries	Vessels that usually carry blood away from the heart toward the tissues
Arterioles	Tiny arteries that deliver blood to capillaries
Arthralgia	Pain in a joint
Arthrology	The study of joints
Articulation	Point of contact between two bones, commonly called a joint
Atony	Lack of muscle tone
Atrioventricular valves	Valves lying between the atria and ventricles that prevent the backflow of blood
Atrium	Receiving chamber of the heart
Atrophy	Wasting away of muscles
Auditory ossicles	Three tiny bones extending across the middle ear: the malleus, incus, and stapes
Auditory tube	See Eustachian tube
Auricle	The part of the ear that we see
Autonomic nervous system (ANS)	Part of the nervous system that controls all processes that are automatic or involuntary
Autorhythmic cells	Muscle or nerve cells that generate an impulse without an external stimulus; i.e., they are self-excitable
Avascular	Lacking blood vessels
Axial skeleton	Part of the skeleton comprising the bones found in the center of the body
Axilla	Armpit
Axon	Transmitting portion of a neuron
Axon terminal	Area found at the end of the axon that contains membrane-enclosed sacs called synaptic vesicles

B

B cells	Cells of the immune system that develop into plasma cells and are able to synthesise and secrete antibodies
Ball-and-socket joint	Synovial joint in which a ball-shaped bone fits into the cup-shaped socket of another bone
Baroreceptors	Sensory nerve endings that monitor blood pressure changes in the arteries and veins
Basophils	Type of white blood cell that contains histamine and is capable of ingesting foreign particles
Benign	Not harmful, non-cancerous
Bile	Liquid produced by the liver that emulsifies fats; contains water, bile acids, bile salts, cholesterol, phospholipids, bile pigments, and some ions
Blood pressure	Force exerted by blood on the walls of a blood vessel
Bowman's capsule	See glomerular capsule
Brachial	Pertaining to the arm
Bradycardia	Slow heart rate
Brain stem	Continuation of the spinal cord that connects the spinal cord to the diencephalon; consists of the medulla oblongata, pons, and midbrain
Bronchus	Branchlike passageway inside the lungs
Bruise	Discoloration of the skin caused by the escape of blood from underlying vessels
Brush border	Area in the small intestine composed of microvilli that contain digestive enzymes
Buccal cavity	Mouth
Bursa	Sac-like structure made of connective tissue, lined with a synovial membrane, and filled with synovial fluid

C

Cachexia	General ill health and wasting away
Calcitonin (CT)	Hormone secreted by the thyroid gland that lowers blood calcium levels
Calcitriol	Active form of vitamin D
Canaliculus	Very small channel or canal
Cancellous bone tissue	See spongy bone tissue

Capillary	Very small blood vessel that connects arterioles to venules
Carbohydrate	Organic compound composed of units of glucose that contain carbon, hydrogen, and oxygen
Cardiac cycle	All the events associated with a heartbeat
Cardiac muscle	Muscle forming most of the wall of the heart; composed of striated muscle fibers; involuntary
Cardiac output	Amount of blood pumped out of the heart by the left ventricle
Carpal	Pertaining to the wrist
Cartilage	Resilient, strong connective tissue that is less hard but more flexible than bone
Cartilaginous joint	Joint in which bone ends are held together by cartilage and do not have a synovial cavity between them
Catagen	The transitionary stage of the hair cycle
Catalyst	Substance that affects the rate of a chemical reaction without itself being changed by the reaction
Caudal	Away from the head, below
Cecum	2 2/5 in (6 cm) long pouch of the large intestine that receives food from the small intestine via the ileocecal valve
Cellular respiration	Metabolic reaction that uses oxygen and glucose and produces energy in the form of ATP; also called oxidation
Central nervous system (CNS)	The brain and spinal cord
Centriole	Structure found near the nucleus of a cell that plays a role cell division
Centrosome	Area near the nucleus of a cell that contains centrioles and forms the mitotic spindle in dividing cells
Cephalad	Toward the head, above
Cephalic	Pertaining to the head
Cerebellum	Region of the brain located behind the medulla oblongata and pons; functions in producing smooth, coordinated movements as well as posture and balance
Cerebral cortex	Outer, most superficial layer of the cerebrum, consisting of gray matter
Cerebrospinal fluid (CSF)	Fluid that circles the CNS, protecting it and helping to maintain homeostasis
Cerebrum	Largest part of the brain and the area that gives us the ability to read, write, speak, remember, create, and imagine
Cerumen	Earwax
Cervical	Pertaining to the neck
Chemoreceptor	Receptor sensitive to chemicals
Choroid	Lining of most of the internal surface of the sclera
Chromatin	Mass of chromosomes all tangled together in a non-dividing cell
Chromosome	Threadlike structure found in the nucleus of a cell; carries the genes
Chyle	Fluid found inside the lacteals of the small intestine
Chyme	Semifluid contents of the stomach, consisting of partially digested food and gastric secretions
Cilia	Tiny hairlike projections on the surfaces of cells that move the cell or substances along the surface of the cell
Ciliary body	Part of the eye between the iris and choroid
Circumduction	Circular movement of the distal end of a body part; e.g., circling the shoulder joint
Cistern	Channel or tubule in a cell
Clitoris	Small cylindrical mass of erectile tissue and nerves that forms part of the female genitalia
Club hair	Fully grown hair that has detached from the hair bulb during the catagen stage of hair growth
Cochlea	Bony, spiral canal in the inner ear that resembles a snail's shell and houses the organ of Corti (for hearing)
Colic	Acute paroxysmal pain
Colon	Long tube that forms most of the large intestine
Compact bone tissue	Very hard, compact tissue with few spaces within it
Complement system	Group of proteins in the blood that helps antibodies during an immune response
Concentric contraction	Contraction toward a center that results in a movement that shortens the angle at a joint
Conductivity	Ability of cells, such as nerve or muscle cells, to move action potentials along their plasma membranes
Condyloid joint	Joint in which an oval protuberance at the end of a bone fits into an elliptical cavity of another bone
Cones	Photoreceptors that respond to color

Connective tissue	One of the basic tissue types in the body; consists of few cells in a large matrix and functions in support, storage, and protection
Contractility	Ability of muscles to contract and shorten
Cooper's ligaments	*See* suspensory ligaments
Cornea	Avascular, transparent coat that covers the iris; it is curved and helps focus light
Coronal plane	Plane that divides vertically into anterior and posterior portions
Coronary circulation	Circulation that supplies the muscles of the heart with blood
Corpus luteum	Gland formed after a Graafian follicle has discharged its ovum; secretes progesterone, estrogen, relaxin, and inhibin
Cortex	Outer layer of an organ
Corticotropin	*See* adrenocorticotropic hormone
Costal	Pertaining to a rib
Cough	Sudden, explosive movement of air rushing upward through the respiratory passages
Cranial	Toward the head, above, pertaining to the head
Cranium	Hard bones of the skull
Creatinine	Product of muscle activity
Cross-infection	Transfer of infection from one person to another
Cross-section	Division that divides horizontally into inferior and superior portions
Crust (scab)	Accumulation of dried blood, pus, or skin fluids on the surface of the skin; forms where the skin has been damaged
Cutaneous	Pertaining to the skin
Cutaneous membrane	The skin; composed of an epidermis and dermis
Cuticle	Outer layer of cells of a hair or the epidermis of the skin or the base of the nail plate
Cyanosis	Bluish discoloration of the skin or mucous membranes due to reduced oxygen or hemoglobin in the blood
Cyst	Semi-solid or fluid-filled lump above and below the skin
Cytokinesis	Process by which a cell splits into two new cells during cellular division
Cytology	The study of cells
Cytoplasm	Cellular material inside the plasma membrane, excluding the nucleus
Cytosol	Thick, transparent, gel-like fluid inside a cell

D

Deep	Away from the surface of the body
Defecation	Process by which indigestible substances and some bacteria are eliminated from the body
Deglutition	Process of swallowing food
Demineralization	Process through which minerals such as calcium and phosphorus are lost from the bones
Dendrite	Receiving or input portion of a neuron
Dense connective (fibrous) tissue	Contains thick, densely packed fibers and fewer cells than loose connective tissue
Dentes	Teeth
Depolarization	Process by which an action potential is produced
Depression (of the shoulders or jaw)	Dropping the shoulders or jaw downward
Dermatology	Study of the skin
Dermis	Deep layer of the skin; composed of dense irregular connective tissue
Desquamation	Process by which the skin is shed
Diaphysis	Main, central shaft of a long bone
Diarthrosis	Freely movable joint that permits a number of different movements
Diastole	Relaxation of the heart muscle during the cardiac cycle
Diencephalon	Region of the brain that lies above the brain stem, enclosed by the cerebral hemispheres; contains the thalamus, hypothalamus, and epithalamus and has a number of different functions, including housing the pituitary and pineal endocrine glands
Diffusion	Movement of substances from areas of high concentration to areas of low concentration
Digestion	Process by which large molecules of food are broken down into smaller molecules that can enter cells
Digit	Finger or toe
Diploid	Having two complete sets of chromosomes per cell (i.e., 46)

Distal	Farther from its origin or point of attachment of a limb
Distal convoluted tubule	Area furthest from the glomerular capsule; section of the tube where fine-tuning of the filtrate occurs
Diuretic	Substance that increases urine production
Dopamine	Type of neurotransmitter
Dorsal	At the back of the body, behind
Dorsiflexion	Pulling of the foot upward toward the shin, in the direction of the dorsum
Duodenal glands (Brunner's glands)	Glands in the duodenum that secrete an alkaline mucus
Duodenum	First segment of the small intestine; connects the stomach to the ileum
Dura mater	Outer covering of the brain
Dyslipidemia	Abnormal amounts of lipids in the blood
Dyspareunia	Pain experienced during sexual intercourse
Dyspnea	Labored or difficult breathing
Dysuria	Painful or uncomfortable urination

E

Eardrum (tympanic membrane)	Very thin, semi-transparent membrane between the auditory canal and the middle ear; when sound waves hit it, it vibrates, passing the sound waves on to the middle ear
Eccentric contraction	Contraction away from the center
Eccrine gland	Sweat gland; distributed around the body
Edema	Excessive accumulation of interstitial fluid in body tissues
Efferent	Carrying away from a center
Efferent neuron	*See* motor neuron
Elasticity	Ability of a tissue to return to its original shape after stretching, contracting, or extending
Electrolyte	Charged particle (ion) that conducts an electrical current in an aqueous solution
Elevation (of the shoulders or jaw)	Lifting the shoulders or jaw upward
Ellipsoid joint	*See* condyloid joint
Enamel	Extremely hard substance that protects the teeth from being worn down and acts as a barrier against acids

Endocardium	Thin, smooth lining of the inside of the heart
Endocrine glands	Ductless glands that secrete substances into the extracellular space around their cells; these secretions then diffuse into blood capillaries and are transported by the blood to target cells located throughout the body
Endocrinology	Study of the endocrine glands and the hormones they secrete
Endometrium	Mucous membrane lining of the uterus
Endomysium	Connective tissue that surrounds each individual muscle fiber
Endoplasmic reticulum	Network of fluid-filled cisterns within a cell that provides a large surface area for chemical reactions and also transports molecules within the cell
Endosteum	Membrane that lines the medullary cavity of bones
Enteroendocrine cell	Specialized cell that secretes hormones into the intestinal glands
Enzyme	Protein that speeds up a chemical reaction without itself being used up in the reaction
Eosinophils	Type of white blood cell that can destroy certain parasitic worms, phagocytize antigen–antibody complexes, and combat the effects of some inflammatory chemicals
Epicardium	Outer layer of the heart wall; also called the visceral layer of the serous pericardium
Epidermis	Superficial, outer layer of the skin
Epididymis	The organ lying along the posterior border of each testis; composed of a series of coiled ducts; the site of sperm maturation
Epimysium	The outermost layer of connective tissue that encircles an entire muscle
Epinephrine	Hormone secreted by the adrenal medulla that functions in the fight-or-flight response
Epiphyseal plate	A layer of hyaline cartilage in a growing bone that allows the diaphysis to grow in length
Epiphysis	The end of a long bone
Epithelium	Basic tissue type; forms glands, lines internal cavities and vessels, and is the superficial layer of the skin
Equilibrium	Balance
Erythema	Redness of the skin

Erythrocyte	Red blood cell, contains a protein called hemoglobin, which transports oxygen in the blood
Erythropoietin	Hormone secreted by the kidneys that stimulates the production of red blood cells
Essential fatty acid	Fats that are vital for the proper functioning of the body
Estrogens	Hormones secreted by the ovaries that stimulate the development of feminine secondary sex characteristics and, together with progesterone, regulate the female reproductive cycle
Eustachian tube	Tube that connects the middle ear with the upper portion of the throat; equalizes the middle-ear-cavity pressure with the external atmospheric pressure
Eversion	Turning the sole of the foot outward
Excitability	Ability of muscle or nerve cells to respond to stimuli
Excoriation	Removal of the skin caused by scratching or scraping
Excretion	Elimination of waste products
Exocrine glands	Glands that secrete substances into ducts that carry these substances into body cavities or to the outer surface of the body
Extensibility	Ability of muscles to extend and lengthen or stretch
Extension	Straightening movement in which a body part is restored to its anatomical position after being flexed
External auditory canal	Curved tube that carries sound waves from the auricle to the eardrum
External nares	Openings to the nose; commonly called the nostrils
External respiration (pulmonary respiration)	Gaseous exchange between lungs and blood; in external respiration, the blood gains oxygen and loses carbon dioxide

F

Facilitated diffusion	Diffusion in which substances are helped across the plasma membrane by channel or transporter proteins within the membrane
Falciform ligament	Fold of the peritoneum that binds the liver to the anterior abdominal wall and diaphragm and separates the two principal lobes of the liver

Fallopian tubes	Two thin tubes running from the ovaries to the uterus
Fascia	Connective tissue that surrounds and protects organs, lines walls of the body, holds muscles together, and separates muscles
Fascicle	Bundle of 10–100 muscle fibers
Fatigue (of muscles)	A muscle's inability to respond to stimulus or maintain contractions
Feces	Waste material of the digestive system that is eliminated through the anus
Fertilization	Union and fusion of an ovum and a spermatozoon to form a zygote
Fetus	Unborn child in the uterus from the eighth week of development until birth
Fibrosis	Replacement of connective tissue by scar tissue
Fibrous joints	Joints in which bone ends are held together by fibrous connective tissue with no synovial cavity between them
Filtration	Movement of a liquid through a membrane or filter
Fissure	Crack in the skin that penetrates into the dermis
Fixator	Muscle that helps the prime mover by stabilizing and preventing unnecessary movements in surrounding joints
Flagella	Long, whiplike extensions of the cell membrane of certain cells such as sperm or bacteria; they move the cell
Flat bones	Thin bones consisting of a layer of spongy bone enclosed by layers of compact bone
Flexion	Bending of a joint in which the angle between articulating bones decreases; the opposite of extension
Follicle-stimulating hormone (FSH)	Hormone secreted by the anterior pituitary gland that stimulates the development of ova and sperm
Formed elements	Cells and cell fragments found in blood
Free radical	Highly unstable, reactive molecule that damages cells
Frontal plane	*See* coronal plane

G

Gamete	Sex cell (ovum or spermatozoon)
Ganglion	Bundle or knot of nerve cell bodies

Gastric juice	Substance secreted by the gastric glands in the stomach, containing water, hydrochloric acid, intrinsic factor, pepsinogen, and gastric lipase
Gastric lipase	Enzyme that acts on lipids in the stomach, breaking down triglycerides into fatty acids and monoglycerides
Gastrin	Hormone produced by the stomach that stimulates gastric secretions
Gastrointestinal (GI) tract	Tube that runs from the mouth to the anus in which digestion and absorption take place
Gene	Basic unit of genetic material
Germinal matrix	Region of the nail where cell division takes place and growth occurs
Gingivae	Gums
Gliding joint	Joint in which two flat surfaces meet
Glomerular (Bowman's) capsule	Cuplike structure surrounding the glomerulus in a kidney's nephron; forms the closed end of the renal tubule
Glomerulus	Knotted network of capillaries in a kidney's nephron
Glucagon	Hormone produced by the pancreas that raises blood glucose levels
Glucocorticoids	Group of hormones secreted by the adrenal cortex that stimulate metabolism, help the body resist long-term stressors, control the effects of inflammation, and depress immune responses
Glucose	Sugar that is the major energy source for all cells
Gluteal	Pertaining to the buttocks
Glycogen	Carbohydrate consisting of subunits of glucose; the main form in which carbohydrates are stored in the body
Glycolysis	Cellular process through which glucose is split into pyruvic acid and ATP
Goblet cells	Cells that secrete mucus
Golgi apparatus	See Golgi complex
Golgi complex	Cellular structure located near the nucleus that processes, sorts, and packages proteins and lipids for delivery to the plasma membrane; also forms lysosomes and secretory vesicles
Gonad	Male or female reproductive organ in which sex cells are produced
Graafian follicle	Large, fluid-filled follicle that ruptures and releases an ovum during ovulation
Granulocytes	Group of white blood cells containing granules in their cytoplasm (includes neutrophils, eosinophils, and basophils)

Gustation	Sense of taste

H

Hair matrix	Ring of cells that divide to create hair
Hair root	Portion of the hair that penetrates into the dermis
Hair shaft	Superficial end of the hair that projects from the surface of the skin; commonly called the hair strand
Haploid cell	Cell with a single set of chromosomes (23 chromosomes)
Haustra	Pouches on the external surface of the colon
Haversian system	See osteon
Heart rate	Number of times the heart beats in one minute
Hematuria	Presence of red blood cells in the urine
Hemoglobin	Protein found in red blood cells that transports oxygen and gives the blood cells their red color
Hemopoiesis	Production of blood cells and platelets
Hemoptysis	The coughing up of blood
Hemostasis	The stopping of bleeding
Hepatocyte	Specialized cell found in the liver; has many metabolic functions
Hinge joint	Joint in which the convex surface of a bone fits into the concave surface of another bone
Hirsutism	Abnormal and excessive bodily hair growth
Histology	Study of tissues
Hive	See wheal
Homeostasis	Process by which the body maintains a stable internal environment
Hormone	Chemical messenger regulating cellular activity, produced by an endocrine gland and transported in the blood
Human growth hormone (hGH)	Hormone secreted by the anterior pituitary gland that stimulates growth and regulates metabolism
Hydrophilic	Water-loving
Hydrophobic	Water-hating
Hydroxyapatite	Form of calcium phosphate found in bones and teeth
Hymen	Thin membrane that partially covers the opening of the vagina
Hyperextension	Occurs when a body part extends beyond its anatomical position

Hypersecretion	Over- or excessive secretion
Hypertonia	Increase in muscle tone; muscles are described as hypertonic
Hyposecretion	Under-secretion
Hypotonia	Loss of muscle tone; muscles are described as hypotonic
Hypoxia	Inefficient delivery of oxygen to tissues

I

Ileum	Longest segment of the small intestine, which receives food from the jejunum and passes it into the large intestine
Immunity	Ability of the body to resist infection
Inclusions	Diverse group of substances that are temporarily produced by some cells
Inferior	Away from the head, below
Inflammation	Body's response to tissue damage
Ingestion	Process of taking food into the mouth
Inguinal	Pertaining to the groin
Inner ear	System of cavities and ducts that contains the organs of hearing and balance; also called the labyrinth
Insertion	Point where a muscle attaches to the moving bone of a joint
Insulin	Hormone produced by the pancreas that lowers blood glucose levels
Integumentary system	System of the skin and its derivatives (hair, nails, and cutaneous glands)
Internal nares	Openings that connect the nasal cavity to the pharynx
Internal respiration	Gaseous exchange between the blood and tissue cells; in internal respiration the blood loses oxygen and gains carbon dioxide
Interstitial endocrinocytes	Cells in the testes that secrete testosterone; also called Leydig cells
Intestinal juice	Clear yellow fluid that has a slightly alkaline pH and contains water and mucus; helps bring nutrient particles into contact with the microvilli
Intrinsic factor	Substance produced by the stomach and necessary for the absorption of vitamin B12 from the ileum
Inversion	Turning the sole of the foot inward
Ion	Electrically charged molecule or atom
Iris	Colored portion of the eye, suspended between the cornea and lens; contains the pupil

Irregular bones	Bones that have complex shapes and varying amounts of compact and spongy tissues
Irritability	Ability to respond to a stimulus and convert it into an impulse
Ischemia	Reduced or inadequate blood supply to an area
Islets of Langerhans	Clusters of endocrine cells located in the pancreas that secrete hormones including insulin and glucagon
Isometric contraction	Contraction in which the muscle contracts but does not shorten and no movement is generated
Isotonic contraction	Contraction in which muscles shorten and create movement while the tension in the muscle remains constant

J

Jaundice	Yellowing of skin or whites of eyes due to high levels of bilirubin
Jejunum	Portion of the small intestine between the duodenum and the ileum

K

Keratinization	Process in which cells die and become full of the protein keratin
Keratinocytes	Cells that produce keratin; 95% of the cells of the epidermis are keratinocytes
Kinesiology	Study of the motion of the body
Kinetic energy	Energy of motion

L

Labia	Lips
Labia majora	Two longitudinal folds of skin that extend inferiorly and posteriorly from the mons pubis of the female genitalia
Labia minora	Two smaller folds of skin running medially to the labia majora of the female genitalia
Labyrinth	*See* inner ear
Lacrimal gland	Gland that secretes tears
Lactase	Brush-border enzyme that breaks down lactose into glucose and galactose
Lactation	Secretion of milk by mammary glands

Lacteals	Specialized lymphatic vessels found in the villi of the small intestine
Lactiferous	Pertaining to the breasts
Lactogenic hormone	*See* prolactin
Lamellae	Concentric rings of calcified matrix found in compact bone
Lamellated corpuscles	Nerve endings that are sensitive to pressure; also called Pacinian corpuscles
Langerhans cell	A cell that functions in skin immunity
Lanugo hair	Soft hair that begins to cover a fetus from the third month of pregnancy; usually shed by the eighth month of pregnancy
Larynx	Short passageway between the laryngopharynx and the trachea; commonly called the voice box
Lateral	Away from the midline, on the outer side
Lens	Transparent structure of the eye, located behind the iris and responsible for fine-tuning of focusing
Leucocyte	White blood cell; functions primarily in protecting the body against foreign microbes and in immune responses
Ligament	Tough band of connective tissue that attaches bones to bones
Limbic system	Region of the brain that controls the emotional and involuntary aspects of behavior and also functions in memory
Lingual frenulum	Fold of mucous membrane that secures the tongue to the floor of the mouth
Lingual lipase	Enzyme in the mouth that begins the breakdown of lipids from triglycerides into fatty acids and glycerol
Lipid	A fat; fats are organic compounds composed of carbon, hydrogen, and oxygen and they are usually insoluble in water
Long bones	Bones that have a greater length than width and usually contain a longer shaft with two ends
Longitudinal plane	Plane that divides vertically into right and left sides
Loop of Henle	Portion of the renal tubule of a kidney nephron
Loose connective tissue	Tissue that consists of two or more layers of cells; it is durable and functions in protecting underlying tissues in areas of wear and tear

Lumbago	Pain in the muscles and joints of the lower back
Lumbar	Lower back region between the thorax and pelvis
Lumen	Hollow space within a tube-like structure, such as an artery, vein, or intestine
Lunula	Crescent-shaped white area at the proximal end of the nail plate
Luteinizing hormone (LH)	Hormone secreted by the anterior pituitary gland that stimulates ovulation, formation of the corpus luteum, and secretion of estrogens and progesterone in females; also stimulates production of testosterone in males
Lymph	Clear, straw-colored fluid derived from interstitial fluid
Lymphocyte	Type of white blood cell involved in immunity; B cells and T cells are types of lymphocyte
Lymphoid tissue	Tissue where lymphocytes and antibodies are produced; found in lymph nodes, the tonsils, the thymus, the spleen, and as diffuse cells
Lysosomes	Cellular vesicles containing powerful digestive enzymes that can break down and recycle many different molecules
Lysozyme	Enzyme found in certain body secretions such as tears and saliva; catalyzes the breakdown of the cell walls of certain bacteria

M

Macrophage	Scavenger cell that engulfs and destroys microbes
Macule	Small, flat, discolored spot of any shape; e.g., freckles
Malignant (of cells)	Dividing abnormally and uncontrollably, cancerous
Maltase	Brush-border enzyme that breaks down maltose into glucose
Mammary glands	Two modified sudoriferous glands; commonly called the breasts
Marrow cavity	*See* medullary
Mast cells	Large cells in connective tissue that release substances such as histamine during inflammation
Mastication	Process of chewing food

Meatus	*See* external auditory canal
Medial	Toward the midline, on the inner side
Median line	Imaginary line through the middle of the body
Mediastinum	Space in the thorax containing the aorta, heart, trachea, esophagus, and thymus gland; found between the two pleural sacs
Medulla	Inner layer of an organ
Medullary	Space within the diaphysis of a bone; contains yellow bone marrow and is also called the marrow cavity
Meiosis	Reproductive cell division in which four haploid daughter cells are produced
Meissner's corpuscles	Nerve endings that are sensitive to touch
Melanocytes	Melanin-producing cells
Melanocyte-stimulating hormone (MSH)	Hormone secreted by the anterior pituitary gland; exact actions are unknown, but can cause darkening of the skin
Melatonin	Hormone secreted by the pineal gland that causes sleepiness
Membrane	Thin, flexible sheet made up of different tissue layers; membranes cover surfaces, line body cavities, and form protective sheets around organs
Meninges (sing. meninx)	Three connective tissue membranes that enclose the brain and spinal cord
Meniscus	Pad of fibrocartilage that lies between the articular surfaces of bones
Menopause	When a woman stops menstruating and ovulating and can no longer bear children
Menses	*See* menstruation
Menstrual cycle	Cycle in which the endometrium of the uterus is prepared for the arrival of a fertilized ovum
Menstruation	Cyclical, periodic discharge of menstrual flow from the uterus; contains blood, tissue fluid, mucus, and epithelial cells derived from the endometrium
Merkel cells	Cells only found in the stratum basale of hairless skin and attached to keratinocytes; they make contact with nerve cells to form Merkel discs, which function in the sensation of touch
Metabolism	Changes that take place within the body to enable its growth and function
Metastasis	Spread of cancer from its site of origin
Microbe (microorganism)	Organism too small to be seen by the naked eye; microbes include bacteria, viruses, protozoa, and some fungi
Microvilli	Tiny, membrane-covered projections extending into the small intestine and increasing surface area for absorption
Micturition	Urination
Middle ear	Small, air-filled cavity found between the outer ear and the inner ear; contains the three auditory ossicles
Midline	*See* median line
Mineralocorticoids	Group of hormones secreted by the adrenal cortex that regulate the mineral content of the blood
Mitochondria	Powerhouses of the cell where ATP is generated through the process of cellular respiration
Mitosis	Cellular reproduction in which a mother cell divides into two daughter cells, each containing the same genes as the mother cell
Mitral valve	Left atrioventricular valve
Mixed nerve	Nerve containing both sensory and motor fibers
Mole	Small, dark skin growth; a concentrated area of melanin
Monocyte	Type of white blood cell
Mons pubis	Elevation of adipose tissue that cushions the pubic symphysis
Motor neuron	Neuron that conducts impulses from the CNS to muscles and glands
Mucosa	*See* mucous membrane
Mucosa-associated lymphoid tissue (MALT)	Concentrations of lymphatic tissue that are strategically positioned to help protect the body from pathogens that have been inhaled, digested, or have entered via external openings
Mucous membrane	Membrane that lines body cavities that open directly to the exterior; they are wet membranes whose cells secrete mucus
Muscle tissue	Tissue composed of elongated cells that are able to shorten (contract) to produce movement
Muscularis	Muscular layer or coat of an organ
Myalgia	Muscular pain
Myelin sheath	Sheath that protects and insulates a neuron; composed of a white fatty substance called myelin

Myocardium	Middle layer of the heart wall; composed of cardiac muscle tissue and contracts to pump blood
Myofiber	Muscle fiber
Myofibrils	Long, threadlike organelles, the contractile elements of a skeletal muscle fiber
Myofilaments	Filaments found inside myofibrils; there are two types: actin/thin and myosin/thick filaments
Myogenic rhythm	Inherent rhythmicity of certain muscles that does not rely on nervous stimulation; e.g., in cardiac muscle
Myoglobin	Protein that binds with oxygen and carries it to muscle cells
Myology	Study of muscles
Myosin	Protein that functions in muscle contraction
Myositis	Inflammation of muscle tissue
Myopathy	Disease of muscle tissue

N

Nail bed	Area that lies directly beneath the nail plate and secures the nail to the finger or toe
Nail free edge	The part of the nail that extends past the end of the finger or toe; also called the distal edge
Nail grooves	Grooves on the sides of the nail that guide it up the fingers and toes
Nail mantle	The skin that lies directly above the germinal matrix of the nail
Nail plate	The visible body of the nail
Nail wall	The skin that covers the sides of the nail plate and protects the nail grooves
Nasal conchae	Bony shelves projecting from the lateral walls of the nasal cavity
Natural killer cells (NK cells)	Type of lymphocyte that can kill a variety of microbes as well as some tumor cells
Nephron	Functional unit of the kidney where filtration occurs
Nerve fiber	Term referring to the processes that project from a nerve body; e.g., dendrites and axons
Nerve tissue	Tissue made up of neurons and neuroglia; found in the brain, spinal cord, and nerves and functions in communication

Neurofibril node	*See* node of Ranvier
Neuroglia	Supporting cells that insulate, support, and protect neurons
Neurolemmocytes	*See* Schwann cells
Neurology	Study of the nervous system
Neuron	Nerve cell responsible for the sensory, integrative, and motor functions of the nervous system
Neurotransmitter	Chemical that transmits impulses across synapses from one nerve to another
Neutrophil	Type of white blood cell that engulfs and digests foreign particles and removes waste through phagocytosis
Nocturia	Need to urinate regularly at night
Node of Ranvier	Gap along a myelinated nerve fiber
Nodule	Solid bump that may be raised
Noradrenaline	*See* norepinephrine
Norepinephrine	Hormone secreted by the adrenal medulla that functions in the fight-or-flight response
Nucleic acid	Organic compound composed of nucleotides: DNA or RNA
Nucleolus	Spherical body inside the nucleus made up of protein, some DNA, and RNA
Nucleus	Structure in a cell that controls all cellular structure and activities and contains most of the genes

O

Oblique plane	Plane that divides at an angle between a transverse plane and a frontal or sagittal plane
Occipital	Pertaining to the back of the head
Olfaction	Sense of smell
Oliguria	Production of abnormally small amounts of urine
Omentum	Double layer of the peritoneum; covers and links the abdominal organs
Onyx	Nail
Oocyte	Immature ovum
Oogenesis	Production of mature ova in the ovaries
Ophthalmic	Pertaining to the eye
Organelle	Little organ of the cell
Organic compound	Compound containing carbon

Origin	Point where a muscle attaches to the stationary bone of a joint
Osmoreceptor	Receptor sensitive to a decrease in water or an increase in solutes in the blood
Osmosis	Diffusion of water through a selectively permeable membrane from an area of lower solute concentration to an area of higher solute concentration
Osseous tissue	Bone tissue; an exceptionally hard connective tissue that protects and supports other organs of the body
Ossification	Process of bone formation
Osteoblast	Cell that secretes collagen and other organic components to form bones
Osteoclast	Cell found on the surface of bones that destroys or resorbs bone tissue
Osteocyte	Mature bone cell that maintains the daily activities of bone tissue; derived from osteoblasts and the main cells found in bone tissue
Osteology	Study of the structure and function of bones
Osteon	Basic unit of structure of an adult compact bone; consists of a system of interconnecting canals called Haversian canals
Osteoprogenitor cell	Stem cell derived from mesenchyme (the connective tissue found in an embryo) that has the ability to become an osteoblast
Outer ear	External region of the ear that collects and channels sound waves inward; composed of the auricle, external auditory canal, and eardrum
Ova	Mature female sex cells (commonly called eggs)
Ovarian cycle	Cycle in which an oocyte matures until it is ready for ovulation
Ovulation	Event occurring around day 14 of the 28-day cycle; involves the rupture of the mature Graafian follicle and the release of an ovum into the pelvic cavity
Oxidation	*See* cellular respiration
Oxytocin (OT)	Hormone released by the posterior pituitary gland that stimulates contraction of the uterus during labor and stimulates the milk let-down reflex during lactation

P

Pancreatic amylase	Enzyme present in pancreatic juice that completes the breakdown of starches and glycogen
Pancreatic islets	*See* islets of Langerhans
Pancreatic juice	Pancreatic secretion composed of mostly water, some salts, sodium bicarbonate, and some enzymes
Pancreatic lipase	Enzyme present in pancreatic juice; breaks down triglycerides into fatty acids and monoglycerides
Paneth cells	Specialized cells that secrete a bactericidal enzyme called lysozyme into the small intestine
Papillae	Small projections covering the tongue; some papillae house the taste buds
Papillary layer	Undulating membrane that makes up approximately $1/5$ of the thickness of the dermis; composed of areolar connective tissue and fine elastic fibers and has nipple-shaped fingerlike projections called papillae
Papule	Small, solid bump that does not contain fluid; e.g., warts, insect bites, and skin tags
Parasympathetic nervous system	Nervous system that opposes the actions of the sympathetic nervous system by inhibiting activity, thus conserving energy
Parathormone (PTH)	Hormone secreted by the parathyroid glands that increases blood calcium and magnesium levels, decreases blood phosphate levels, and promotes formation of calcitriol by the kidneys
Parathyroid hormone	*See* parathormone
Paresthesia	Abnormal tingling sensations, commonly called pins and needles
Parietal	Relating to the wall of the body or any of its cavities
Pathogen	Disease-causing microorganism
Pathology	Study of the diseases of the body
Pepsin	Enzyme in the stomach that begins the breakdown of proteins
Pepsinogen	Enzyme precursor in the stomach that is converted into pepsin in the acidic environment of gastric juice
Peptidases	Brush-border enzymes that complete the breakdown of proteins into amino acids
Pericardium	Membranous sac that surrounds and protects the heart

Perimysium	Connective tissue that surrounds bundles of 10–100 muscle fibers
Perineum	Diamond-shaped area that contains the external genitals and the anus; located between the thighs and buttocks and present in both males and females
Periosteum	Connective tissue membrane that covers bones
Peripheral	At the surface or outer part of the body
Peripheral nervous system (PNS)	Part of the nervous system connecting the rest of the body to the central nervous system (brain and spinal cord)
Peristalsis	Involuntary wave-like movement that pushes the contents of the gastrointestinal tract forward
Peritoneum	Large serous membrane lining the abdominal cavity
Peroxisomes	Cellular vesicles containing enzymes that detoxify any potentially harmful substances in the cell
Peyer's patches	Patches of mucosa-associated lymphoid tissue located in the lining of the small intestine
Phagocytosis	Engulfment and digestion of foreign particles by phagocytes
Phagocyte	Cell that can engulf and digest microbes; phagocytes include macrophages and some types of white blood cells
Phalanges	Bones of the fingers and toes
Pharynx	Funnel-shaped tube whose walls are made up of skeletal muscles lined by mucous membrane and cilia; commonly called the throat
Photoreceptors	Specialized cells that convert light into nerve impulses
Physiology	Study of the functions of the body
Pia mater	Thin inner covering of the brain; dips into all the folds and spaces of the brain tissue
Pivot joint	Joint in which a rounded/pointed surface of a bone fits into a ring-shaped bone
Plane	Imaginary flat surface that divides the body or organs into parts
Plane joint	*See* gliding joint
Plantar	Pertaining to the sole of the foot
Plantar flexion	Pointing of the foot downward, in the direction of the plantar surface

Plaque	Large, flat, raised bump or group of bumps
Plasma	Liquid portion of blood
Plasma cell	Cell that develops from a B cell (type of lymphocyte) and produces antibodies
Plasma membrane	Barrier that surrounds a cell and regulates the movement of all substances into and out of it
Platelet	*See* thrombocyte
Plexus	Network of nerves or blood vessels
Polyuria	Production of more than 3 liters of urine per day
Popliteal	Relating to the hollow space behind the knee
Posterior	At the back of the body, behind
Postovulatory phase	Phase starting 14 days after ovulation in which the endometrium awaits the arrival of a fertilized ovum
Pregnancy	Sequence of fertilization, implantation, embryonic growth, and fetal growth
Preovulatory phase	Time between menstruation and ovulation; in a 28-day cycle it can vary from 6 to 13 days in length and is the time when a mature Graafian follicle forms and the endometrium proliferates
Priapism	Persistent erection of penis without sexual desire
Prime mover	Muscle responsible for causing a movement
Process	Bony projection or prominence
Progesterone	Hormone secreted by the ovaries that, together with estrogens, regulates the female reproductive cycle and helps maintain pregnancy
Prolactin (PRL)	Hormone secreted by the anterior pituitary gland that stimulates the secretion of milk from the breasts
Proliferative phase	*See* preovulatory phase
Pronation	Movement involving turning the palm posteriorly or inferiorly
Proprioceptor	Specialized nerve receptor located in muscles, joints, and tendons that provides sensory information regarding body position and movements
Prostate gland	Gland surrounding the prostatic urethra; secretes a milky, slightly acidic fluid that contributes to sperm mobility and viability

Protein	Organic compound made up of amino acids and containing carbon, hydrogen, oxygen, and nitrogen; the main building material of cells
Proteinuria	Presence of protein in urine
Protraction	Drawing the shoulders or jaw forward
Proximal	Closer to its origin or point of attachment of a limb
Proximal convoluted tubule	Portion of the renal tubule closest to the glomerular capsule of a kidney nephron; where the reabsorption of most substances takes place
Pruritis	Itching
Puberty	Time at which a person develops secondary sexual characteristics and becomes able to reproduce
Pulmonary circulation	Circulatory system in which the right side of the heart receives deoxygenated blood from the body and pumps it to the lungs where it is oxygenated
Pulmonary respiration	*See* external respiration
Pulmonary ventilation	Process in which air is inspired or breathed into the lungs and expired or breathed out of the lungs
Pupil	Hole in the center of the iris through which light enters the eye
Pustule	Lump containing pus

Q

Quadrant	Region of the abdominopelvic cavity

R

Rectum	Last portion of the gastrointestinal tract
Reflex	Automatic response to a stimulus
Remodeling	Process through which new bone tissue replaces old, worn-out, or injured bone tissue
Renal	Pertaining to the kidneys
Renin	Enzyme produced by the kidneys that functions in raising blood pressure
Rennin	Enzyme found only in the stomachs of infants; begins the digestion of milk by converting the protein caseinogen into casein

Respiration	Exchange of gases between the atmosphere, blood, and cells
Retina	Innermost layer of the wall of the eyeball; consists of a non-visual pigmented portion and a neural portion
Retraction	Drawing the shoulders or jaw backward
Rheumatism	Pain, stiffness, and inflammation in the joints and/or muscles
Ribosomes	Tiny granules that are sites of protein synthesis in the cell
Rima glottidis	Vocal folds
Rods	Photoreceptors that respond to different shades of gray only
Rotation	Movement of a bone in a single plane around its longitudinal axis
Rugae	Folds in the mucous lining of a hollow organ; found in the stomach and vagina

S

Saddle joint	Joint in which a surface shaped like the legs of a rider fits into the saddle-shaped surface of another bone
Sagittal plane	Plane that divides vertically into right and left sides
Salivary amylase	Enzyme present in saliva that begins the breakdown of large carbohydrate molecules
Sarcolemma	Plasma membrane of a muscle fiber
Sarcomere	Basic functional unit of a skeletal muscle
Sarcoplasm	Cytoplasm of a muscle fiber
Scales	Areas of dried, flaky cells; e.g., in psoriasis or dandruff
Scar	Area where normal skin has been replaced by fibrous tissue; forms after an injury
Schwann cells	Cells that wrap around the axon of a neuron to form a myelin sheath
Sclera	White of the eye; made up of dense connective tissue; protects the eyeball and gives it its shape and rigidity
Scrotum	Sac of loose skin and superficial fascia in which lie the testes
Sebaceous oil gland	Exocrine gland that secretes sebum; usually associated with a hair follicle

Sebum	Oily substance secreted by sebaceous glands
Secretion	Substance released from a gland cell; secretions are usually useful substances as opposed to waste products
Secretory phase	*See* postovulatory phase
Segmentation	Main movement in the small intestine; involves localized contractions that move food back and forth
Semen (seminal fluid)	Fluid containing sperm and a mixture of fluids secreted by the reproductive glands
Semicircular canals	Three semicircular canals that project from the vestibule in the ear and contain receptors for equilibrium
Semilunar valves	Valves lying between the ventricles and the arteries that prevent the backflow of blood
Seminal fluid	*See* semen
Seminal vesicles	Paired, pouch-like structures located at the base of the bladder that secrete a viscous alkaline fluid
Seminiferous tubules	Tightly coiled tubules located in the testes, where sperm are formed
Sensory neurons (afferent neurons)	Neurons that conduct impulses from sensory receptors to the CNS
Sepsis	Extreme inflammatory response to infection
Septicemia	Presence of bacteria in the blood
Serous membrane	Membrane lining body cavities that do not open directly to the exterior and covering the organs that lie within those cavities
Sesamoid bones	Oval bones that develop in tendons where there is considerable pressure
Short bones	Cube-shaped bones that are nearly equal in length and width
Simple epithelium	Single layer of cells; usually very thin and functions in absorption, secretion, and filtration
Sinoatrial node	The heart's pacemaker (SA node)
Skeletal muscle tissue	Muscle tissue attached to bones that is composed of long, cylindrical fibers that are striated and under voluntary control
Smooth muscle tissue	Muscle tissue that contains non-striated (smooth) fibers and is regulated by the autonomic nervous system
Solvent	Medium (usually a liquid) in which substances (solutes) can be dissolved
Somatic cell	Any cell except the reproductive cells
Somatic cell division	Process of nuclear division called mitosis; a single diploid parent cell duplicates to produce two identical daughter cells
Somatic nervous system (voluntary nervous system)	Part of the nervous system that allows us to control our skeletal muscles; also called the voluntary nervous system
Somatostatin	Hormone secreted by the pancreas that inhibits insulin and glucagon release
Somatotropin	*See* human growth hormone
Spermatogenesis	Production of sperm in the testes
Spermatozoa	Mature male sex cells (commonly called sperm)
Spinal nerves	Nerves emerging from the spinal cord that carry impulses to and from the rest of the body
Spongy bone tissue	Light bone tissue with many spaces within it and a sponge-like appearance; does not contain osteons
Sputum	Material coughed up from the respiratory tract
Stratified epithelium	Consists of two or more layers of cells; durable; protects underlying tissues in areas of wear and tear
Stratum basale	Deepest layer of the epidermis and the base from where new cells germinate or sprout
Stratum corneum	Outermost layer of the skin, consisting of dead, tough cells
Stratum functionalis	Deep layer of the endometrium of the uterus; shed during menstruation
Stratum germinativum	*See* stratum basale
Stratum granulosum	Epidermal layer of degenerating cells that are becoming increasingly filled with little grains or granules of keratin
Stratum lucidum	Epidermal waterproof layer of dead, clear cells
Stratum spinosum	Epidermal layer of prickly cells that are beginning to go through the process of keratinization
Stretchmarks	Small tears in the dermis caused by the skin stretching beyond its ability
Striated	Having the appearance of light and dark bands or striations
Stridor	High-pitched wheezing sound when breathing
Subcutaneous	Beneath the skin
Substrate	Substance on which an enzyme acts

Sucrase	Brush-border enzyme that breaks down sucrose into glucose and fructose
Sudoriferous gland	Gland that excretes sweat onto the surface of the skin
Superficial	Toward the surface of the body
Superior	Toward the head, above
Supination	Movement involving turning the palm anteriorly or superiorly
Suspensory (Cooper's) ligaments	Strands of connective tissue that support a breast
Sympathetic nervous system	Part of the nervous system that reacts to changes in the environment by stimulating activity, thereby using energy
Synapse	Gap at the end of a nerve fiber that an impulse crosses to pass from one neuron to the next
Synaptic vesicle	Sac that stores neurotransmitters and is located in a synaptic end bulb at the distal end of an axon terminal
Synarthrosis	Immovable joint
Syncope	Temporary loss of consciousness, commonly called fainting
Synergist	Muscle that helps the prime mover
Synovial joint	Freely movable joint in which a cavity is present between the articulating bones
Synovial membrane	Membrane composed of areolar connective tissue that lines freely movable joints and secretes synovial fluid
Systemic circulation	Type of circulation in which the left side of the heart receives oxygenated blood from the lungs and pumps it to the rest of the body
Systole	Contraction of the heart muscle during the cardiac cycle

T

T cell	Lymphocyte that matures in the thymus gland and functions in cell-mediated immunity
Tachycardia	Abnormally fast heart rate
Taeniae coli	Three thickened bands of longitudinal smooth muscle running the length of the colon
Taste bud	A receptor for taste
Telangiectasia	A localized collection of blood vessels in the skin; characterized by a red spot that can be spidery in appearance and that blanches under pressure

Telogen	Resting phase of the hair cycle in which the follicle is inactive until stimulated to develop another hair
Tendon	Strong cord of dense connective tissue that attaches muscles to bones, to the skin, or to other muscles
Terminal hair	Hair found on the head, eyebrows, eyelashes, under the arms, and in the pubic area
Testes	Gonads of the male reproductive system
Testosterone	Hormone secreted by the testes that stimulates the development of masculine secondary sex characteristics and libido
Thermogenesis	Generation of heat in the body
Thorax	The chest
Thrombocyte	Type of white blood cell that functions in hemostasis and blood clotting
Thymosin	Hormone secreted by the thymus gland that promotes the growth of T cells
Thyroid hormone	Hormone secreted by the thyroid gland that functions in metabolism, growth, and development
Thyroid-stimulating hormone (TSH)	Hormone secreted by the anterior pituitary gland that controls the thyroid gland
Thyrotropin	*See* thyroid-stimulating hormone
Thyroxine	*See* thyroid hormone
Tissue respiration	*See* internal respiration
Tone (tonus)	Partial contraction of a resting muscle
Trachea	Long, tubular passageway that transports air from the larynx into the bronchi; commonly called the windpipe
Tract	Bundle of nerve fibers that is not surrounded by connective tissue
Transverse plane	Plane that divides horizontally into inferior and superior portions
Tricuspid valve	Right atrioventricular valve
Trimester	Period of three months; pregnancy is divided into three trimesters
Trypsin	Enzyme secreted by the pancreas that continues the breakdown of proteins
Tubercle	Solid lump that is larger than a papule
Tumor	An abnormal growth of tissue
Tympanic membrane	*See* eardrum

U

Ulcer	A deep, open lesion on the skin; ulcers penetrate the dermis
Unguis	Nail
Urea	Main product of protein metabolism
Uric acid	Product of nucleic acid metabolism
Urobilinogen	Bile pigment derived from the breakdown of hemoglobin
Urology	Study of the urinary system
Uterine cycle	*See* menstrual cycle
Uterus	The womb
Uvula	Fingerlike projection hanging from the soft palate at the back of the mouth

V

Vacuole	Space within the cytoplasm of a cell that contains material taken in by the cell
Vas deferens	Long duct running from the epididymis to the urethra; transports sperm via peristaltic contractions
Vascular tissue	Blood; a type of connective tissue whose matrix is made of a fluid called blood plasma
Vasoconstriction	Constriction of blood vessels
Vasodilation	Dilation of blood vessels
Vasopressin	*See* antidiuretic hormone
Veins	Vessels that usually carry blood away from the tissues toward the heart
Vellus hair	Soft and downy hair that is found all over the body except the palms of the hands, soles of the feet, eyelids, lips, and nipples
Ventral	At the front of the body, in front of
Ventricle (brain)	Fluid-filled cavity in the brain; there are four of them

Ventricle (heart)	Delivery chamber of the heart that pumps blood into the blood vessels
Venule	Small vein; it drains blood away from capillaries
Vesicle	Small, fluid-filled sac
Vesicular ovarian follicle	*See* Graafian follicle
Vesicular transport	Type of transport across the plasma membrane of a cell in which vesicles (small sacs) carry particles
Vestibule (ear)	Central portion of the bony labyrinth of the ear; contains receptors for equilibrium.
Vestibule (female genitalia)	Entire region between the labia minora, consisting of the vaginal orifice and external urethral orifice
Villi	Fingerlike projections of intestinal mucosa cells that increase the total surface area of the small intestine
Virilization	Development of masculine physical characteristics
Viscera	Organs of the abdominal body cavity
Visceral	Relating to the internal organs of the body
Vitreous body	Jelly-like substance that helps produce intraocular pressure in the eye
Voluntary nervous system	*See* somatic nervous system

W

Wheal	Common allergic reaction in which there is swelling with an elevated, soft area
Wheezing	Whistling sound produced when the airways are partially obstructed

Z

Zygote	A fertilized ovum

Index

Note: *f* = figure, *c* = chart, *b* = boxed information